Comparative Biology
of Skin

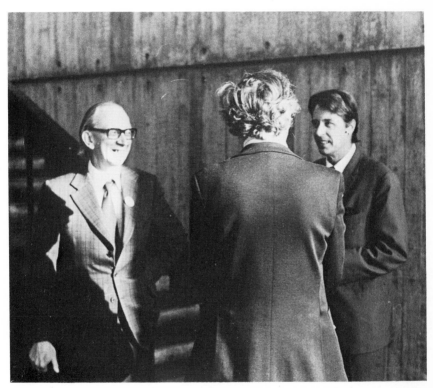

FRONTISPIECE: T. E. Weis-Fogh (Cambridge) on right in discussion with M. Abercrombie (Cambridge), left, and R. T. Tregear (Oxford), centre.

SYMPOSIA OF THE ZOOLOGICAL SOCIETY OF LONDON

NUMBER 39

Comparative Biology of Skin

(The Proceedings of a Symposium held at The Zoological Society of London on 30 and 31 October 1975)

Edited by

R. I. C. SPEARMAN

Department of Dermatology, University College Hospital Medical School, London, England

Published for

THE ZOOLOGICAL SOCIETY OF LONDON

BY

ACADEMIC PRESS

1977

ACADEMIC PRESS INC. (LONDON) LTD

24/28 Oval Road

London NW1

U.S. Edition published by

ACADEMIC PRESS INC.

111 Fifth Avenue,

New York, New York 10003

Library of Congress Catalog Card Number: 74–5683

ISBN: 0–12–613339–5

PRINTED IN GREAT BRITAIN BY
J. W. ARROWSMITH LTD, BRISTOL

CONTRIBUTORS

ANDERSEN, S. O., *Zoophysiological Laboratory C, August Krogh Institute, University of Copenhagen, Universitetsparken 13, DK-2100, Copenhagen ∅, Denmark* (p. 7)

BUDTZ, POVL E., *Zoophysiological Laboratory A, August Krogh Institute, University of Copenhagen, Universitetsparken 13, DK-2100, Copenhagen ∅, Denmark* (p. 317)

COLLETTE, BRUCE B., *Systematics Laboratory, National Marine Fisheries Service, National Museum of Natural History, Washington DC 20560, USA (p. 225)*

FOX, H., *Department of Zoology, University College London, Gower Street, London WC1E 6BT, England* (p. 269)

GEORGE, J. DAVID, *Department of Zoology, British Museum (Natural History), Cromwell Road, London SW7 5BD, England* (p. 195)

GRAHAM, A., *Department of Zoology, The University, Whiteknights, Reading RG6 2AJ, England* (p.1)

JOHNSON, ELIZABETH, *Department of Zoology, The University, Whiteknights, Reading RG6 2AJ, England* (p. 373)

LEE, D. L., *Department of Pure and Applied Zoology, Agricultural Sciences Building, The University, Leeds LS2 9JT, England* (p. 145)

LYONS, KATHLEEN M., *Bryanston School, Blandford Forum, Dorset, England* (p. 97)

RICHARDS, K. SYLVIA, *Department of Biology, The University, Keele, Staffs ST5 5BG, England* (p. 171)

RILEY, P. A., *Department of Biochemical Pathology, University College Hospital Medical School, London WC1E 6JJ, England* (p. 77)

SIMKISS, K., *Department of Zoology, The University, Whiteknights, Reading RG6 2AJ, England* (p. 35)

SPEARMAN, R. I. C., *Department of Dermatology, University College Hospital Medical School, London WC1E 6JJ, England* (pp. 335, 405)

WHITEAR, MARY, *Department of Zoology, University College London, Gower Street, London WC1E 6BT, England* (p. 291)

WIGGLESWORTH, V. B., *Department of Zoology, The University, Downing Street, Cambridge CB2 3EJ, England* (p. 33)

WILBUR, K. M., *Department of Zoology, Duke University, Durham, North Carolina 27706, USA* (p. 35)

WRENCH, ROSANNE, *Department of Dermatology, University College Hospital Medical School, London WC1 6JJ, England* (p. 353)

ORGANIZER AND CHAIRMEN

ORGANIZER

R. I. C. SPEARMAN on behalf of The Zoological Society of London

CHAIRMEN OF SESSIONS

M. ABERCROMBIE, *Strangeways Research Laboratory, Worts Causeway, Cambridge CB1 4RN, England*

T. E. HUGHES, *Cox Green Cottage, Rudgwick, near Horsham, Sussex, England* (p. 223)

A. JARRETT, *Department of Dermatology, University College Hospital Medical School, London WC1E 6JJ, England* (p. 315)

R. I. C. SPEARMAN, *Department of Dermatology, University College Hospital Medical School, London WC1E 6JJ, England*

T. E. WEIS-FOGH, *Department of Zoology, The University, Downing Street, Cambridge CB2 3EJ, England*

DEDICATION

This volume is dedicated by the contributors to Torkel Weis-Fogh 1922–1975.

Distinguished in the field of comparative physiology and in particular for his research on the insect cuticle, his breadth of interest was immense, and the discussion in both the invertebrate and vertebrate sessions of this symposium was enlivened by his brilliance.

PREFACE

In the last 20 years there have been numerous symposia dealing with advances in mammalian skin biology but, apart from occasional papers in these works on reptilian and avian skin, no attempt has been made to bring together findings on skin in other groups of animals—with the exception of the arthropod integument which has been the subject of several recent works. Investigations on skins of arthropods and mammals have a connecting link in the biochemistry of melanin, quinones and catechols; important in all groups of animals whether for pigmentation or for cross-bonding of structural proteins.

The present volume is the proceedings of a symposium at which investigators, active in skin research on various groups of invertebrates and vertebrates, reviewed recent advances in their areas, mainly on epidermal functions, with additional contributions on bony contact organs of fishes, on melanogenesis and on epidermal sensory cells. The contributors are authorities in their subjects and they have succeeded in integrating their work so that articles do not appear in isolation from each other as can so easily happen in a broadly based symposium. This was achieved because speakers were told over a year before the conference what each of the other contributors would be dealing with and common ground could be worked out. In such a broadly based work it may seem difficult to believe that there is a connection between those peculiar deep-sea worms, the Pogonophora, and mammals, but themes such as structural proteins and their variation, mucus and its functions and transport through the skin run through the text. Therefore, I suggest to specialized readers that they would benefit from reading contributions in addition to those in their own fields of study or of immediate interest.

In this time of recession with contraction of research and additional difficulty in obtaining funds to invite speakers from abroad it is becoming increasingly difficult to organize symposia in this country and indeed in some specialized fields it is no longer possible. The broad basis of this symposium made selection an easier matter. Contributors are engaged on research which is active in the United Kingdom and Denmark with help from the USA. Many interesting groups are left out but the recent spurt of research on amphibian skin is the subject of three papers.

PREFACE

Most symposia overlap with other works in their contents but the present volume is only the second to be published on comparative skin biology in any language, the first being an introductory text (Spearman, 1973 *The integument* London: Cambridge U.P.). In particular, work on invertebrate skins apart from arthropods is scattered in research papers and is here brought together for the first time.

In the preparation of this work we wish to acknowledge the help of Dr H. G. Vevers and Miss Unity McDonnell of the Zoological Society of London and the assistance of Dr H. Fox with the editing. We are grateful to Mrs Anne Ephgrave of Academic Press for her care in the arrangement of this volume. We are also indebted to the Wellcome Trust for their provision of a travel grant.

London   R. I. C. SPEARMAN
August 1977

CONTENTS

Introduction

A. GRAHAM

Arthropod Cuticles: Their Composition Properties and Functions

S. O. ANDERSEN

The Waterproofing Layer of the Insect Cuticle

V. B. WIGGLESWORTH

CONTENTS

The Molluscan Epidermis and its Secretions

K. SIMKISS and K. M. WILBUR

The Mechanism of Melanogenesis

P. A. RILEY

Epidermal Adaptations of Parasitic Platyhelminths

KATHLEEN M. LYONS

The Nematode Epidermis and Collagenous Cuticle, its Formation and Ecdysis

D. L. LEE

Structure and Function in the Oligochaete Epidermis (Annelida)

K. SYLVIA RICHARDS

The Pogonophore Epidermis, its Structure, Functions and Affinities

J. DAVID GEORGE

Chairman's Summing up on Lower Animals

T. E. HUGHES

Epidermal Breeding Tubercles and Bony Contact Organs in Fishes

BRUCE B. COLLETTE

The Anuran Tadpole Skin: Changes Occurring in it During Metamorphosis and Some Comparisons with that of the Adult

H. FOX

A Functional Comparison Between the Epidermis of Fish and of Amphibians

MARY WHITEAR

Chairman's Summing up on Higher Animals

A. JARRETT

Aspects of Moulting in Anurans and its Control

POVL E. BUDTZ

Keratins and Keratinization

R. I. C. SPEARMAN

Changes in Mouse Tail Epidermal Keratinization Induced by Tar Derivatives

ROSANNE WRENCH

Seasonal Changes in the Skin of Mammals

ELIZABETH JOHNSON

Conclusions from the Discussion

R. I. C. SPEARMAN

Symp. zool. Soc. Lond. (1977) No. 39, 1–5

INTRODUCTION

A. GRAHAM

Department of Zoology, The University, Whiteknights, Reading, England

Of the importance of an animal's skin there can be no doubt: my skin is the end of me and the beginning of the rest of the universe. In too many parts of the world its colour decides what I may do or not do, where I may go or not go; its adolescent spottiness causes me intolerable social embarrassment, though the softness and smoothness of my girl friend's skin and the look and texture of her hair give me a great deal of gratification—and give her the same too, I guess later, when she is my wife, and I discover how much time, energy and money she spends in maintaining these characteristics. However, we are getting involved in a symposium on the sociology of skin and that is not the title of this one.

On one side of my skin lies the apparatus of life, the elaboration of structure and the delicate regulation of physical and chemical circumstances within which alone life is possible; on the other extends the vastness of the universe existing either at the fantastically high temperatures of the stars or the abysmally low ones of interstellar space, both too extreme to support life, and pulsating with radiations that would soon destroy it. Even within the kindly confines of Earth where these extremes are softened, the external medium is often still hostile—too wet, too dry, too hot, too cold, too deficient in the right kind of ion, too rich in the wrong kind—to allow direct and uncontrolled contact with living substance. The first role of the skin thus emerges as a boundary, a barrier between the living and the non-living, the microcosm and the macrocosm, though the latter has none of the life with which Paracelsus endowed it.

Yet the organism cannot isolate itself from this external world, cannot shut itself within an impermeable shell and live the life of a recluse. It has evolved in relation to it; it depends upon it for food, for oxygen, for water; it must be aware of what goes on in it to eat and to avoid being eaten; to select a habitat in which it may flourish and avoid circumstances detrimental to its well-being. The same skin which protects the animal against external conditions must also inform it about these in order that it may survive. Skin is therefore in the paradoxical condition of being the organ which isolates animal from environment and at the same time the organ

1

which binds animal to environment. It must perform both roles simultaneously and must not let efficiency in the one impair efficiency in the other.

I could, I suppose, at this point make a case for counting both gut and nervous system as skin on the grounds that, first, from the evolutionary point of view, they are derived from the original external covering of the animal, and, second, from the functional point of view, they share in one of these major activities of skin—its traffic with the environment. I think, however, I read the mind of the organizer correctly in confining myself to the narrower but more customary meaning of the word, the layer of tissue which forms the outer surfaces of animals.

A naïve approach to the subject would suppose all skins homologous: the embryologist would describe them as ectodermal, and this supposition, indeed, seems largely true. Yet some observations in the phylum Platyhelminthes make one hesitate to accept it as universally valid. The epidermal cells of free-living flatworms all contain the kind of structures known as rhabdites, rod-shaped bodies which, when discharged in quantity, give rise to a sheet of gelatinous consistency perhaps acting as a food-trap or as a defensive layer or even as an excretory product. Skaer (1965) showed in *Polycelis tenuis*—but it is likely to be true of all turbellarians—that rhabdites develop within cells belonging to the parenchyma and that as the rhabdites mature the cells migrate to take up their station within the epidermis. As every epidermal cell contains rhabdites one may conclude that the whole layer has arisen in this way and that the original ectodermal skin has been replaced by one of "mesodermal" origin.

Further, it may be right to see in the tegument of the parasitic platyhelminth classes something of the same nature. This is a secondary skin replacing the original which is cast off when the miracidium larva, for example, has successfully found the host in which it will establish itself. If this is true the phylum Platyhelminthes would then prove a genetic unity with a skin different from that of other phyla. One phylum approaches them in part, for Prenant showed half a century ago that the gland cells of the molluscan foot originate within the parenchyma-like connective tissue of that organ. At Reading one of my research students, Dr B. Pande (1958), was able to show that, after cauterization of the skin of the foot of *Helix aspersa*, the epidermis is replaced by cells immigrating from the edge of the damaged area but that the glands (one kind excepted which grows inwards from the epidermis) arise from connective tissue cells deep in the foot that extend long necks outwards to the surface. This suggests a link at cellular level between the two phyla which supports many more at organ level.

One lesson which zoologists have learned, perhaps more thoroughly in recent years, is to expect convergence of structure where there is similarity of function. It may make life less exciting to find superficially identical solutions to the same functional problem in unrelated stocks but it should not perhaps surprise us when we consider the essential similarities of organisms—and, though alike, the solutions are never truly identical. This may be illustrated by seeing how skin gives protection against adverse external conditions. This could be achieved almost entirely by metabolic activity of the skin cells but this would be very extravagant. It is much more economical of energy to cover the body with a cuticle which will mechanically reduce movement of materials from one side of the skin to the other. Many kinds of animal, so to speak, have had this idea and have usually elaborated it by adding some skeletal to the protective function. Arthropods, nematodes, molluscs and vertebrates all illustrate this principle. But though similar in general, their arrangements differ in detail—in arthropods the cuticle is made of chitin and proteins but has no collagen; it may be strengthened by the addition of calcareous salts and waxed to decrease its permeability and it gives attachment to muscles; in nematodes a cuticle, so superficially similar to that of arthropods that it was at one time used to buttress the idea of a close relationship between the groups, turns out to be chemically quite unlike—devoid of chitin but rich in collagen, and, though it gives no direct attachment to muscle fibres, its elasticity lets it act as antagonist to the longitudinal ones that are the only muscles the nematode possesses.

In the phylum Mollusca a fundamentally similar device appears in the shell and operculum, cuticular secretions strengthened by deposition of calcareous salts and used as the origin of many muscles. In both nematodes and arthropods the cuticle inhibits growth and an elaborate system has had to be devised under hormonal control to cast off the old cuticle periodically and produce a new one. The molluscan shell and operculum, however, can grow continuously—day by day in many species—and retain the same fundamental shape, preserving for the observant a record of growth and appearance from the embryonic and larval stages of last spring to the adult of today. The vertebrates achieve the same ends by still different means though a kind of calcareous shell may occur in the scales of fish or the scutes of reptiles. Their covering, however, is unique. Unlike that of all other animals their epidermis is a stratified epithelium, the outer layers of which die and keratinize as they are moved away from the living and dividing ones within.

Protection, physical and chemical, from the environment, information about the environment, adjustment to the environment: these are the primary integumental functions. But in some animals others supervene. When I was an undergraduate one topic discussed was Pütter's theory (1909) that at least some of the nutritive matter available to marine animals came from organic molecules in solution in sea-water. We were then led to believe that this was unlikely, yet within the last decade work by Stephens (1963), Ferguson (1967), and Taylor (1969) has given convincing proof of the uptake of organic solutes through the epidermis of animals in nearly every phylum. Arthropods form an apparent exception—doubtless their thick cuticle makes it impossible. In the polychaete worm *Clymenella torquata*, an abundant little animal of muddy shores, the uptake of amino acids ($c.2.5$ μg h^{-1} per worm) has been shown to be at a level which, if maintained, would require more than the measured oxygen consumption of the animal for its respiratory oxidation. It has further been shown that in the water in which the worm lives there is the necessary amount of amino acids in solution ($c.$ 75 μmol l^{-1}) to support such an uptake. There is no suggestion that *Clymenella* obtains all its amino acids in this way and that its gut is functionless but the role of skin as a route for the uptake of some fraction of the animal's food seems well grounded. Indeed Ferguson (1967) has suggested that the starfish *Henricia* has two more or less equivalent sites of uptake—the gut absorbs what is required for its own metabolic activity and for the ripening of the gonads; the skin is responsible for all the rest of the body—the creature is a kind of double organism with gut and skin equally active. This leads on to those extraordinary deep-water animals, the Pogonophora, the length of whose body is never less than 100 times and may be 600 times its breadth, as in *Siboglinum minutum* which is 55 mm long and only 100 μm in breadth. In addition to these very unusual dimensions the animals have no gut so that when they were first found they were believed to be the tentacles, shorn off by the dredge, of some elusive burrowing creature the body of which was never captured.

If *Clymenella* can supplement what it derives from its gut by what it obtains through its skin; if *Henricia* can run half its body on foodstuffs taken through the body wall, perhaps pogonophorans can dispense with a gut altogether—after all they have plenty of skin. But are they gutless because their dimensions gave them great surface area, or did a trend towards loss of gut compel these bizarre dimensions?

Pogonophorans, of course, are not the only gutless animals—so too are tapeworms. Here it seems that the skin must again be the main route for food uptake. They show rather more complexity in their arrangements, however. The cestodes and some trematodes like the strigeoid flukes (all gut parasites) have been shown to erode the gut epithelium and establish an association with the underlying vascular submucous layer which can be compared to that between the trophoblast of a developing mammal and the wall of the uterus. Has this ability any relationship to the special nature of platyhelminth skin?

Man, poor creature, has perhaps always felt that, so far as skin goes, he has had a raw deal from Nature. Like all animals he has a protective skin, he has a sensitive skin; he has a skin useful in temperature regulation and to some extent apparently absorptive. But by comparison with other animals how bald it is, how plain, how lacking in decorative effect; by comparison with other creatures—tropical fish, snakes, birds, even his close relation the mandrill—how lacking in striking colour. How imperative it has seemed throughout the ages to add woad, or rouge, or henna, how essential to use lipstick or eye shadow! But to pursue that theme would call for a whole symposium and my time is up.

REFERENCES

Ferguson, J. C. (1967). Utilization of dissolved exogenous nutrients by the starfishes, *Asterias forbesi* and *Henricia sanguinolenta*. *Biol. Bull. mar. biol. Lab. Woods Hole* **132**: 161–173.

Pande, B. (1958). *Wound healing and regeneration in the snail* Helix aspersa *O. F. Müller and the earthworm* Lumbricus terrestris *L.* Ph. D. thesis, University of Reading.

Pütter, A. (1909). *Die Ernährung des Wassertiere und der Stoffgehalt der Gewasser.* Jena: Fischer.

Skaer, R. J. (1965). The origin and continuous replacement of epidermal cells in the planarian *Polycelis tenuis* (Iijima). *J. Embryol. exp. Morph.* **13**: 129–139.

Stephens, G. C. (1963). Uptake of organic material by aquatic invertebrates. II. Accumulation of amino acids by the bamboo worm, *Clymenella torquata*. *Comp. Biochem. Physiol.* **10**: 191–209.

Taylor, A. G. (1969). The direct uptake of amino acids and other small molecules from seawater by *Nereis virens* Sars. *Comp. Biochem. Physiol.* **29**: 243–250.

Symp. zool. Soc. Lond. (1977) No. 39, 7–32.

ARTHROPOD CUTICLES: THEIR COMPOSITION, PROPERTIES AND FUNCTIONS

S. O. ANDERSEN

August Krogh Institute, University of Copenhagen, Copenhagen, Denmark

SYNOPSIS

The main components of most arthropod cuticles are chitin and proteins. Collagen is completely absent from the cuticles, although it is present in other parts of the body such as basement membranes. The chitin molecules are organized into microfibrils 2·8 nm in diameter, and these microfibrils are embedded in a protein matrix. The proteins are presumably globular and not organized into fibres. We do not know the amino acid composition of any single protein from an insect cuticle, whereas it has been possible to isolate and charcterize the individual proteins in *Limulus* (Merostomata) cuticle. There are minor differences in amino acid composition of cuticles from insect species of the same order and pronounced differences between orders. Material from the same developmental stage was used for the comparisons. The compositions of different types of cuticle from a single animal differ in a characteristic manner.

The mechanical properties of cuticles depend partly upon the organization of the chitin microfibrils and partly upon the degree of interaction between protein molecules. Solid cuticle is obtained by sclerotization, i.e. the introduction of covalent cross-linkages between proteins. Several types of cross-linking mechanisms have been described. Their characteristic features are discussed and tentatively related to the physical properties of the cuticles.

INTRODUCTION

The integument of arthropods consist of a single layer of epidermal cells with some associated extracellular materials: a collagen-containing basement membrane which separates the epidermis from the haemocoel, and the cuticle which separates the epidermis, and thereby the whole animal, from the outside world. The cuticle is formed by the epidermal cells, and although it is an extracellular structure it remains in close contact with the cells, and after it has been deposited several of its properties can be controlled by the cells. The cuticle has several functions: it serves as an exoskeleton for attachment of muscles and so is of prime importance for the movements of the animal whether it walks, flies or swims. The cuticle also serves as a barrier between the animal and its surroundings, and it is often highly impermeable to many compounds, for instance water. An intact cuticle is essential for protecting insects from rapid dehydration.

Some functions are common to all or most of the cuticle of a given animal, whereas other functions are connected with highly restricted and specialized areas. Modified cuticle is thus an integral part of many sense organs, for instance sound- and mechanoreceptors, ocelli and compound eyes. It is therefore not surprising that one meets an apparently endless variation in types and properties of cuticle. They all appear to be constructed according to a single fundamental scheme and it is surprising that Nature has been able to form such a variety of structures by relatively slight modifications of the components involved.

An excellent review of nearly all aspects of cuticle biology, covering both biophysics, biochemistry, ultrastructure, physiology and development, has recently been published (Neville, 1975) and should be consulted for more detailed information than I can supply here.

SUBLAYERS OF THE CUTICLE

The epicuticle

Apparently all cuticles consist of two fundamentally different parts: epicuticle and procuticle (Fig. 1). The epicuticle is a very thin

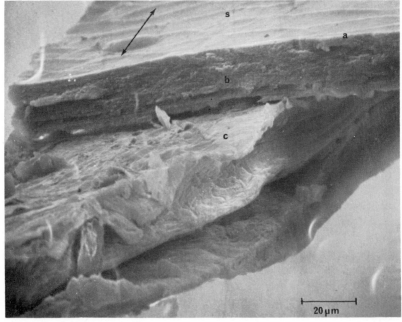

FIG. 1. Scanning electron photomicrograph of fractured locust femur sclerite. Abbreviations: s, outer surface; a, epicuticle; b, exocuticle; c, endocuticle. The specimen was fractured by applying tension in the direction indicated by the arrow. Courtesy of H. R. Hepburn & I. Joffe. (1974). *J. Insect Physiol.* **20**: 631. Pergamon Press.

layer which covers all types of cuticle, both soft and solid. Both in the light microscope and in the electron microscope epicuticle can be seen to consist of several layers, but some doubts remain about how to correlate the layers seen with the two instruments. The main part of the epicuticle is also the structural part and the part which is laid down at an early stage of cuticle deposition. It has been subdivided in various ways, but I can recommend the terms outer and inner epicuticle (Weis-Fogh, 1970) to avoid the confusion caused by the various uses of the term cuticulin. Shortly before ecdysis a wax layer is deposited on the outside of the epicuticle, thereby making it much less permeable for water, and soon after ecdysis the wax layer is in many insects covered by a cement layer, produced by dermal glands. The cement layer is assumed to have a protective function and to resemble shellac in composition. Little has been established about its chemistry, whereas the wax layers of many insects have been relatively well characterized. They contain a number of long chain hydrocarbons, alcohols, fatty acids and waxes, and each species appears to have its own characteristic blend of components.

Our ignorance is also great with regard to the composition of the structural part of the epicuticle; this is partly due to its complete insolubility and partly to the extremely small amounts of material which it contains. On the basis of staining reactions it is assumed to consist of tightly cross-linked lipids and proteins and to contain no chitin, but as emphasized by Neville (1975) the absence of chitin needs to be confirmed by more reliable methods.

Although it is thin and only represents a small fraction of the total mass of the cuticle the epicuticle constitutes an essential part of the cuticle. Not only is it impermeable to water but it is also the first part to be deposited during the formation of a new cuticle. Usually the surface area of the new cuticle is larger than that of the old, and before ecdysis the new cuticle is present in a highly folded state beneath the old cuticle. How much it is folded is determined by how much epicuticle is deposited, which again is determined by the epidermal cells. The chitin-containing cuticle is deposited beneath the epicuticle and follows it closely in all its folding. After ecdysis, when the remnants of the old cuticle have been discarded, and the new one is brought into use, it becomes stretched as the animal pumps itself up to a larger volume by swallowing air or water and by muscular contractions to press blood out into the extremities. In some insects the cuticle is stretched until the folds of the epicuticle have been flattened, but in other insects the stretching stops before that, and the epicuticle remains thrown into folds.

If the procuticle beneath the epicuticle stays plastic or can later be made plastic, these folds will allow continued growth and expansion of the cuticle. The epicuticle itself has been reported to be brittle and only slightly stretchable (Hepburn & Joffe, 1976), so expansion beyond the area of the original epicuticle should not be possible.

Microstructure of the procuticle

The bulk properties of the cuticle, such as the mechanical properties, reside in the procuticle, which is all the cuticle located between the epicuticle and the epidermal cells. The procuticle has been subdivided in various ways, mainly based upon the microscopical appearance and upon staining reactions. The subdivisions are of practical use for describing cuticles, but one should be careful not to place too much reliance upon them. They can both represent different types of molecular architecture and different degrees of post-depositional modification (sclerotization), and their differences are not as essential as the difference between epicuticle and procuticle. The outermost layer of the procuticle, the exocuticle, is characterized by being refractory towards staining by Mallory's method and it is often darkly coloured. An exocuticle is not always present. Exocuticle will usually correspond to that part of the cuticle which is deposited before ecdysis.

Beneath the exocuticle there is often a layer that stains red by Mallory's method, and which has been called mesocuticle. The innermost layer staining blue by Mallory's method is called endocuticle (Fig. 1). This term is also used for the red- and blue-staining layers together and endocuticle will then roughly correspond to the part of the procuticle which is deposited after ecdysis.

CHEMICAL COMPOSITION OF THE PROCUTICLE

Common to the whole procuticle is that it consists of two types of macromolecules: chitin and proteins. Chitin is present as microfibrils which are embedded in a protein matrix, and the properties of the cuticles will depend upon both the molecular arrangements of the two types of molecules and their interactions with each other and with their own kind. A third factor which is of great importance is water, but little is known about the hydration of cuticle and whether it can be regulated. Reynolds (1975b) has suggested that hydration and mechanical properties of *Rhodnius* abdominal cuticle can be controlled by changes in intracuticular pH. Lipids can also be found in procuticle, but presumably it is not of the same importance as in the epicuticle.

The chitin microfibrils

Chitin is present as long microfibrils which according to electron microscopy and X-ray evidence (Neville, 1975) are about 2·8 nm in diameter and of indefinite length. Owing to its low solubility it is not possible to bring the chitin into solution without some risk of degradation, and the exact molecular weight is not known. There is no reason to assume that all the chains have the same length, and the average length may well vary between various types of cuticle. According to the dimensions of the molecule about 18–20 chitin molecules can be arranged in parallel within a microfibril (Rudall & Kenchington, 1973; Neville, 1975). The microfibrils are packed or arranged in various ways in the protein matrix in the cuticle. The arrangement is nearly always parallel to the surface but the direction within the plane of the cuticle can vary.

The microfibrils are commonly arranged in the helicoidal pattern which was first described by Bouligand (1965) and investigated in detail by Neville (1967b). In this arrangement the microfibrils are parallel to their neighbours in the same plane, but run at a slight angle to the fibrils in the planes immediately above and below. It appears that the angle, on going from one plane to the next, can vary considerably, but the rotation, with a few exceptions, is always in the same direction (anticlockwise). When such a packing arrangement is cut obliquely and viewed in the electron microscope, the microfibrils give the appearance of being arranged in a parabolic pattern. Such parabolic patterns have been observed in a number of cuticles. It is possible that they are not always caused by a helicoidal arrangement (Dennell, 1973, 1974). A perfect helicoidal arrangement of chitin filaments will give a procuticle which is isotropic in the plane of the cuticle, since filaments are running in all directions although not at random.

A highly anisotropic arrangement is found where the chitin microfibrils all run parallel to each other in a preferred direction. The preferred direction in the cuticle is often parallel to the long axis of a leg or some other body part, but it may be at right angles to the body axis, for instance in some intersegmental membranes.

In some insects a third arrangement has been described which consists of relatively thick layers where all chitin microfibrils are parallel to each other within each layer, but the directions in any two neighbouring layers are at nearly right angles to each other. The structure is thus somewhat like plywood. It has been found that the change in direction between two layers is not abrupt but that a thin stretch of cuticle with a helicoidal arrangement of microfibrils is interspersed (Neville & Luke, 1969; Neville, 1975).

Cuticles are not always composed of only one of these patterns, but several of them can occur in the same piece of cuticle. Neville (1967b) has for instance shown that in the cuticle of locust hind leg tibia there are layers with microfibrils arranged in a preferred direction alternating with layers with microfibrils arranged in a helicoidal pattern. External factors, such as temperature and light, may determine whether the chitin microfibrils are deposited in one or the other arrangement. The locust preferably deposits the helicoidal pattern during night conditions and the preferred orientation during day conditions (Neville, 1967b).

The matrix proteins

As mentioned above the chitin microfibrils, whatever their arrangement, are placed in a protein matrix. The chitin content of whole cuticles varies from about 20% to about 60% of the dry weight, and the rest is mainly made up of proteins. To the best of my knowledge a cuticle has not yet been found which contains only a single type of protein. From all the cuticles which have been investigated a mixture of several proteins has been extracted. Some of the proteins may have enzyme activities but the main part consists probably of proteins which have a passive structural role.

When one compares the various results which have been obtained in separating proteins in cuticular extracts it is important to consider whether completely unsclerotized cuticle or more or less sclerotized cuticle has been used. Only completely unsclerotized cuticle can be expected to give reliable results, as just a few covalent cross-links formed during sclerotization will result in a mixture of various protein dimers, trimers, and higher polymers, and an original heterogeneous mixture of protein molecules will thus become more complicated.

The proteins in soft cuticles can be divided into groups by successively extracting the cuticles with solvents of increasing ability to dissolve proteins. In one of the more detailed investigations of this type Hackman (1972) extracted cuticle from larvae of the beetle, *Agrianome spinicollis*, successively with water, 0.5 M potassium chloride, 7 M urea and 1 M sodium hydroxide. Each fraction was subjected to polyacrylamide electrophoresis, both with and without sodium dodecylsulphate (SDS) in the gels, to isoelectric focusing in polyacrylamide gels, and to thin layer gel filtration. He found that each of the fractions contained a number of proteins and that the compositions of the fractions were different. The major components in each fraction had molecular weights below 18 000 and isoelectric points between pH 3·35 and 5·7.

The extracts obtained from a given cuticle with the various solvents also show differences in amino acid composition, which confirms that they contain different types of proteins. However, none of the proteins in an insect cuticle has yet been purified and characterized, so we do not know how pronounced the differences are. I have attempted the isolation of single protein species from unhardened locust (*Schistocerca gregaria*) cuticle, but although I have obtained highly purified fractions, I have not obtained preparations which gave only a single band on polyacrylamide electrophoresis. It became clear, however, that unhardened locust cuticle contains a large number of proteins which are very similar in properties and composition. Separation by means of SDS-gel electrophoresis or gel filtration on Sephadex G-100 indicates the presence of between 20 and 30 proteins, and as these methods separate according to molecular size, the protein mixture must be heterogeneous with respect to molecular weight. When the amino acid compositions of the various fractions obtained by gel filtration were determined it was found that irrespective of molecular weight the amino acid compositions of the proteins were nearly identical. Small differences were observed but they were not as pronounced as reported for fractions obtained from soft cuticles. That locust cuticular proteins are homogeneous in composition but heterogeneous in size (and also in isoelectric points according to electrofocusing) can be explained by assuming that only a few proteins are present in the cuticle and that some cross-linking has already taken place, so that what is separated is a mixture of oligomeric proteins. If this explanation is correct, it will mean that cross-linking starts in the new cuticle before ecdysis, since the animals used for the preparations were caught just as they had initiated ecdysis. It must also be another type of cross-linking than the one which occurs after ecdysis, since no trace of ketocatechols could be obtained from these cuticles. The relationship between sclerotization and ketocatechols will be discussed below.

Another explanation for the homogeneity in composition and heterogeneity in size of the cuticular proteins could be that a pronounced gene duplication has occurred, and that the collection of genes for cuticular proteins thus formed has not diverged very much in their base sequences. In that case one should expect pronounced sequence homologies between the individual proteins and also between various parts of the same protein especially among those belonging to the higher molecular weight class. Hackman (1972) has suggested that the presence of a number of similar but non-identical proteins in cuticle will result in a plastic structure which will have little tendency to crystallize, and could have a favourable effect on the mechanical properties.

Larsen (1975) has succeeded in purifying the major part of the proteins in the endocuticle of *Limulus polyphemus* and has determined their molecular weights, isoelectric points, and amino acid compositions. He finds that they are only superficially similar: they are small, their molecular weights are in the range 4000 to 16 000; they have alkaline isoelectric points, between pH 7 and pH 10; they are devoid of sulphur-containing amino acids; and they are rich in tyrosine (ranging from 12 to 24% of the total number of amino acid residues). The *Limulus* proteins are neither specially enriched in small or in hydrophobic amino acid residues as has been described for other cuticles.

When the various cuticular amino acid analyses which have been published are compared certain trends can be seen in the compositions, but the total number of analyses is too small to allow any far-reaching conclusions. It appears that different species within a given order tend to have a similar cuticular composition when they are at the same developmental stage.

Amino acid analyses of puparia from six different species of Diptera have been published, and there are only minor differences between them. The species which have been analysed are: *Lucilia cuprina* (Hackman & Goldberg, 1971; Gilby & McKellar, 1970), *Calliphora augur* (Hackman & Goldberg, 1971), *Musca domestica* and *Musca autumnalis* (Bodnaryk, 1972), *Drosophila virilis* (Fukushi & Seki, 1965) and *Drosophila melanogaster* (Fukushi, 1967). It is interesting that all the puparia except that from *M. autumnalis* contain significant amounts of beta-alanine. This beta-amino acid is assumed to play a role in the sclerotization of some cuticles, as will be discussed later, and the puparium of *M. autumnalis* is calcified and not sclerotized.

The various larvae of Lepidoptera which have been analysed resemble each other too in cuticular amino acid composition. The species which have been analysed are: *Bombyx mori* (Hackman & Goldberg, 1971), *Sphinx ligustri*, *Hyalophora cecropia* and *Aglais urticae* (E. Palm, pers. comm.). Welinder (1974) has analysed the cuticle of five species of Crustacea (*Astacus fluviatilis, Cancer pagurus, Carcinus maenas, Nephrops norvegicus* and *Penaeus duorarum*), and he found only minor differences between them.

Adult cuticle from three species of beetle, *Xylotrupes gideon* (Hackman & Goldberg, 1971), *Tenebrio molitor* (Andersen, Chase & Willis, 1973) and *Pachynoda epphipiata* (Andersen, 1975), have similar amino acid compositions, whereas there are significant differences between *Tenebrio* larval cuticle and larval cuticle from *P. epphipiata* (Andersen, 1975) and *Agrianome spinicollis* (Hackman & Goldberg, 1971). The larval cuticle of *Tenebrio* differs also from that of the two other species in its mechanical properties, it is much more hard and solid, and the proteins are presumably more stabilized. This must be seen in relation to the different external conditions in which the larvae live. It is interesting that solid cuticle from larval and adult locusts, *Schistocerca gregaria*, has an amino acid composition (Andersen, 1971b, 1973) which resembles that of the cockroach *Periplaneta americana* (Hackman & Goldberg, 1971).

I have collected in Table I some data from various analyses to compare "solid" cuticles with "soft" cuticles. I use the term "solid" for those cuticles which are not easily deformed, and "soft" for those which can be deformed by applying slight forces. This classification is not based on precise measurements, but on a subjective estimate of how easily they are deformed when handling them. Quantitative measurements have been performed on a number of cuticles (Hepburn & Joffe, 1976), but I believe it is too early to relate amino acid composition to the quantitative measurement of the stiffness.

I consider the cuticles obtained from pupal and adult stages as well as from larvae of *Tenebrio molitor* as "solid", whereas the cuticles from all the other larvae are classified as "soft". Among the "soft" cuticles I have also included the dipteran puparia, as these cuticles are transformed "soft" larval cuticle.

It appears that those cuticles which I have grouped as "solid" are generally poorer in amino acid residues with polar side chains than are the "soft" cuticles. The latter are, on the other hand, poorer in the small amino acids (glycine, alanine, serine) than the former type of cuticle. This indicates that the "soft" cuticles are more hygroscopic than the "solid" cuticles and thefore *in vivo* will contain more water, and that the proteins in the "solid" cuticles will be able to be packed closer owing to the large amount of small residues. How they are packed will depend upon the

TABLE I

Composition of various insect cuticles

	Proline	Residues with small side-chains	Residues with polar side-chains	Beta-alanine	Type of cuticle
LEPIDOPTERA					
Adults					
Xylophasia monoglypha[a]	7	40	38	present	solid
Sphinx ligustri[b]	8	44	39	?	solid
Pupae					
Bombyx mori[c]	10	21	38	14	solid
Sphinx ligustri[b]	12	38	41	?	solid
Larvae					
Bombyx mori[d]	10	31	47	nil	soft
Sphinx ligustri[b]	9	28	51	?	soft
Hyalophora cecropia[b]	10	29	50	?	soft
Aglais urticae[b]	9	29	52	?	soft
COLEOPTERA					
Adults					
Xylotrupes gideon[d]	8	47	25	1	solid
Tenebrio molitor[e]	9	42	27	?	solid
Pachynoda epthipiata[f]	7	50	29	trace	solid
Tenebrio molitor[e]	7	42	36	?	solid
Pupae					
Pachynoda epthipiata[f]	10	38	42	trace	solid
Agrianome spinicollis[d]	10	32	43	nil	soft
Tenebrio molitor[e]	9	40	36	?	solid
Pachynoda epthipiata[f]	8	37	45	nil	soft
DIPTERA					
Larvae					
Lucilia cuprina[d]	9	29	43	nil	soft
Lucilia cuprina[d]	9	28	46	9	soft
Calliphora augur[d]	7	28	47	11	soft
Drosophila melanogaster[g]	5	26	47	1	soft
Puparia					
Drosophila virilis[c]	11	22	46	3	soft
Musca domestica[c]	7	32	38	6	soft
Musca domestica[h]	6	25	51	9	soft
Musca autumnalis[h]	7	26	52	nil	soft
Average for solid cuticles	8·7	40·2	35·1		
Average for soft cuticles	8·4	28·7	47·0		

The results are expressed as residues of amino acids per 100 residues.

[a] Hunt (1971); [b] E. Palm (pers. comm.); [c] Fukushi & Seki (1965); [d] Hackman & Goldberg (1971); [e] Andersen, Chase & Willis (1973); [f] Andersen (1975); [g] Fukushi (1967); [h] Bodnaryk (1972).

configurations of the protein chains, whether they are in the extended beta-configuration or whether they are globular. The relatively large amount of proline which is found in all cuticles, both "solid" and "soft", should make alpha-helices improbable. We do not know the configuration of the proteins in the intact cuticles, both beta-configuration and globular structure have been suggested, but the evidence is only tentative. It is difficult to obtain conclusive evidence from intact cuticle owing to the presence of the chitin crystallites, and it is dangerous to conclude anything about their configuration inside the cuticle from the configuration of proteins in the extracted state, as the surrounding of the protein molecules will be different in the two cases.

Relationship between chitin and proteins

This leads on to the question of the relationship between the proteins and the chitin structure in cuticle. Are the chitin microfibrils just imbedded in a homogeneous matrix of proteins? Or are there specific bonds between chitin molecules and some of the proteins? Definitive answers can not yet be given to the questions. One thing which complicates the issue is that unspecific bonds between chitin and protein molecules are probably introduced during sclerotization, but not even this is known for certain. As a slight degree of sclerotization can also occur in "soft" cuticles, it is difficult to be sure whether chitin–protein linkages which may be present are linking specific proteins to the chitin or whether they are of a secondary, unspecific nature. When "soft" cuticles are extracted with various solvents a certain fraction of the proteins is always non-extractable, and it has been implied that this is due to chitin–protein linkages. Hydrolysis of cuticle, which removes proteins and leaves the chitin more or less intact, leaves a few amino acid residues firmly attached to the chitin. Hackman (1960) found that aspartyl and histidyl residues were the most resistant towards alkaline hydrolysis and he suggested that they might be involved in linking protein to chitin.

By extracting non-hardened locust cuticle with formamide I have been able to remove about 90% of the proteins (Andersen, 1971b), and the remaining 10% has an amino acid composition quite distinct from that of the extracted fraction (Table II). The composition of the insoluble part is such that one should expect it to be readily soluble, and formamide is usually a good solvent for proteins. A similar difference in the composition of the formamide

TABLE II

Amino acid compositions of fractions obtained by extracting two types of locust cuticle with pure formamide

	Unhardened femur cuticle			Intersegmental membrane[a]		
	Unextracted cuticle	Residue	Extract	Unextracted cuticle	Residue	Extract
Aspartic acid	3·9	4·0	3·9	8·4	4·5	9·6
Threonine	2·3	3·3	1·9	4·6	3·7	4·5
Serine	4·7	5·9	4·2	6·1	6·3	5·6
Glutamic acid	3·0	4·9	3·3	9·6	6·1	10·7
Proline	11·1	12·6	11·2	13·2	11·9	11·9
Glycine	7·4	17·4	6·5	18·0	30·1	14·5
Alanine	35·7	18·7	39·1	9·5	7·4	12·7
Valine	8·4	11·3	7·5	6·3	8·5	6·5
Half-cystine	nil	nil	nil	nil	nil	nil
Methionine	nil	nil	nil	nil	nil	nil
Isoleucine	3·6	3·9	3·6	4·5	4·3	4·8
Leucine	4·7	5·8	4·1	5·1	6·3	4·7
Tyrosine	7·1	1·8	7·6	2·2	0·5	2·5
Phenylalanine	0·8	1·7	0·8	3·0	2·0	3·4
Lysine	1·5	2·1	1·3	3·4	2·9	2·8
Histidine	2·1	2·4	1·7	1·8	2·3	1·5
Arginine	3·8	4·3	3·3	4·5	3·5	4·2

The results are expressed as residues of amino acids per 100 residues.
[a] From Andersen (1971b).

extractable fraction and the insoluble residue has been reported for locust intersegmental membranes (Andersen, 1971b). The insoluble fraction may be prevented from going into solution by being covalently bound to chitin. The evidence is inconclusive, and the problem deserves a much more critical investigation.

MECHANICAL PROPERTIES OF THE CUTICLE

Until recently only a few measurements of the mechanical properties of cuticle have been published, and the most important of these were the measurements of Jensen & Weis-Fogh (1962) on locust cuticle and the measurements on resilin by Weis-Fogh (1961). The latter showed resilin to be a nearly perfect rubber as the change in internal energy upon stretching was virtually nil and the elastic force was solely due to the entropy decrease caused by pulling randomly coiled peptide chains into a less random configuration. The resilin tendon from dragonflies could be extended about 300% before breaking.

The measurements on solid cuticle (Jensen & Weis-Fogh, 1962) where locust tibia was used demonstrated that this material is much less extensible, it could be extended 2 to 3% before breaking. The elastic modulus in extension was found to 9400 N/mm^2 and the tensile strength to 94 N/mm^2, whereas the corresponding values for pure resilin from dragonflies were 2 N/mm^2 and 3 N/mm^2, respectively. During the last few years these measurements have been extended by a series of measurements on the tensile properties of a wide range of arthropod cuticles (Hepburn & Joffe, 1976). They find that the mechanical properties of arthropod cuticles span a very wide range, from soft, plastic, highly extensible cuticles, as found in some larvae, to very stiff, brittle cuticles as found in some beetles and in *Limulus*. Most cuticles fall somewhere in between these extremes, and no sharp transition from "soft" to "solid" cuticle can be found. Typical values for the elastic modulus are 90 N/mm^2 for larval cuticle of *Bombyx mori* and 15 000–20 000 N/mm^2 for beetle elytra (Hepburn & Joffe, 1976). The larval cuticle of *Bombyx mori* also shows a pronounced plastic flow upon stretching in contrast to brittle cuticle. In typical "solid" cuticles, consisting of sclerotized exocuticle and non-sclerotized or little-sclerotized endocuticle, it was observed that after the exocuticle had broken in a brittle manner the endocuticle then carried the force and was deformed by plastic flow before it also broke. Cuticles where the chitin microfibrils are arranged in a cross-plied manner were clearly mechanically anisotropic, the tensile behaviour depended upon whether the tensile force was applied parallel to some of the chitin microfibrils and at right angles to the other or whether it was applied at 45° to all the microfibrils (Hepburn & Ball, 1973). Cuticles where the chitin microfibrils are mainly in a helocoidal orientation behaved mechanically isotropic in the plane of the cuticle (Hepburn & Joffe, 1976). The authors interpret the results as indicating that the mechanical properties of the lepidopteran larval cuticle are mainly determined by the chitin skeleton, and that the proteins contribute only little to the tensile strength. At the other extreme, in the brittle cuticles, the contribution from the chitin microfibrils is negligible and the properties are determined by the sclerotized matrix. In a "typical" cuticle both components will contribute, the hardened matrix will be the most important component of the exocuticle and the chitin microfibrils will contribute relatively more to the properties of the endocuticle.

When some cuticles, such as untanned locust femur cuticle, are repeatedly stretched they become gradually more stiff (Hepburn & Joffe, 1976). This so called work-hardening may be due to stretch-induced reorientation of molecules so that they can interact more firmly. The phenomenon may be of physiological importance, as it indicates that a fully stretched but still unsclerotized cuticle will be stiffer than when unstretched.

The opposite phenomenon, work-softening, has also been reported from cuticle (Vincent, 1975). The abdominal intersegmental membranes of mature female locusts are very soft and stretchable, they can be stretched elastically up to about 15 times their resting length. This enables the females to lay their eggs at a depth of 8 to 9 cm below the surface while the normal length of their abdomen is about 2·5 cm (Vincent & Prentice, 1973). Stress softening allows the locusts to extend the membranes elastically and thereafter to hold the membranes extended with the use of a relatively small extension force (Vincent, 1975).

In the blood-sucking bug, *Rhodnius prolixus*, the abdominal cuticle becomes greatly distended during a meal to accommodate a large amount of blood. Before a meal the cuticle is relatively stiff, but becomes softer as soon as the animal starts feeding. Reynolds (1975a) reports a modulus of 62 N/mm^2 for the unplasticized cuticle while the plasticized cuticle showed a modulus of 2·5 N/mm^2. The animals are thus able to change the mechanical properties of the abdominal cuticle according to their needs. The results of Reynolds (1975b) indicate that this change is brought about by changes in the cuticular pH. The mechanical properties of isolated pieces of cuticle are pH-dependent, and the extensibility increases much when the pH of the medium is lowered to about pH 6. It has not been possible to measure the intracuticular pH directly, but from observations of drops of indicator solutions in which small pieces of plasticized or unplasticized cuticle were placed, Reynolds (1975b) concluded that the pH in the plasticized cuticle is less than pH 6 whereas in the non-plasticized cuticles it is higher than pH 6.

CROSS-LINKS BETWEEN CUTICULAR PROTEINS

A characteristic feature of the cuticle of many insects (mainly in adults but also in many larvae) is that large regions of the cuticle are heavily stabilized by various types of cross-links between the protein molecules. The proteins have become less soluble and more resistant towards enzymatic degradation, and the cuticle has become more firm and solid. The various types of sclerotization have been reviewed several times, and I do not intend to discuss them in all details. I shall mainly describe their characteristic features, and compare them with respect to the properties of the final product, the fully formed cuticle.

The most common cross-link in proteins is the disulphide-linkage of cystine, so well known from keratins. Cuticular proteins are generally poor in sulphur-containing amino acids, and quantitatively such cross-links can only be of minor importance. Hackman (1971) has suggested that disulphide-linkages can play a role in stabilizing the pre-sclerotized cuticle, and they have also been implied in the stabilization of cuticle from arthropods other than insects. The problem requires more detailed investigation, before the importance of disulphide-linkages in cuticles can be considered established.

Rubber-like cuticle

Some specialized regions of cuticle are stabilized by cross-links formed by joining tyrosine residues together to give dityrosine and tertyrosine (formerly called trityrosine) residues (Andersen, 1966). These amino acids were first found in the rubber-like type of cuticle containing resilin, but they have since been demonstrated in various types of cuticle, and also in other structural proteins. The cross-link can be formed *in vitro* by treatment of proteins with oxidants, which will oxidize tyrosine residues to free radicals, and the cross-linking of solubilized silk fibroin by treatment with peroxidase and hydrogen peroxide has been reported (Andersen,1966). The biosynthesis of the cross-links occurs presumably by a similar reaction, but it has not been experimentally confirmed. The cross-links are very stable, and once formed they are apparently not broken again *in vivo*.

In resilin the cross-links are formed soon after the protein has been secreted from the cells, and both secretion and cross-linking are continuous processes lasting at least some weeks. There is never a measurable quantity of uncross-linked resilin present, and the isolation and characterization of the proresilin molecule is extremely difficult (Coles, 1966). The degree of cross-linking in resilin depends to some extent upon the external conditions. The cross-links are strongly fluorescent, and in resilin from animals grown under alternating day and night conditions one can see alternating layers with different degrees of fluorescence (Neville, 1963). Strongly fluorescent resilin is deposited during day conditions and less fluorescent resilin is deposited during night conditions (Neville, 1967a).

Solid cuticle

During cross-linking of solid cuticle amino acid residues in neighbouring protein molecules are not linked directly together as in resilin; they are linked together by means of a small molecule which is able to react with several groups. Two different reactions have been proposed for the process and both can apparently occur in a given piece of cuticle. The final properties of the cuticle will depend upon which of the two is the dominating reaction.

Quinone sclerotization

According to the classical scheme, which is based upon Pryor (1940) and contributions from a number of other investigators, a polyphenoloxidase is present in the outer layer of the cuticle, the epicuticle. When sclerotization is about to be initiated a low molecular weight *ortho*-diphenol, *N*-acetyldopamine, is secreted into the cuticle from the epidermal cells. Presumably it passes through the cuticle via the pore canals and reaches the enzyme in the epicuticle. The enzyme catalyses the oxidation of the compound to the corresponding *ortho*-quinone, and the oxygen needed for this process comes also from the inside of the animal. Although the enzyme is located less than a micron from the surrounding air the oxygen present here cannot get access to the enzyme owing to the impermeability of the epicuticle.

Quinones are highly reactive compounds and react spontaneously with a number of groups, such as sulphydryl groups, amino groups, phenolic groups, and even with water. They can also react with each other and form quinone polymers. When such a reactive molecule is continuously generated inside a protein matrix it will first react with the groups available in the immediate vicinity and thereafter diffuse further and further into the cuticle, with the result that the cuticle gradually becomes sclerotized from outside and inwards. When a quinone molecule reacts with a group on a protein the catechol structure is re-formed, and it will not be able to react with other groups before it has been reoxidized to the quinone stage. This oxidation does not need to be catalysed enzymatically. The presence of a surplus of free quinones is enough to ensure that the protein-linked derivatives are reoxidized and therefore capable of reacting with more groups. The process will eventually stop either due to inactivation of the enzyme or to exhaustion of available substrate. In the fully hardened cuticle one can imagine that residues derived from N-acetyldopamine will be bound to most of the amino and phenolic groups on the proteins, some of the residues will be in the reduced state as catechol derivates and others will be present as quinones. Some will only be connected with a single group and will therefore not act as cross-links, but will influence the solubility properties of the proteins. Some of the residues will be connected with two or more groups and can thus act as cross-links, making the proteins insoluble and hindering their movements relative to each other. Some of the quinones may also have polymerized to large polymers, whereby they will be able to act as cross-links over large distances and also act as filling material between the protein molecules. It is also possible that some of the quinones will react with the chitin molecules and thereby establish a firm connection between proteins and chitin.

The formula (Fig.2) shows a highly simplified picture of a quinone-derived cross-link:

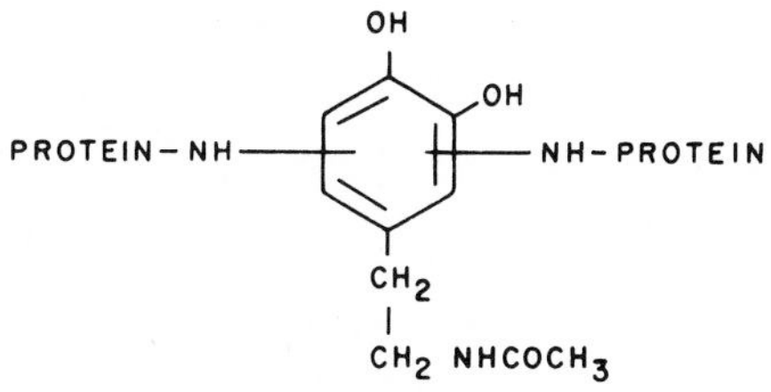

Fig. 2.

Several features which presumably make the actual cross-links more complex have not been included in the formula. It has been drawn without regard to polymer formation or to the possibility that groups other than amino groups can be involved, or that the ring may be in the oxidized, quinoid state.

The picture of the quinone-sclerotized cuticle is, moreover, mainly based upon circumstantial evidence, partly obtained from the behaviour of simple quinones in model experiments and partly from a study of the tanning of the egg-capsules of cockroaches. In the latter case there is hardly any doubt that a quinone is formed which reacts with some groups in the oothecal proteins. It has been demonstrated that lysine residues in the proteins disappear during the sclerotization of the egg-capsules (Hackman & Goldberg, 1963), but the nature of the cross-links has never been established. Our knowledge of the reactions in cuticle is also rather incomplete. An enzyme capable of oxidizing various diphenols has been shown to be present, but the nature of the products formed by oxidation of the substrate has never been established; it has just been assumed that it is a quinone. All attempts to isolate either quinone-derived cross-links or degradation products of such cross-links from hydrolysates of cuticle have to my knowledge been fruitless, but if the structure of a quinone-tanned cuticle is as I outlined above, then it must be exceedingly difficult to isolate well defined degradation products from the cross-links owing to their highly diverse structures. The lack of firm, conclusive evidence for quinone tanning is therefore due to the complexity of the reactions involved, and I hope that it will be possible to obtain better evidence by means of modern fractionation and identification techniques, such as various forms for chromatography combined with mass spectrometry.

Beta-Sclerotization

The other mechanism which has been suggested for hardening of insect cuticle resembles in many respects the scheme for quinone sclerotization; the main difference is that *ortho*-quinones are not involved. The alternative scheme has been called beta-sclerotization, as the beta-position in the side-chain of *N*-acetyldopamine is involved in connecting the compound to the cuticular proteins (Andersen & Barrett, 1971; Andersen, 1971a). According to the scheme, *N*-acetyldopamine is secreted from the epidermal cells into the cuticle where it encounters an enzyme in the epicuticle which oxidizes it in such a way that the beta-position becomes reactive and forms connections to available amino and phenolic groups (Andersen, 1972). When it becomes connected to more than one group cross-links are established between protein molecules. Polymers of N-acetyldopamine can also be formed, as the beta-position of one molecule can form links to the phenolic groups of other molecules. *In vitro* we have obtained a dimer of N-acetyldopamine by incubating locust cuticle with excess of substrate. In the dimer both phenolic groups of one residue of N-acetyldopamine are connected to the beta-position of the other residue (Andersen, 1972).

The formula shows a simplified picture of the type of cross-link which is assumed to be formed during beta-sclerotization:

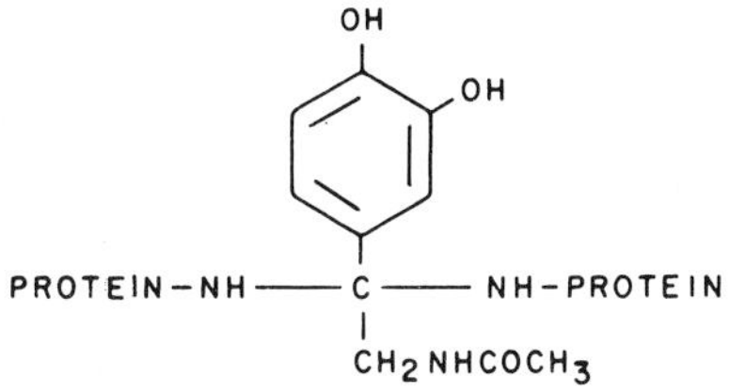

FIG. 3.

Several features which presumably make the actual cross-links more complex have not been included in the formula. It has been drawn without regard to polymer formation or to the possibility that groups other than amino groups can be involved.

The evidence for beta-sclerotization is obtained from studies of incorporation of labelled precursors, studies of the cuticular enzymes, and from isolation and characterization of degradation products of the cross-links.

When locust cuticle is subjected to acid hydrolysis a number of phenolic compounds are liberated. They can easily be separated by column chromatography and several have been identified (Andersen, 1970, 1971a; Andersen & Barrett, 1971). They are ketocatechols and have the general structure seen in Fig. 4.

The nature of the side-chain (R) depends upon the conditions of hydrolysis: reflux with 1M hydrochloric acid gives as main product a compound where R is CH_2OH, reflux with 6M hydrochloric acid gives mainly arterenone, where R is CH_2NH_2, and hydrolysis in conc. hydrochloric acid at room temperature or reflux in methanolic hydrochloric acid gives significant amounts of N-acetylarterenone ($R = CH_2NHCOCH_3$). This compound is pre-

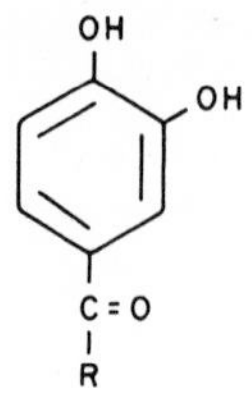

Fig. 4.

sumably the one which has suffered least degradation on being liberated from the cuticle.

If locusts are injected with labelled tyrosine, dopa, dopamine or N-acetyldopamine, part of the label is incorporated into the cuticle in insoluble form and can afterwards be recovered as ketocatechols (Andersen & Barrett, 1971; Andersen, 1971a). The best precursor is N-acetyldopamine, where about 80% of the injected radioactivity was recovered in the ketocatechol fraction. If tritiated N-acetyldopamine is injected it makes no difference whether the tritium is located in the acetyl group or on the dopamine moiety, as long as it is not present on the beta-carbon atom of the side-chain. From this position the tritium is lost, and the loss does not occur during hydrolysis but in the animal, since no label can be found in intact cuticle.

Material which contains the bound N-acetyldopamine derivative can be brought into solution by digestion of fully hardened locust cuticle by proteolytic enzymes (Andersen, 1970). We have not succeeded in isolating a pure compound which contains the derivative, but the phenolic material appears to be inseparable from peptide material, indicating that covalent bonds exist between the N-acetyldopamine derivative and peptides. The keto group of the ketocatechols is not present in the solubilized material, but when the digest is treated with acid the characteristic ketocatechol spectrum gradually appears, and the same ketocatechols can be isolated from the hydrolysate as from untreated cuticle.

No ketocatechols can be obtained from completely un-sclerotized locust femur cuticle, but as the animals grow older larger and larger amounts of ketocatechols can be obtained (Andersen & Barrett, 1971), and a significant decrease in the number of free amino groups occurs at the same time (Andersen, 1972). The solubility of the proteins decreases drastically during the same period. Although the three phenomena—increase in ketocatechol precursor, amino group disappearance and loss of protein solubility—occur simultaneously they need not be causally connected; but this is the simplest explanation.

It is not only intact animals which will incorporate labelled *N*-acetyldopamine into the cuticle. Pieces of cuticle, completely devoid of epidermal cells, can manage the incorporation without addition of any cofactors (Andersen, 1972). Not only is *N*-acetyldopamine incorporated, but the product is indistinguishable from the natural product. Hydrolysis of artificially sclerotized cuticle gives the same ketocatechols as can be obtained from normal cuticle, and the solubility of the cuticular proteins decreases with the amount of *N*-acetyldopamine which is incorporated *in vitro*.

When pieces of locust cuticle are incubated with *N*-acetyldopamine labelled with tritium on the beta-carbon atom of the side-chain the tritium is gradually released from the substrate and can be recovered as tritiated water, whereas tritium in other positions is released much more slowly or not at all. The catalysed release of tritium from the ring is between 10 and 20 times slower than the release from the beta-position (Andersen, 1974). The cuticular component which catalyses the release is apparently an enzyme, and the rate of the release of tritium has been used as a measure for the amount of enzyme which is present (Andersen, 1972, 1976). The enzyme is rather thermostable, about half the activity survives heating the cuticle to 80°C for 5 min. The pH-optimum is between pH 5·0 and 5·5, and the enzyme is firmly bound to the cuticular structure. It is not possible to extract it, even from completely unsclerotized cuticle, and it has only been brought into solution by digestion of such cuticles with trypsin (Andersen, 1976). The full amount of enzyme activity is already present in the cuticle at emergence of the adult from the exuviae. Since the cuticle grows considerably in thickness after emergence the amount of enzyme per mg cuticle decreases with age, but the amount of enzyme per mm^2 cuticle stays constant. This indicates that neither is the enzyme destroyed during sclerotization nor is more enzyme deposited during the maturation period.

Most of the results concerning beta-sclerotization have been obtained from the desert locust, *Schistocerca gregaria*. They have, however, been supplemented by results from a number of other arthropods, and this type of sclerotization has been found to occur in all insect species investigated, but not in any other arthropod group.

It appears that I was lucky when I chose the locust as experimental animal, since sclerotization of its cuticle is a simpler process than that of the cuticles of many other insect species. Beta-sclerotization is the all-important mechanism for stabilizing the cuticle of locusts, whereas both beta-sclerotization and quinone tanning are important for many other insects.

I have used the release of tritium from the beta-position of N-acetyldopamine as a measure for the beta-sclerotizing enzyme, and in a similar way one can use the release of tritium from the aromatic ring of N-acetyldopamine as a measure for the formation. of quinones. While locust cuticle has little tendency to release ring-located tritium, other cuticles such as *H. cecropia* pupal cuticle, *Tenebrio* adult cuticle, and *Calliphora* puparia, show considerable activity towards tritium in this position (Andersen, 1974, 1976). These cuticles are also active towards beta-located tritium. It is characteristic that the cuticles which contain both activities become dark brown during sclerotization whereas those which only contain the beta-directed activity stay lightly coloured.

Our knowledge of the enzymes involved in sclerotization is still limited, with regard to their number, their nature, and their quantitative importance. The cuticle of mature blowfly larvae (*Calliphora erythrocephala*) appears to have at least three different enzymes which could be involved in sclerotization of the puparium: a soluble enzyme, described by Hackman & Goldberg (1967), and two insoluble enzymes, one of which will release tritium from the aromatic ring of N-acetyldopamine; the other is active towards the beta-position of the same molecule (Andersen, 1976). A fourth enzyme, present as an inactive proenzyme in the haemolymph, occurs also in many insects, but this enzyme is presumably not involved in cuticle sclerotization. To make the situation more complicated it appears that blowfly larval cuticle not only uses N-acetyldopamine as sclerotizing agent, as first suggested by Karlson & Sekeris (1962), but that it also uses a compound derived from beta-alanyltyrosine. Beta-alanyltyrosine occurs in the haemolymph of some species of blowflies, and both the beta-alanyl moiety and the tyrosine moiety are incorporated into the puparium during the sclerotization process (Bodnaryk & Levenbook, 1969; Bodnaryk,1971). It is possible that the compound *in vivo* is transformed to beta-alanyldopamine which could be the actual sclerotization agent. In our laboratory N. J. Larsen (unpub. obs.) has found that the soluble phenoloxidase from *Calliphora* larval cuticle will readily hydroxylate beta-alanyltyramine to beta-alanyldopamine, and that the latter is then further oxidized. When intact cuticles were incubated with ^{14}C-labelled beta-alanyldopamine radioactivity was incorporated into the cuticle which at the same time went slightly brown. Acid hydrolysis of these cuticles liberated a part of the labelled material as ketocatechols, indicating that the beta-sclerotizing mechanism can use beta-alanyldopamine as substrate.

Now we have to decide how many sclerotizing agents are used for cuticle stabilization, how many enzymes are involved and how we can determine the relative importance of the various substrates and enzymes. This leads up to the important question: how are the properties of the sclerotized cuticle influenced by the nature of the substrate and by the type of enzyme involved? There is no convincing evidence that compounds other than N-acetyldopamine and beta-alanyl derivatives are involved in cuticle sclerotization. If isolation of N-acetylarterenone is accepted as evidence for the utilization of N-acetyldopamine during sclerotization and the isolation of beta-alanine as evidence for the utilization of beta-alanyltyrosine (or some derivative of it) then both compounds are commonly used among insects as sclerotizing agents. The main difference between the two compounds is that the beta-alanyl derivative carries a free amino group, which during sclerotization can be used for the attachment of more quinones or beta-activated dopamine derivatives. It can therefore be assumed that polymer formation from the sclerotizing agent will be more pronounced with beta-alanyl derivatives than with N-acetyldopamine.

We do not know the importance of polymer formation for the properties of cuticle, and we do not know how to measure it, but I shall suggest that much more phenolic material can be incorporated into the cuticle when polymer production is pronounced, and that the cuticle will become much more hard and brittle when all available space in the cuticular matrix has become filled with such a material.

It was mentioned above that one difference between cuticle sclerotized by the beta-mechanism and cuticle sclerotized by quinone tanning is that of colour: beta-sclerotization gives lightly coloured cuticle and quinone tanning gives brown cuticle. However, the two reactions are often going on simultaneously in the same cuticle, and the outcome will be the result of a competition among the enzymes for the available substrate(s). It can therefore be assumed that the polymers which are formed will be mixed polymers, where both mechanisms have contributed. This will not make their composition simpler to unravel, and I believe that what has been true until now, that the exploration of insect cuticle has mainly been hampered by the lack of proper methods for analysing the structure, will also be true for the future. But I hope we shall soon be able to answer some of the questions mentioned above.

REFERENCES

Andersen, S. O. (1966). Covalent cross-links in a structural protein, resilin. *Acta physiol. scand.* **66**: suppl. 263, 1–81.

Andersen, S. O. (1970). Isolation of arterenone (2-amino-3',4'-dihydroxyaceto-phenone) from hydrolysates of sclerotized insect cuticle. *J. Insect Physiol.* **16**:1951–1959.

Andersen, S. O. (1971a). Phenolic compounds isolated from insect hard cuticle and their relationship to the sclerotization process. *Insect Biochem.* **1**: 157–170.

Andersen, S. O. (1971b). Resilin. In *Comprehensive biochemistry* **26C**: 633–657. Florkin, M. & Stotz, E. H. (eds). Amsterdam: Elsevier.

Andersen, S. O. (1972). An enzyme from locust cuticle involved in the formation of crosslinks from N-acetyldopamine. *J. Insect Physiol.* **18**: 527–540.

Andersen, S. O. (1973). Comparison between the sclerotization of adult and larval cuticle in *Schistocerca gregaria*. *J. Insect Physiol.* **19**: 1603–1614.

Andersen, S. O. (1974). Evidence for two mechanisms of sclerotization in insect cuticle. *Nature, Lond.* **251**: 507–508.

Andersen, S. O. (1975). Cuticular sclerotization in beetles, *Pachynoda epphipiata* and *Tenebrio molitor*. *J. Insect Physiol.* **21**: 1225–1232.

Andersen, S. O. (1976). Cuticular enzymes and sclerotization in insects. In *The insect integument.* Hepburn, H. R. (ed.). Amsterdam: Elsevier.

Andersen, S. O. & Barrett, F. M. (1971). The isolation of ketocatechols from insect cuticle and their possible role in sclerotization. *J. Insect Physiol.* **17**: 69–83.

Andersen, S. O., Chase, A. M. & Willis, J. H. (1973). The amino acid composition of cuticles from *Tenebrio molitor* with special reference to the action of juvenile hormone. *Insect Biochem.* **3**: 171–180.

Bodnaryk, R. P. (1971). Studies on the incorporation of β-alanine into the puparium of the fly, *Sarcophaga bullata*. *J. Insect Physiol.***17**: 1201–1210.

Bodnaryk, R. P. (1972). Amino-acid composition of the calcified puparium of *Musca autumnalis* and the sclerotized puparium of *Musca domestica*. *Insect Biochem.* **2**: 119–122.

Bodnaryk, R. P. & Levenbook, L. (1969). The role of β-alanyl-L-tyrosine (sar-cophagine) in puparium formation in the fleshfly *Sarcophaga bullata*. *Comp. Biochem. Physiol.* **30**: 909–921.

Bouligand, Y. (1965). Sur une architecture torsadée répandue dans de nom-breuses cuticules d'arthropodes. *C. r. hebd. Séanc. Acad. Sci., Paris* **261**: 3665–3668.

Coles, G. C. (1966). Studies on resilin biosynthesis. *J. Insect Physiol.* **12**: 679–691.

Dennell, R. (1973). The structure of the cuticle of the shore-crab *Carcinus maenas* (L.). *Zool. J. Linn. Soc.* **52**: 159–163.

Dennell, R. (1974). The cuticle of the crabs *Cancer pagurus* L. and *Carcinus maenas* (L.). *Zool. J. Linn. Soc.* **54**: 241–245.

Fukushi, Y. (1967). Genetic and biochemical studies on amino acid compositions and colour manifestation in pupal sheaths of insects. *Jap. J. Genet.* **42**: 11–21.

Fukushi, Y. & Seki, T. (1965). Differences in amino acid compositions of pupal sheaths between wild and black pupa strains in some species of insects. *Jap. J. Genet.* **40**: 203–208.

Gilby, A. R. & McKellar, J. W. (1970). The composition of the empty puparia of a blowfly. *J. Insect Physiol.* **16**: 1517–1529.

Hackman, R. H. (1960). Studies on chitin. IV. The occurrence of complexes in which chitin and protein are covalently linked. *Aust. J. Biol. Sci.* **13**: 560–577.

Hackman, R. H. (1971). Distribution of cystine in a blowfly larval cuticle and stabilization of the cuticle by disulphide bonds. *J. Insect Physiol.* **17**: 1065–1071.

Hackman, R. H. (1972). Gel electrophoresis and Sephadex thin-layer studies of protein from an insect cuticle, *Agrianome spinicollis*(Coleoptera). *Insect Biochem.* **2**: 235–242.

Hackman, R. H. & Goldberg, M. (1963). Phenolic compounds in the cockroach ootheca. *Biochim. biophys. Acta* **71**: 738–740.

Hackman, R. H. & Goldberg, M. (1967). The o-diphenoloxidases of fly larvae. *J. Insect Physiol.* **13**: 531–544.

Hackman, R. H. & Goldberg, M. (1971). Studies on the hardening and darkening of insect cuticles. *J. Insect Physiol.* **17**: 335–347.

Hepburn, H. R. & Ball, A. (1973). On the structure and mechanical properties of beetle shells. *J. Materials Sci.* **8**: 618–623.

Hepburn, H. R. & Joffe, I. (1976). On the material properties of insect exoskeletons. In *The insect integument.* Hepburn, H. R. (ed.). Amsterdam: Elsevier.

Hunt, S. (1971). Composition of scales from the moth *Xylophasia monoglypha. Experientia* **27**: 1030–1031.

Jensen, M. & Weis-Fogh, T. (1962). Biology and physics of locust flight. V. Strength and elasticity of locust cuticle. *Phil. Trans. R. Soc. (B)* **245**: 137–169.

Karlson, P. & Sekeris, C. E. (1962). N-acetyl-dopamine as sclerotizing agent of the insect cuticle. *Nature, Lond.* **195**: 183–184.

Larsen, N. J. (1975). Isolation and characterization of proteins from the cuticle of *Limulus polyphemus* L. *Comp. Biochem. Physiol.* **51B**: 323–329.

Neville, A. C. (1963). Daily growth layers in locust rubber-like cuticle influenced by an external rhythm. *J. Insect Physiol.* **9**: 177–186.

Neville, A. C. (1967a). Factors affecting the tertiary structure of resilin in locusts. *J. Cell Sci.* **2**: 273–280.

Neville, A. C. (1967b). Chitin orientation in cuticle and its control. *Adv. Insect Physiol.* **4**: 213–286.

Neville, A. C. (1975). *Biology of the arthropod cuticle.* Berlin: Springer-Verlag.

Neville, A. C. & Luke, B. M. (1969). A two-system model for chitin–protein complexes in insect cuticles. *Tissue and Cell* **1**: 689–707.

Pryor, M. G. M. (1940). On the hardening of the cuticle of insects. *Proc. R. Soc.* (B) **128**: 393–407.

Reynolds, S. E. (1975a). The mechanical properties of the abdominal cuticle of *Rhodnius* larvae. *J. exp. Biol.* **62**: 69–80.

Reynolds, S. E. (1975b). The mechanism of plasticization of the abdominal cuticle in *Rhodnius. J. exp. Biol.* **62**: 81–98.

Rudall, K. M. & Kenchington, W. (1973). The chitin system. *Biol. Rev.* **48**: 597–636.

Vincent, J. F. V. (1975). Locust oviposition: stress softening of the extensible intersegmental membranes. *Proc. R. Soc.* (B) **188**: 189–201.

Vincent, J. F. V. & Prentice, J. H. (1973). Rheological properties of the extensible intersegmental membrane of the adult female locust. *J. Materials Sci.* **8**: 624–630.

Weis-Fogh, T. (1961). Thermodynamic properties of resilin, a rubber-like protein. *J. Molec. Biol.* **3**: 520–531.

Weis-Fogh, T. (1970). Structure and formation of insect cuticle. *Symp. R. ent. Soc. Lond.* **5**: 165–185.

Welinder, B. S. (1974). The crustacean cuticle. I. Studies on the composition of the cuticle. *Comp. Biochem. Physiol.* **47A**: 779–787.

Symp. zool. Soc. Lond. (1977) No. 39, 33–34.

THE WATERPROOFING LAYER
OF THE INSECT CUTICLE

V. B. WIGGLESWORTH

Department of Zoology, University of Cambridge, Cambridge, England

Andersen in the previous article has concentrated mainly on the skeletal properties of the insect cuticle. Equally important in terrestrial insects are its waterproofing properties. Forty years ago Ramsay (1935) showed that the waterproofing of the cockroach is due to a mobile layer of free lipid on its surface; and some years later (Wigglesworth, 1945) I found that all the insects studied were waterproofed by a superficial layer of wax, the hardness of the wax varying with the environment of the insect in question. Extracts of the wax from cast cuticles by Beament (1945) suggested that it formed a layer about 0·25 μm thick.

I was interested in the formation and deposition of this layer during moulting. In those days the cuticle was known to be traversed by vertical pore canals; but these appeared to end blindly below an impermeable epicuticle, some 0·5–1 μm thick. But I found that, in the larval stages of *Rhodnius*, if the old cuticle was stripped away shortly before ecdysis and the insect, so exposed in its new cuticle, was immersed in ammoniacal silver, this formed minute brown spots over the surface, from each of which a fine silver-containing channel ran through the epicuticle to the pore canals.

The silver-binding material was described as exuding from the tips of these epicuticular channels and spreading to form a continuous layer on the surface. It was regarded as a proteinaceous material rich in phenolic groups. I got into the habit of calling it (wrongly) a "polyphenol layer". When newly formed it was readily wetted by water. But shortly before ecdysis the surface of this layer became hydrofuge: I concluded that the wax layer was crystallizing out on its surface and covering up the silver reacting layer. Finally, within 0·5–1 h after ecdysis the surface became hydrophil again: that was shown to be due to the pouring out of secretion from the distended dermal glands to form a covering "cement layer".

I had come increasingly to doubt the details of this description, particularly the persistence of the successive layers on the surface, and I have recently reinvestigated the matter with the help of the electron microscope (Wigglesworth, 1975). It appears that the silver-binding material is indeed discharged by way of the pore canals and the fine epicuticular channels; and it does form a very thin layer on the surface. But most of this material impregnates the substance of the inner epicuticle, escaping from the epicuticular channel just below the outer epicuticle and spreading radially to join up with material from neighbouring channels. Then the lipid is exuded from the same channels and spreads over the surface, and unites to form a continuous layer; it then hardens or polymerizes and no longer stains with Sudan black.

After ecdysis the dermal gland secretion is poured out and stains a brilliant blue green with alcian blue: the cement layer appears to be a mucopolysaccharide. Finally, in the course of a day or two, the surface becomes hydrophobe again. I imagine that the whole extra-cuticular structure is by now permeated by the waxy lipid. In the electron microscope the composite layer outside the epicuticle is seen to be only about 30–100 nm thick. It seems likely that the thicker wax layers, inferred in earlier work, resulted from reserve wax extracted from the cast cuticles.

In short, the waterproofing layer consists of the proteinaceous silver-binding layer, covered by the mucopolysaccharide cement layer and permeated throughout by wax. The silver-binding material is thought to represent precursor substances which become involved in the sclerotization processes described by Andersen.

REFERENCES

Beament, J. W. L. (1945). The cuticular lipoids of insects. *J. exp. Biol.* **21**: 115–131.
Ramsay, J. A. (1935). The evaporation of water from the cockroach. *J. exp. Biol.* **12**: 373–383.
Wigglesworth, V. B. (1945). Transpiration through the cuticle of insects. *J. exp. Biol.* **21**: 97–114.
Wigglesworth, V. B. (1975). Incorporation of lipid into the epicuticle of *Rhodnius* (Hemiptera). *J. Cell Sci.* **19**: 459–485.

Symp. zool. Soc. Lond. (1977) No. 39, 35–76.

THE MOLLUSCAN EPIDERMIS
AND ITS SECRETIONS

K. SIMKISS and K. M. WILBUR

Department of Zoology, The University, Whiteknights, Reading, England and
Department of Zoology, Duke University, Durham, North Carolina, USA

SYNOPSIS

The structure of the skin is briefly reviewed. It is a ciliated epithelium containing epidermal cells with microvilli and numerous gland cells.

Experimental evidence is discussed which indicates that this epithelium may be permeable to a large number of molecules up to at least m.w. 68 000. Influx and efflux measurements are given for a number of ions and related to transepithelial potential differences. The possible effect of this permeability on a number of physiological functions in the Mollusca is briefly considered.

The epidermis also secretes a wide variety of substances including the tanned proteins of the byssus threads, operculum and periostracum; the elastic protein of the bivalve hinge; the calcified shell; and the viscoelastic mucus. The production of these secretions is discussed and a hypothesis is proposed for calcium deposition which is compatible with the observed fluxes of calcium and bicarbonate ions and the cellular distribution of carbonic anhydrase. The effects of phenolic tanning are indicated in a number of systems and are also related to shell formation. The physical properties of snail mucus are briefly outlined in relation to the collecting and locomotory functions of molluscs. The formation of the "mucus trail" by gastropods is investigated experimentally and also described ultrastructurally.

INTRODUCTION

The skin represents one of the main interfaces between the external and internal environments of an animal. It provides one of the main regions for contact with the outside world while at the same time it must protect the animal from the rigours of its surroundings. It is, therefore, a paradoxical structure in that the more effectively it carries out one of its functions the less effectively can it carry out its other main activity (Graham, 1957).

In most molluscs the epidermis is involved in respiratory exchanges, water fluxes and probably ion regulation. It is well innervated and contains a number of sense organs so that it is obviously of great importance to the mollusc in making contacts with the outside world. It protects the animal with mucus and a shell, both of which are characteristic secretions of the molluscan epidermis. Many molluscs also secrete a variety of substances ranging from acids to aromatic esters which may have protective functions as may many of the pigments in the skin and shell. It will be clear, therefore, that the molluscan epidermis performs a wide variety of functions and rather than list all these we have decided to concentrate on two main themes. These are (a) the transfer of water and electrolytes across the epidermis and (b) the function of the secretory products produced by it. In order to understand either of these, however, it is first necessary to consider briefly the structure of the molluscan epidermis.

THE STRUCTURE OF THE EPIDERMIS

The fundamental structure of the molluscan epidermis is a single layered epithelium of columnar cells resting on a basement membrane. It is supported by a mat of connective tissue through which run muscle fibres.

Three main types of cells have been described in the gastropod and lamellibranch skin. These are: epidermal cells, bearing a well developed microvillus layer on their outer surface; ciliated cells of various sorts; and numerous types of glands many of which produce mucus (Campion, 1961; Lane, 1963; Wondrak, 1968, 1969; Zylstra, 1972a).

The microvilli on the surface of the epidermal cells of *Helix aspersa* may increase its area by up to 15-fold (Lane, 1963), but there is often a covering layer of "slime" surrounding them forming what is sometimes confusingly referred to as a "cuticle". The size of the microvilli varies according to the region of the skin and they are usually well developed in exposed regions (1–1·5 μm high on the exposed epidermis of *Lymnaea stagnalis*) but only about half this size on the outer mantle epithelium. Beneath the microvilli are a large number of vesicles and this has generally been interpreted as indicating that either endocytotic or exocytotic activity is occurring (Wondrak, 1968). The epidermal cells are rich in microfilaments and there are numerous mitochondria, Golgi bodies and lysosomes in the cytoplasm (Zylstra, 1972a).

The ciliated cells vary greatly in their occurrence. On much of the epidermis they are relatively sparse with poorly developed rootlets. They are always well developed, however, around the foot, pneumostome and mouth of gastropods (Campion, 1961; Zylstra, 1972a) and around the palps and gills of bivalves (Satir & Gilula, 1970). Here the basal bodies are well developed and actually make contact with neighbouring cilia in a way that may be important in co-ordinating the ciliary beat. In some regions of the foot epidermal cells bear both cilia and microvilli (Rogers, 1971).

Typically, the skin of a mollusc is covered with a layer of mucus produced by various glands. In the snail *Helix aspersa* Campion (1961) identified eight types of unicellular glands discharging by pores between the epidermal cells. Four of these glands produced various kinds of mucus, one secreted protein, one calcium carbonate granules, one fat globules and one a pigmented secretion. In *Lymnaea stagnalis* Zylstra (1972a) described at least 13 types of gland cell many of which were localized in specific regions of the epidermis. The histochemical properties and regional distributions of these glands are very varied and will not be described in detail, although Fig. 1 is typical of the types of data that are available.

In some regions of the skin, the epidermal cells become specialized and folded into the connective tissue to produce more complex glands. Examples of this may be seen in the cells producing the resistant quinone-tanned proteins of the periostracum, operculum and byssus threads of various molluscs (pp. 53–55). In the gastropods, well developed mucus glands are often found—such as the anterior and posterior pedal glands which open onto the sole of the foot, and the ventral pedal gland which moulds the egg capsules of some prosobranchs (Fretter, 1941). Within the

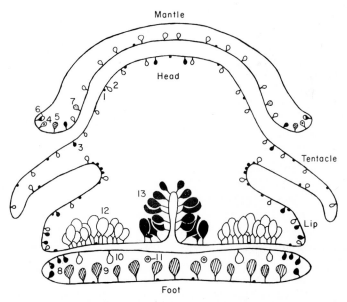

FIG. 1. Schematic drawing of 13 different types of gland cells in the skin of the snail *Lymnaea stagnalis* (redrawn from Zylstra, 1972a).

mantle lies the hypobranchial gland and around the mantle edge are a variety of glandular cells, some of which produce sticky, coloured and apparently toxic secretions (Graham, 1957).

Little is known about the mechanisms underlying the control of the discharge of these epithelial glands. The haemocoel often surrounds the bases of the mucus glands and it has been suggested that changes in blood pressure cause the release of mucus during normal locomotion (Machin, 1964a). There must, however, be other mechanisms in regions away from the sole where changes in blood pressure are less marked, and Campion (1961) has described a network of fine muscle fibres around a number of glands. The possible neural or endocrine systems which control the activities of the epidermal glands are an unexplored problem. There are, however, numerous descriptions of the nerves and sensory cells in the epidermis of molluscs (Bullock & Horridge, 1965). These provide information on both the general innervation of the skin and on the specific innervation of sensory cells. Such studies have included investigations on the tentacles of prosobranchs, the palps and tentacles of bivalves and the suckers of cephalopods. The basic localization of chemoreceptors, mechanoreceptors and photo-receptors in the epidermis has been considered both as regards their innervation (de Vlieger, 1968) and their ultrastructure (Zylstra, 1972c). The receptor cells are primary sensory nerve cells with the cell bodies lying below the epidermis. Dendrites extend from these cell bodies between the epidermal cells and form at least six different types of free nerve endings. In *Lymnaea stagnalis* these sensory cells are restricted primarily to the tentacles, lips, front edge of the foot, pneumostome and mantle edge (Zylstra, 1972c).

The protective functions of the molluscan epidermis are, there-fore, clearly served by its glandular secretions and sensory innerva-tion. If the skin is damaged the wound is closed by muscular contraction and plugged by a clot of blood amoebocytes. Thin tubercles (c.20 nm) can then be seen in this region possibly repres-enting a blood clotting system, and within a few days the differenti-ation of the amoebocytes occurs to form the flattened cells of the healing surface (Sminia, Pietersma & Scheeloom, 1973). The per-meability of the damaged epithelium is presumably soon returned to normal by the development of zonula adherens junctions at the cell apex below which zonula septata occur (Wondrak, 1968; Zylstra, 1972a). There is considerable speculation at the present time about the role which septate junctions perform in controlling the permeability between cells and across epithelia (Gilula, Bran-ton & Satir, 1970). In addition, a number of workers have pointed out that the microvillus structure of the molluscan epithelial cells is more typical of an absorptive epithelium than of a protective layer (Newell, 1973; Zylstra, 1972a) and this leads naturally from these histological studies to a general consideration of the physiological properties of the molluscan skin.

Osmotic and ionic relations

The osmotic relationships of the Mollusca are similar to those of other phyla, such as the Crustacea, in that marine species are approximately isosmotic with their environment (e.g. 645 mosmol/kg H_2O in *Siphonaria pectinata*) whereas freshwater species are hyperosmotic but tend to have a lower salt content in their blood (e.g. 125 mosmol/kg H_2O in *Lymnaea stagnalis*). Terrestrial pulmonates have a more variable and often higher haemolymph concentration (128–312 mosmol/kg H_2O in *Helix pomatia*). This variation is generally thought to reflect environmental changes in humidity and the availability of free water. It has been argued, for instance, that the high blood osmotic pressure of 430 mosmol/kg H_2O in the slug *Agriolimax reticulatus* would reduce the rate of evaporative water loss, but, in fact, concentration changes of this sort have relatively small effects on the vapour pressure of water and they are probably the results of water loss rather than an adaptation to prevent it. Most pulmonates are only in equilibrium with air at relative humidities of over 96% at 20°C (Machin, 1975).

Undoubtedly one of the main osmoregulatory structures in the molluscs is the kidney and much has been learnt about its ultrafiltration and resorption systems in the past decade (Martin, Stewart & Harrison, 1965; Andrews & Little, 1971; Newell & Skelding, 1973). In some species part of the resorption of ions occurs in the mantle (Table I) or in the ureter which in *Viviparus* is derived from it (Little, 1965). This implies, of course, the transport of ions across parts of the epidermis, and Krogh (1939) observed that many freshwater molluscs could in fact take up chloride ions from very dilute solutions. More recent evidence from the freshwater snail *Lymnaea stagnalis* suggests that sodium must be actively transported into the blood although about 40% of the sodium influx from water containing 0·35 mmol/l was due to an exchange component (Greenaway, 1970). Similar results were obtained by Chaisemartin, Martin & Bernard (1968) on the bivalve *Margaritana margaritifera* where it was shown that sodium and chloride influx

TABLE I

Composition of fluids from the excretory system of the terrestrial snail Eutrochatella tankervillei

	Osmotic pressure as NaCl (mmol/l)
Haemolymph	36·8
Distal kidney	25·0
Bladder	15·3
Mantle	7·2

Data from Little, 1972.

rates were related in a non-linear way to the external ion concentrations with a maximum uptake from solutions of about 1 mmol/l.

Calcium is also actively absorbed across the epidermis of the freshwater snail *Lymnaea stagnalis* (van der Borght & van Puymbroeck, 1964) although the quantitative importance of this phenomenon has been questioned (van der Borght & van Puymbroeck, 1966). At concentrations below 0·5 mmol/l, the uptake was against a small electrochemical gradient but at higher concentrations it was not necessary to invoke an active mechanism (Greenaway, 1971). A similar passive effect of calcium upon the transepithelial potential of the mantle of the bivalves *Anodonta grandis* and *Amblema costata* was found by Istin & Kirschner (1968) and Istin & Fossat (1972), implying that this tissue was permeable to calcium but impermeable to corresponding anions.

Water movement across the skin

An animal in isosmotic equilibrium with its environment would not, of course, be expected to show any net water fluxes across its skin. Most of the interest in this subject has, therefore, centred upon terrestrial pulmonates and Machin's extensive work on this subject has revealed several important phenomena.

In his early work, Machin (1964a,b) showed that the osmotic permeability of the skin was a limiting factor in the rate at which water could leave the animal. Experimental comparisons between living and freshly killed tissues of *Helix aspersa* led him to the conclusion that mucus secretion was a fundamental mechanism for the transfer of water to the evaporating surface. In the absence of mucus, the skin dries to a parchment-like texture but in its presence it remains pliant and acts as a free-water surface. The mucus normally accumulates in grooves in the epidermis, which act as reservoirs from which it is spread by muscular activity. Fresh mucus secretion occurs if the hydrostatic pressure on the skin is increased by about 10 cm H_2O (Machin, 1964a).

Some support for this concept of mucus formation has been proposed by Burton (1965) who analysed the blood and slime of the snail *Helix pomatia* and concluded that there must be two phases in mucus secretion. First, ions such as potassium and magnesium, which are normally accumulated within cells, would become associated with the macromolecules of mucus and would be extruded with them. Second, a watery component, rich in sodium and chloride ions, was considered to be added to this secretion as an ultrafiltrate of blood. The variations found in mucus composition could thus be accounted for by variations in the ratios of thick and thin components. From what is known about the mechanisms of mucus secretion these suggestions seem very plausible but it may be important to recognize that the second component may also contain some renal fluids (Table I) or pallial fluid as described by Blinn (1964).

A theoretically more important aspect of Machin's studies has come from his investigations on the nature of the permeability barrier of the skin. Surfaces covered with freshly secreted mucus lose water by evaporation at a rate of about $2 \cdot 5$ mg/cm^2/h/mmHg. When the snail withdraws within the shell this water loss falls dramatically and this has often been ascribed to the impermeability of the epiphragm. The epiphragm, however, has a considerable permeability to water and although it is undoubtedly of value in reducing air currents, it does not account for the very low water loss of inactive snails (Table II). It appears instead that the mantle collar has a mechanism for reducing water loss to very low values similar, in fact, to those of insect cuticles. This has led to speculation as to whether there is an active water pump in the mantle collar (Andrewartha, 1964) or what is more likely, a passive impermeable barrier over this region of the epidermis. The site of this impermeability has been the source of considerable speculation (Machin, 1965, 1972) but Machin has now produced evidence for a relatively enormous osmotic gradient of 2000–3000 mosmol/kg H_2O across the microvilli of the epithelial cells in this region (Machin, 1974).

Observations on the efflux of materials across the epidermis

It would appear from the evidence in the literature that the molluscan epidermis is permeable to various ions and aqueous

TABLE II

Water loss from Helix aspersa *under various conditions together with comparable data for the cockroach* (Periplaneta) *and desert locust* (Schistocerca)

Species	Conditions	Transfer coefficient (mg $H_2O/cm^2/h/mmHg$)
Helix aspersa	Shell filled with water (control)	2·3
Helix aspersa	Dorsal body in still air	2·5
Helix aspersa	Withdrawn, secreting mucus	2·6
Helix aspersa	Withdrawn, regulating water loss	0·039
Periplaneta	—	0·049
Schistocerca	—	0·022
Helix aspersa	Shell with epiphragm	16·97 mg H_2O/day
Helix aspersa	Shell without epiphragm	28·56 mg H_2O/day

Partly after Machin, 1975.

solutions. Preliminary experiments performed by us indicated that the skin is also permeable to ^{45}Ca and a number of other substances. We therefore have attempted to answer three specific questions.

(i) What materials will pass onto the surface of the mollusc from the blood? In particular are they limited by a particular molecular size which might indicate the dimensions of a pore in the epidermis?

(ii) By what avenues do materials pass onto the skin?

(iii) How are these substances transported and, in particular, how do ion fluxes relate to transepithelial potential differences?

Movement of substances from the blood to the body surface

In approaching the first of these questions, namely the outward movement of large molecules from the blood, we have studied the snail *Helix aspera* obtained commercially or collected near Reading, England. The animals were kept in moist aquarium tanks and fed on lettuce and carrots. The basic technique consisted of cannulating the right optic tentacle with plastic tubing so that 200 μl of saline could be injected directly into the blood sinuses. When the cannula is withdrawn the circular musculature of the tentacle contracts sealing off the cut end. In critical experiments the tentacle was ligatured and carefully washed but this was not normally necessary. Blood for analysis was obtained by cracking the shell and taking samples directly from the heart. If serial samples were required however the left optic tentacle was cannulated and the tubing sealed with modelling clay between collections.

All injections were made with a snail saline containing NaCl, 48 mmol/l; NaHCO$_3$, 20 mmol/l; KCl, 3 mmol/l; CaCl$_2$, 4·5 mmol/l; MgCl$_2$, 3·3 mmol/l. In the first series of experiments, hydroxy-^{14}C-methyl inulin (m.w. approximately 5000); sperm whale myoglobin (m.w. 17 000) and beef haemoglobin (m.w. approximately 68 000) were injected in the saline. The snails were then allowed to move normally within a glass beaker and blood samples were taken initially at 5-min and then at 30-min intervals throughout the experiment. Every 30 min the snails were transferred to a clean beaker and the one that had contained them was carefully washed out with 5 ml of distilled water using a "rubber policeman". The resulting washings were counted for ^{14}C activity or their absorption was measured in a spectrophotometer at 450 and 408 nm (myoglobin) or 450 and 404 nm (haemoglobin). Total protein was also measured at 325 and 280 nm. The results were compared with standards prepared from the injection solutions and with blood samples taken throughout the experiment.

The blood sample taken after 5 min was used to calculate the distribution volume (presumably equal to blood volume) of the injected materials. There was no significant difference in the distribution volume of the three materials in the animals used. The results were then standardized by expressing them as the percentage of the total injected load which was lost from the sole of the snail during the next 90 min. The results for 12 individuals are shown in Fig. 2. It is immediately apparent that the values of loss of

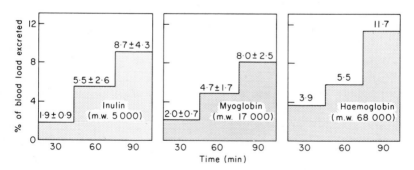

FIG. 2. Rate of loss of substances of various molecular weights after their injection into *Helix aspersa*. Values are means ±s.d. except for haemoglobin which represents only a single experiment.

these three materials are very similar and show no significant variation despite a 12-fold change in molecular weight. This suggests that these substances are lost by a mechanism resembling bulk-flow rather than diffusion through some critically sized pore. Another aspect of interest in these results is the magnitude of the effect. A snail moving for 12 h would on this basis completely lose the equivalent of its total blood volume across its epidermis.

The fact that substances the size of haemoglobin were leaking out of the snail and being left in the slime trail was something of a surprise although it has been known for some time that phenol red and similar substances behaved in this way (Martin, Stewart & Harrison, 1965). It appeared at least a possibility, however, that this loss was from the kidney leaking urine via the pneumostome onto the foot and thus incorporating material in the mucus without it passing through the epidermis of the foot. This possibility was investigated by attaching a rubber sheet around the body at the base of the shell so that the pneumostome was on the opposite side of the rubber from the head and foot. Shreds of absorbent paper were packed around the opening of the pneumostome so that the duct of the kidney was in close contact with them. The animals were then injected with saline containing both hydroxy-^{14}C-methyl inulin and haemoglobin, and the animals were allowed to crawl within clean glass beakers. At 30-min intervals, the absorbent paper was changed and the animals placed in fresh beakers. In six experiments of this type it was found that 76% of the haemoglobin and 79% of the inulin originated from the kidney and only 24 or 21% came from the foot. Furthermore, when the ratio of ^{14}C-inulin:haemoglobin was compared for the two sources, the ratios of foot:kidney were $1 \cdot 57$, $0 \cdot 71$, $0 \cdot 90$ and $1 \cdot 14$ with a mean of $1 \cdot 08$. This suggests that there is no clear distinction between the rate at which the two substances are lost from the foot and the kidney. It therefore appears that urine may be a major source of the blood components which appear in the mucus of the snail. It may, in fact, be the only source, for the alternative hypothesis would be that the two routes (urine and exudate) show no difference in discrimination between haemoglobin and inulin. Unfortunately, our data do not allow a complete answer to this problem but they do clearly show that the ionic content of the mucus cannot be regarded as representing purely the local secretion resulting from epidermal movements (cf. Burton, 1965).

Effects of ions on skin potentials

In the first of these experiments, agar/KCl salt bridges were inserted down the tentacles of the snails into the blood sinus. A second salt bridge was placed in the experimental solution into which the snail was then lowered. The salt bridges were connected through calomel half cells to a high impedance Keighley millivoltmeter. The potential difference across the snail epidermis was then measured in a variety of solutions. Diffusion potentials across the electrodes were found to be negligible and corrections were made for asymmetry potentials .

Four main sets of results are of interest. These deal with snails exposed to:

(i) calcium chloride solutions ranging from 0·1 to 10 mmol/l in water;

(ii) calcium chloride solutions ranging from 0·1 to 10 mmol/l in 70 mmol/l sodium chloride;

(iii) sodium concentrations from 0·7 to 70·0 mmol/l with choline substituted to give a constant chloride concentration of 70 mmol/1;

(iv) chloride concentrations from 0·7 to 70·0 mmol/l with sulphate substituted to give constant sodium concentrations of 70 mmol/l.

The results of these experiments are shown in Fig. 3.

The potential difference (p.d.) across a semi-permeable membrane can be calculated from the concentration gradient of the permeant ions according to Nernst's equation

$$\text{p.d.} = \frac{RT}{nF} \ln \frac{C_1}{C_2}$$

where R is the gas constant, T is the absolute temperature, n is the charge on the ion, F is Faraday's constant, and C_1 and C_2 are the concentrations on the two sides of the membrane.

The concentrations of ions in *Helix aspersa* blood are approximately as follows: Ca^{2+}, 4·5 mmol/l; Na^+, 70 mmol/l; Cl^-, 60 mmol/l. Thus for external concentrations of 0·45 mmol/l Ca^{2+} one would expect a potential difference of 29 mV, for 7 mmol/l Na^+ a potential of 58 mV and for 6 mmol/l Cl a potential of 58 mV. It is clear from Fig. 3 that these predicted results are only found for Ca^{2+} in water. For the other mixtures of ions the ratio of actual: expected = 0·28 for Ca^{2+}, 0·11 for Na^+ and 0·05 for Cl^-.

Calcium in water causes the skin to behave like a calcium electrode, implying a selective and free permeability to calcium ions without a corresponding anion movement. Under these conditions the potential obeys the predictions of Nernst's equation. This, however, only occurs if sodium ions are excluded from the outside solution, and if they are replaced in the normal blood concentration the calcium potential almost disappears. The differences in the ratios of expected to observed potentials in the various

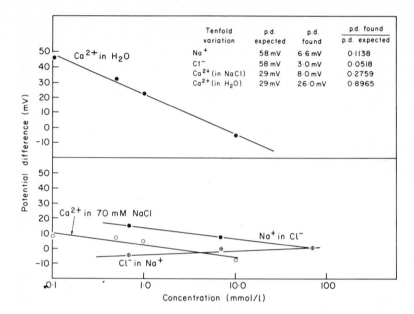

FIG. 3. Potential differences between blood and external solutions surrounding the snail *Helix aspersa*..The results shown in the top graph are for calcium chloride in distilled water. The lower graphs show the effects of other ions when the total concentrations are similar to those of snail blood. The table compares the potential expected, based on Nernst's equation, and those actually found. The signs on the potential difference axis refer to the outside surface.

solutions are presumably due to the different relative per-meabilities of the ions (Fig. 3). If the results are therefore nor-malized, the relative permeabilities for $Ca^{2+}:Na^+:Cl^-$ are $1\cdot00:0\cdot40:0\cdot18$. This indicates that the epidermis may be perme-able not only to calcium but also to a lesser extent to sodium and possibly also chloride ions.

A somewhat similar phenomenon has been found in fish gills where an apparent calcium potential can be demonstrated (Eddy, 1975). In this case, however, the observed potential is the resultant of a high sodium efflux (128 μmol/100g/h) partly balanced by a chloride efflux (110 μmol/100 g/h). In the presence of 10 mmol/1 calcium ions, both flux rates fall but sodium to a greater extent (18·6 μmol/100 g/h) than chloride (28·2 μmol/100 g/h). Through-out these changes the calcium efflux is negligible at about 1 μmol/100 g/h. Thus, although calcium ions produce large changes in the potential across fish gills, they do so not by a "calcium electrode" effect but by preferentially changing the fluxes of sodium and chloride ions. On this basis the calcium potential would not be apparent if there were no differences in sodium and chloride ion concentrations on the two sides of the membrane. This model would clearly explain the results shown in Fig. 3, and for this reason it was decided to try and measure efflux of sodium and calcium ions across the snail foot *in vivo*. There is, however, an experimental problem here for we have already seen that renal excretion could be a major source of ions onto the sole of the snail. We have therefore approached the problem in two ways.

Ion fluxes across the epidermis

In the first technique, the snail was injected down the optic tentacle with saline containing either ^{24}Na or ^{45}Ca. The animal was then inverted and eight discs of filter paper, each 6 mm in diameter, were placed along the length of the sole. The normal locomotory waves carried these discs backwards along the foot and they were then removed with forceps and reapplied to the anterior end. Thus, during an experiment eight discs of paper were in continual motion over the foot and they were renewed every 10 minutes. The radioactivity which had accumulated on the paper during this time was then determined by scintillation counting.

This technique has two advantages. First, it provides a reasonable guarantee that the material collected on the discs has not come from the kidney since inverting the animal will tend to make urine drain away from the foot. Second, it is possible to soak the filter paper discs in a variety of solutions and thus study their effect on the efflux of material from a reasonably constant area of the skin. Experiments of this sort were carried out for 30 min on each animal using solutions containing 0·45 mmol/l Ca^{2+} in water, 4·5 mmol/l Ca^{2+} in water and 4·5 mmol/l Ca^{2+} in snail saline as described previously. Samples of blood were collected at the end of the experiment and the specific activity of ^{24}Na or ^{45}Ca was determined.

The second technique involved injecting the snail as previously and then placing it in 25 ml of 0·45 mmol/l Ca^{2+}, 4·5 mmol/l Ca^{2+} or snail saline for 15 min. An aliquot of the solution was then counted for ^{24}Na or ^{45}Ca as required and again compared with the blood specific activity. It was hoped that by keeping the animals in the solution for only 15 min urinary contamination would be kept to a minimum and that the method could then provide a reasonable check upon the more controlled but less physiologically normal data from the paper disc experiments.

The results of these experiments are shown in Table III where efflux has been expressed as μmol/h/foot. The area of the sole of the foot was estimated as $6\,cm^2$ and the discs had an area of $2\cdot25\,cm^2$. It is therefore possible to convert these data into the more usual efflux values of μmol/h/cm^2 by dividing by approximately $2\cdot5$, but this involves a large number of assumptions. The results have therefore deliberately been left in the simple form shown in Table III.

TABLE III

The efflux of $^{24}Na^+$ and $^{45}Ca^{2+}$ in μmol/h from the foot of Helix aspersa *in various solutions*

Isotope	Method of collection	Solutions		
		0·45 mmol/l Ca$_2$$^+$	4·5 mmol/l Ca^{2+}	Snail saline
$^{24}Na^+$	Paper discs	2·10 ± 1·21	1·46 ± 0·47	7·75 ± 2·36
	Solution	1·87 ± 0·46	0·59 ± 0·25	5·43 ± 0·67
$^{45}Ca^{2+}$	Paper discs	0·67 ± 0·16	0·60 ± 0·06	1·82 ± 0·54
	Solution	1·56 ± 0·21	2·58 ± 0·62	2·36 ± 0·40

Values are means ± s.d. for four animals/treatment.

As might be expected, the results show considerable variation between individuals but considering the different assumptions in the two techniques they are remarkably consistent. Two deductions seem to be justified, namely:
(i) Ca^{2+} tends to decrease the efflux of $^{24}Na^+$;
(ii) physiological snail saline enhances the efflux of $^{24}Na^+$.
In addition, the presence of Ca^{2+} and the presence of the other ions in physiological saline does not inhibit and, in fact, often seems to favour the efflux of $^{45}Ca^{2+}$ from the snail.

Two conclusions follow from these observations. The first is that the occurrence of a calcium electrode effect across the molluscan epidermis (Fig. 3) may not necessarily imply that it is entirely due to the movement of calcium ions (cf. Istin & Kirschner, 1968; Greenaway, 1971). The potential could be due to the variations in permeability of other anions and cations (Eddy, 1975). Unfortunately one cannot be more precise than this since the second conclusion from our data is that there may be a major component in the ion movements which is due to an exchange mechanism. Thus other ions appear to facilitate the efflux of Na^+ and Ca^{2+} ions and this will clearly upset simple conclusions based solely on comparing fluxes and potentials on one-ion species. On a simple ion permeability concept, one would expect the presence of a snail saline outside the animal to reduce the net efflux of both [24]Na and [45]Ca since it effectively removes the concentration gradients across the skin. In fact, the saline enhances the efflux of both ions. Presumably the same explanation accounts for the increase in [45]Ca efflux when more concentrated solutions of ions are placed outside the epidermis.

Observations on the influx across the epidermis

The suggestion that there may be an ion exchange system operating across the epidermis of the snail foot clearly provides the possibility that material may be taken into the animal by this route. A number of experiments have therefore been undertaken to investigate this possibility.

In the first experiment a snail was used with the "paper disc" preparation except that the tentacle was cannulated to enable blood samples to be collected and the paper discs that were put on the foot were soaked in snail saline containing [45]Ca. Blood samples were collected at 10-min intervals for one half-hour and corrected for total [45]Ca content on the assumptions, first, that the label did not leave the blood stream, and second, that the total blood volume of a 5-g snail was approximately 2·5 ml. The accumulated dose is shown in Fig. 4. The results show that calcium was clearly able to enter the snail across the epidermis and does so linearly at a rate of about 0·6 μmol/h.

This experiment was elaborated upon by applying the [45]Ca on paper discs using similar solutions to those used in our previous efflux studies, namely 0·45 mmol/l $CaCl_2$, 4·5 mmol/l $CaCl_2$ and a complete snail saline. The animals used were also digested in Soluene (Packard Inst.) at the end of the experiment to get a better estimate of the total [45]Ca uptake by the whole body. The results are shown in Table IV. The total uptake of 0·86 μmol/h for 4·5 mmol/l and snail saline is similar to the results obtained in the previous experiment and is about 5·6 times greater than the uptake from 0·45 mmol/l.

Similar experiments have been performed with hydroxy-[14]-C-methyl inulin in either water or snail saline. From the specific activity of the inulin it was possible to estimate not only the rate at which it entered the animal but also the equivalent volume of fluid being taken up by the foot. In the case of inulin in water, 8·4 μl of fluid were absorbed per hour whilst the equivalent measurement for saline was $3\cdot6$ μl.

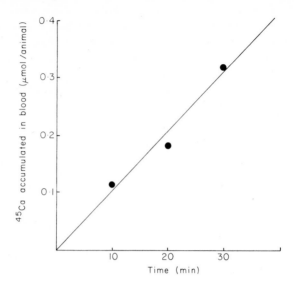

FIG. 4. The influx of calcium into the blood of *Helix aspersa* when the ion is applied to the foot of the snail.

TABLE IV

Distribution and rate of uptake of ^{45}Ca by the foot of the snail Helix aspersa

Tissue	Solution		
	0·45 mmol/l Ca	4·5 mmol/l Ca	Snail saline
Blood	70%	57%	62%
Soft tissues	13%	21%	19%
Foot	10%	17%	13%
Shell	7%	5%	6%
Total uptake	0·154 μmol/h	0·860 μmol/h	0·863 μmol/h

Two animals/treatment.

Conclusions

It is difficult to escape the conclusion that the epidermis of *Helix aspersa* is a relatively permeable structure. If one tries to put some dimensions to this permeability, one gets different results according to one's terms of reference. Taking the animal as a whole, one can say that molecules as large as haemoglobin (m.w. 68 000) will be lost from the animal's blood system and will appear on the skin and in mucus trail within minutes of being introduced into the snail. The loss via this route is sufficient to deplete the total blood volume within a day. What this means in terms of energetics is not clear. It is, however, noteworthy that the amino acid content of snail blood is lower than that of most animals (Kerkut & Cottrell, 1962) and the respiratory pigment is haemocyanin with a molecular weight of several million. Undoubtedly, part of this loss from the animal occurs via the kidney but there is good evidence for considering that it may also occur directly across the epidermis.

We have confined most of our direct observations on the epidermis to *in vivo* work since *in vitro* preparations are in our experience difficult to manipulate and to interpret. The epidermis is closely attached to the underlying tissues which show much muscular activity so that there is no simple way of circulating saline through the preparation. Our *in vivo* observations on potential differences indicate that with water outside, the skin has a greater permeability to calcium than sodium ions by the ratio of $1:0\cdot4$. Efflux measurements suggest that sodium passed out about three times faster than calcium (Table III). This is not necessarily a contradiction of the potential measurements since the blood sodium concentration (60–70 mmol/l) is many times greater than blood calcium ($4\cdot5$ mmol/l). In fact if one multiplies the concentration gradient by the apparent permeability as indicated by potential difference measurements one gets roughly the observed flux ratio, i.e.

$$\frac{60 \times 0\cdot4}{4\cdot5 \times 1} \simeq 5.$$

This treatment is, of course, far too simple to be more than just suggestive since it ignores the effects of transepithelial potentials upon flux rates and also assumes that the potential differences recorded arise from the general epidermis and not from some specialized region.

Our observations with ^{45}Ca indicate that calcium can move in both directions across the epithelium of the foot. At a concentration of $4\cdot5$ mmol/l the influx was about 1 mg/day. This at one and the same time supports the contention of Frick (1965) that the mucus of snails can dissolve marble and thus absorb calcium across the foot while at the same time raising a serious doubt as to whether the quantities involved are likely to be physiologically important.

Obviously flux rates at higher calcium concentrations would be of interest. The other effect of calcium appears to be to reduce the general permeability of the skin. This, of course, is a well documented effect in biology (see e.g. Weil & Pantin, 1931; Heilbrunn, 1952) but it would be interesting to investigate the phenomenon further in calciophilic species. Finally, one should consider the possibility that there may be recycling of materials lost onto the epidermis either from urine, the general permeability of the surface or from secretions such as mucus. The ultrastructure of the epidermis with its numerous microvilli (p. 36) suggests that uptake is a possibility and the absorption of neutral and basic amino acids has been studied in the gill of the common cockle (*Cerastoderma edule*) and shown to occur by a carrier-mediated mechanism (Bamford & McCrea, 1973). Similarly both gastropods (Zylstra, 1972b) and bivalves (Bevelander & Nakahara, 1966; Nakahara & Bevelander, 1967) are capable of taking up particulate matter across the epithelia of the head and mantle by a form of endocytosis. Our observations on *Helix aspersa* indicate that about 5% of the blood constituents may be lost onto the skin per hour while the fluid absorption by the foot is about 10 μl/h for a 5–6 g snail. Although from our data uptake was less than 10% of the loss, further study into possibilities of recycling is needed.

SECRETIONS OF THE EPIDERMIS

The epidermis of molluscs secretes a large number of compounds many of which are not very well understood.

> It may be, of course, that whilst the skin glands of an opisthobranch like *Acteon* are simply dangerous to small predators the skin glands of a nudibranch are simply the cause of a bad taste and the glands which occur on the sides of the foot of *Diodora* or *Helix* are antiseptic rather than truly repugnatorial. (Graham, 1957.)

Some of the secretions may act as pheromones and quite a large number of species can produce strong "sulphate containing" acids (Edmonds, 1968; Thompson, 1969). Unfortunately, relatively little is known about the chemistry of these secretions and rather than try to catalogue them in relation to speculative functions, we have decided on the alternative approach of considering the physical properties of some of the more conspicuous secretions. Some of these properties are readily appreciated. Thus, the radula of gastropods is basically a tough rasping structure which consists of chitin and protein when initially formed (Rudall, 1955) but may later become cross-linked and impregnated with iron and silicon oxides to produce an extremely hard structure (Runham, Thornton, Shaw & Wayte, 1969). Embryologically, the cells which form the radula are derived from the epidermis but in this review we will concentrate on the products of the more external parts of the skin.

Tanned proteins

Many bivalves secrete a bundle of protein fibres from the foot. These threads are unusual in that they contain large amounts of secreted collagen (Pujol, Rolland, Lasry & Vinet, 1970) and they normally attach the mollusc to the substratum. They have been collected and woven into textiles since biblical times (I Chronicles 4:21; 15:27) and have thus been named byssus threads (byssus, L. fine linen).

Three glands are involved in forming the byssus threads. The largest, or white, gland secretes the bulk of the protein. A second purple or polyphenol gland produces a quinone which is the cross-linking component and this is probably activated by the products of the third or enzyme gland (Smyth, 1954; Rudall, 1955). These three secretions are, of course, the basis of the classical tanned protein system of many invertebrates. They are released into a groove running lengthwise along the bivalve's foot. The end of the fibre is applied to the substratum and it may be stretched as the foot withdraws. When first formed, the thread is a creamy white colour but it slowly turns yellow and darkens as the polyphenol tanning system develops and produces melanin-like products (Mercer, 1952, 1972).

The effect of tanning is to turn soluble proteins into insoluble structures by cross-linking the chains and making a more resistant and less extensible structure. The same process occurs in the formation of the outer part of the shell, or periostracum. During the last decade the periostracum has attracted considerable interest both as regards amino acid composition (Wilbur & Simkiss, 1968; Meenakshi, Hare, Watabe & Wilbur, 1969) and function as a substratum in deposition of the outermost crystal layer of shell (Taylor & Kennedy, 1969; Meenakshi, Donnay, Blackwelder & Wilbur, 1974). Some most remarkable findings have, however, come from electron microscopy of the mantle edge where the periostracum is formed in a special groove or fold. In bivalves there are particular basal cells at the bottom of this groove which produce precursor units that are then assembled extracellularly to form the pellicle. The periostracum is elaborated upon this by the addition of a granular region from the intermediate cells on the outer side of the fold and is thickened by the addition of amorphous material from the cells forming the middle mantle fold (Bevelander & Nakahara, 1967; Neff, 1972).

In gastropods the formation of the periostracum has been studied in *Littorina littorea* (Bevelander & Nakahara, 1970); *Lymnaea stagnalis* (Kniprath, 1972); *Helisoma duryi* (Saleuddin, 1975) and *Helix aspersa* (Saleuddin, 1976). Typically the structure arises from between the mantle folds where, in *Helisoma*, Saleuddin (1975) was able to distinguish two types of cells. One, the light cell, extruded preformed periostracal membrane units into the base of the periostracal groove where they became aligned into a single row to form the lamellar covering. The other, dark cells, contributed to the initial formation of the periostracum while the mantle edge cells were responsible for its thickening (Fig. 5). The secretion of "precursor units" which polymerize and cross-link extracellularly appears to be a common observation in all these studies and it is frequently possible to observe these units in the Golgi cisternae of cells (Bevelander & Nakahara, 1970; Saleuddin, 1975, 1976) (Fig. 5).

The quinone-tanned proteins or sclerotins of the periostracum have been demonstrated histochemically in a large number of species (Brown, 1952; Beedham, 1958; Hillman, 1961; Meenakshi, Hare, Watabe *et al.*, 1969; Bubel, 1973) but little is known about their syntheses. In insects, phenoloxidases are involved in sclerotization of the cuticle by the formation of quinones which then bring about cross-linking of the proteins.

Phenoloxidase has been extracted from the larvae of the molluscan borer *Lyrodus pedicellatus* and from both the mantle and the periostracum of the bivalve *Modiolus demissus* (J. H. Waite, unpublished). Interestingly, the mantle phenoloxidase is present in an inactive form whereas in the periostracum 50–60% is in an active form. Activation can be brought about by chymotrypsin (Waite & Wilbur, 1976). Gel electrophoresis of the periostracum after solubilization in sodium dodecyl sulphate demonstrated the presence of five bands, two of which exhibited phenoloxidase activity. The phenoloxidase in the periostracum presumably catalyses the formation of *ortho*-quinones which cross-link the proteins. If such cross-linking reactions occurred within the mantle cells it would obviously be highly deleterious and the presence within the cell of the inactive form of phenoloxidase would appear to be a favourable adaptation. Since insect phenoloxidases are activated by

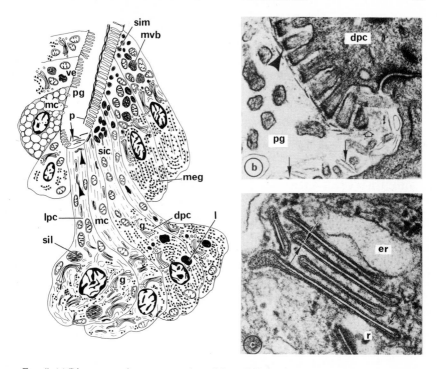

FIG. 5. (a) Diagrammatic representation of the cells lining the periostracal groove (pg) of the snail *Helisoma*. Note the beginning of the periostracum (p) at the base of the groove. Isolated periostracal units (arrowed) can be seen both in the groove [shown also in electronmicrograph (b)], and in the vesicles of the light periostracal cell (lpc) [shown in electronmicrograph (c)]. Other abbreviations: dpc, dark periostracal cell; er, endoplasmic reticulum; g, Golgi complex; l, lysosome; mc, mucus cell; meg, mantle edge gland cell; mvb, multivesicular body; r, ribosomes; sic, secretory inclusion dark cells; sil, secretory inclusion light cells; sim, secretory inclusion mantle edge gland cells; ve, ventral epithelium. (Electron-micrographs by A. S. M. Saleuddin, 1975. Reprinted from *Calc. Tiss. Res.*)

proteolytic enzymes (Karlson & Liebau, 1961; Munn & Bufton, 1973; Dohke, 1973) and chymotrypsin has a similar action on *Modiolus* phenoloxidase, we can expect to find a proteolytic enzyme secreted by the mantle which activates the phenoloxidase of the periostracum.

Elastic proteins

In bivalves the two valves of the shell are joined together by a hinge ligament which is secreted by the mantle epithelium and, as with the rest of the shell, covered by the periostracum (Fig. 6). The outer layer of the hinge is characteristically a hard dark brown material with all the characteristics of a tanned protein (Beedham, 1958; Trueman, 1964). The inner layer consists of a rubbery protein termed resilium or abductin which has now been analysed in detail (Kirshenbaum, 1973). It is an elastic material which stores energy when compressed by the closing of the shell. Thus, when the adductor muscles relax, the abductin recoils and forces the shell open again.

Three main types of rubbery proteins have been studied in animals; namely, elastin in vertebrates, resilin in insects and abductin in bivalves. All three have a low stiffness, the ability to withstand large strains and an almost perfect elasticity although they are all very different in composition. If compressed and allowed to extend again they return between 97% (resilin) and 91% (abductin) of the work put into them (Alexander, 1966). This is because they act as cross-linked amorphous polymers and in the case of the bivalves this cross-linking again appears to be due to quinone tanning. A comparison of the efficiency of the hinge ligaments of various bivalves has been undertaken by Trueman (1964) who showed that the work loss from the hinge was particularly low in the Pectinidae which frequently swim by clapping their valves together.

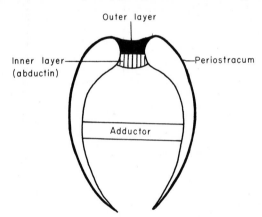

FIG. 6. The abductin layer of the bivalve hinge which is elastic and antagonizes the effect of the adductor muscle.

The calcified shell

The mechanical properties of molluscan shells have only recently attracted attention. It has been known since Bøggild's (1930) structural classification that the crystals forming the shell occur in many different arrangements, namely nacreous, foliate, prismatic, cross-lamellar, cross-foliated and homogeneous structures

(Taylor, Kennedy & Hall, 1969, 1973). Using species of a wide variety of molluscs, Currey & Taylor (1974) and Currey (1976) have investigated the mechanical behaviour of these various shell forms. In tensile tests only prismatic and nacreous structures exceeded a strength of 60 MNm^{-2}. The nacre performed best in modulus of rupture tests and it remains an unsolved problem as to why nacreous shells, which evolved early in the history of molluscs and which appear to perform so well in many mechanical tests, are not more widely represented in modern forms.

Prismatic and nacreous shells have a larger amount of organic matrix than others and it is quite likely that this is important mechanically. The organic matrix is important in the organization of shell and surrounds the individual crystals so that any cracks that do form do not pass through the brittle mineral. The major portion of the shell proteins is present within and between the calcium carbonate crystals. These proteins, the so-called matrix proteins, can be divided into soluble and insoluble fractions (Wilbur & Simkiss, 1968; Voss-Foucart, Laurent & Gregoire, 1969; Crenshaw, 1971; Meenakshi, Hare & Wilbur, 1971). The soluble fraction contains a protein which specifically binds calcium (Crenshaw, 1971), and it appears that this fraction is the medium in which crystal nucleation and growth takes place. As the crystals grow, soluble protein becomes incorporated within the crystals (Watabe, 1965; Crenshaw, 1971). The insoluble protein fraction surrounds the crystals and is present between the laminae of crystals (see Wilbur, 1972). The amino acid composition of the soluble and insoluble fractions is quite different, the insoluble fraction having a higher content of glycine, phenylalanine and tyrosine (Meenakshi, Hare & Wilbur, 1971). The higher content of tyrosine and phenylalanine in the insoluble fraction may contribute to its hydrophobicity and insolubility. In addition, it seems likely that phenoloxidase, secreted by the mantle and then activated, may well result in the cross-linking of matrix as well as periostracal proteins. Such cross-linking would make the matrix proteins insoluble and so limit crystal growth. Considering the soluble and insoluble protein fractions, let us suppose that the following sequence takes place (Meenakshi, Hare & Wilbur, 1971): (1) secretion of soluble protein which initiates crystal nucleation; (2) crystal growth within the soluble protein; (3) secretion of a second protein fraction which becomes insoluble, inhibiting crystal growth; (4) secretion of soluble protein, etc. The result would be the formation of successive laminae of crystals in which the laminae would be separated by insoluble protein and this type of shell structure is a common feature of many molluscan shells (Taylor & Kennedy, 1969; Taylor, 1973; Kennedy, Morris & Taylor, 1970). It will be apparent that this sequencing would require a control mechanism which would alternate the secretion of the two protein fractions and inhibit any phenoloxidase activity in the insoluble protein fraction prior to secretion of the subsequent soluble protein fraction in which crystallization takes place.

The analysis of the mechanism of calcium carbonate deposition is somewhat inhibited by the absence of a generally accepted model. Considerations of central importance in formulating a model are the flux rates across the mantle tissue and the mechanisms of crystal nucleation and growth.

Bicarbonate and carbonate ions have been of special interest in experiments on calcification because of the dramatic effects which inhibitors of the enzyme carbonic anhydrase have upon the process (see Wilbur, 1972). The intracellular distribution of this enzyme in the mantle of the oyster *Crassostrea virginica* has recently been examined by Wheeler (1975) using zonal centrifugation and marker enzymes. Carbonic anhydrase was found on a membrane fraction thought to be the plasma membrane of the epithelial cells and possibly also in the soluble phase of mantle homogenates. By comparing the enzyme content of the mantle after first removing the outer or inner epithelium, it could be shown that the outer epithelium had the higher specific activity.

Flux measurements of ^{14}C-bicarbonate were also made for the whole mantle of the oyster *Crassostrea virginica* and it was estimated that the movement of bicarbonate from the medium could account for almost all the carbonate required for shell growth (Wheeler, pers. comm.; cf. Wilbur & Jodrey, 1952). That the medium may also supply bicarbonate in the scallop *Argopecten erradians* is indicated by deposition of ^{45}Ca and ^{14}C-bicarbonate on the shell from the medium in a ratio of approximately 1 : 1 (Wheeler, Blackwelder & Wilbur, 1975). These results do not, however, preclude the participation of metabolic carbon dioxide and bicarbonate in the deposition of shell carbonate (Campbell & Speeg, 1969). In the case of calcium, Istin & Maetz (1964) found in the freshwater bivalve *Anodonta* that the outer membrane of the mantle was more permeable than the inner membrane. This would favour the movement of calcium towards the site of deposition presumably along a concentration gradient. In contrast to this, Wheeler (1975) found that the bicarbonate fluxes across the whole mantle of the marine oyster *Crassostrea* were not statistically different in the two directions. The efflux away from the shell was however different in separate epithelia from the two sides of the mantle. The inner epithelium had a flux rate about twice that of the outer epithelium. Furthermore, the inhibition of carbonic anhydrase with acetazolamide had little effect on the movement of bicarbonate towards the shell but strongly inhibited the efflux in the opposite direction. These results suggest that carbonic anhydrase is involved in the movement of bicarbonate from the extrapallial fluid into the mantle but not in the opposite direction. Such a polarized effect, together with the finding of carbonic anhydrase in a membrane fraction, might be taken to suggest that the enzyme is attached to the outer face of the epidermis in this region, although trypsin treatment of that surface does not reduce the enzyme specific activity (Wheeler, 1975).

Carbonic anhydrase has been presumed to assist in shell formation by catalysing the conversion of carbon dioxide to bicarbonate (Wilbur, 1972). The enzyme and flux studies just mentioned suggest a new model for shell formation. The inhibition of calcification by the inhibitors mentioned above points to CO_2 hydration–dehydration and bicarbonate as limiting factors in the calcification process. Since acetazolamide inhibits movement of $H^{14}CO_3$ across the mantle away from, but not toward, the shell surface (Wheeler, 1975), movement from the extrapallial fluid into the mantle tissue appears to be critical. This may be related to the carbon dioxide gradient which favours movement outward from the extrapallial fluid. We can reasonably assume that as haemolymph flows from the base of the mantle toward its edge, substances including carbon dioxide and bicarbonate pass into the extrapallial fluid (Crenshaw, 1972). The net movement of carbon dioxide will then be away from the shell because the inner mantle epithelium is exposed to the outer medium with a lower carbon dioxide pressure. Carbonic anhydrase will catalyse the conversion of bicarbonate to carbon dioxide. The carbon dioxide may be expected to pass from the extrapallial through the mantle cells more rapidly than bicarbonate. The effect of carbon anhydrase will be to increase the rate of movement of carbonic dioxide out of the extrapallial fluid. There are two possible sites where the enzyme might accomplish this. One is the lining surface of the outer epithelium or within the extrapallial fluid; and the other is the cytoplasm of the outer epithelium. We do not have information which will permit us to decide which site of catalysis may be involved, but the presence of carbonic anhydrase on the cell membrane and possibly in the soluble phase of the cytoplasm (Wheeler, 1975) suggests that these portions of the epithelial cells may be involved. Wheeler (1975) has suggested as a possibility that carbonic anhydrase on the epithelial surface in contact with the extrapallial fluid may catalyse the conversion of bicarbonate ions to carbon dioxide in an unstirred layer and so increase the rate of diffusion of bicarbonate into that layer. As a consequence, a more rapid movement of carbon dioxide out of the extrapallial fluid would occur. The effect of the enzyme, whether extracellular or intracellular, would be to decrease the hydrogen ion concentration of the extrapallial fluid. This change, in turn, would increase the relative proportions of bicarbonate and carbonate and so favour calcium carbonate deposition and crystal growth (Wheeler, 1975). One other possible mechanism favourable to calcification is perhaps worth mentioning. Bicarbonate ATPase is present in the mantle; and some of the enzyme is associated with a membrane fraction, presumably the cell membrane (Wheeler, 1975). This enzyme could involve energy in moving ions against a gradient, and it therefore provides another possible way in which the ion fluxes and secretory activities of the mantle epidermis may be related to the formulation of the molluscan shell.

Mucus

The ability to secrete mucus over the epidermis is one of the most conspicuous properties of the snail's skin. The mucus which is produced in any one region is frequently a mixture of materials from various glands together with a general exudate from the epithelial cells. It undoubtedly differs from region to region (see pp. 37–38) and all that can be done by way of summarizing its functions in this article is to point out two main topics of interest.

First, it is generally accepted that ciliated surfaces are characteristically covered by a mucus sheet which acts as a vehicle for moving particles across the epithelium. The current concept is that the secreted mucus forms a thick layer or blanket over the tops of the cilia while beneath this there is a thinner, more watery secretion. The activity of the cilia results in the movement of the thicker outer layer across the epithelium (Sadé, Eliezer, Silberberg & Nevo, 1970) (Fig. 7). In the absence of mucus, the ciliary beating has little effect on the transport of materials over the surface but the properties of mucus from diverse sources seem to be similar enough to enable them all to replace this function. Thus, mucus

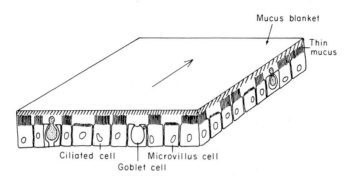

FIG. 7. The concept of a semi-solid mucus blanket passing over a thin mucus layer in which ciliated cells are beating. The thin mucus layer may represent either a general epithelial secretion of different consistency or shear thinning of normal mucus by the activities of the ciliated cells.

from the frog palate, cat trachea or bovine cervix are all inter-changeable and capable of maintaining the clearance of material when used on another species (Eliezer, 1974). The function of mucus sheets, used in this way, is a major part of the ciliary feeding, cleaning and transporting systems described in most standard textbooks (e.g. Nicol, 1960).

The second major function of mucus in molluscs is in locomo-tion. This function is seen most clearly in the pulmonates where a trail of "slime" is left behind the foot. It has been suggested that a "high viscosity" mucus is produced by the suprapedal glands while a "low viscosity" mucus from the sole fills the cavities caused by the muscular pedal waves (Parker, 1911). During normal locomotion in the snail *Helix aspersa*, the sole of the foot remains stationary until a pedal wave approaches from behind. This region of the foot is then raised and moved forwards before being put down again (Fig. 8). There may be some slight forward or backward slip of the foot between waves and the overall forces involved have been analysed by both Lissmann (1945, 1946) and Jones (1975). The role of the mucus in this form of locomotion has not been analysed in detail. The cilia normally beat backwards and this is interpreted as indicating that the mucus needs to be evenly distributed. The viscosity of the mucus appears to vary with the season (Jones, 1973) and is probably an important factor in locomotion. Thus, *Helix aspersa* can drag 50 times its own weight on a horizontal surface and nine times its own weight on a vertical surface. In each case the limiting factor appears to be the adhesive power of the mucus rather than the musculature of the foot (Jones, 1975).

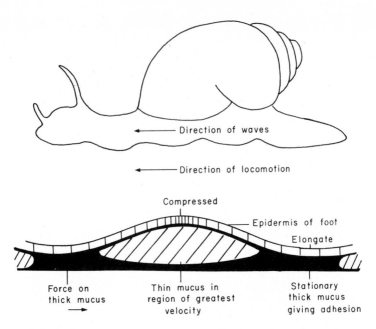

FIG. 8. The concept of thick and thin mucus originally proposed by Parker (1911) to account for snail locomotion. If two forms of mucus exist they may either be secreted by different cells or represent a single source which is modified by the forces put upon it.

From these two brief descriptions of the functions of epidermal mucus it will be apparent that a major gap in our understanding relates to the physical properties of mucus and the way it reacts to the various stresses placed upon it. Mucus comes into the category of materials called viscoelastic fluids. When a liquid is subjected to a shearing force it will flow, and the resistance to this flow is called its viscosity. If a solid is subjected to the same conditions it will deform and, if it has elastic properties, it will resist the shearing force so that when this is removed it returns to its original shape. Viscoelastic materials combine these two effects in that they deform and then flow. They are often difficult to study in that they are often shear-sensitive structures which therefore degrade while being tested. With biological materials there are additional problems of sample size, inhomogeneities and biodegradation. Despite this a number of studies have been made especially on the mucus from the hypobranchial glands of *Busycon canaliculatum* and *Buccinum undatum* (Ronkin, 1955; Kwart & Shashoua, 1957; Hunt & Jevons, 1963, 1966). Mucus can be drawn from these glands in thick ropey strands. If pooled, such samples form compact masses which on stirring shows the Weisman effect, i.e. a strong elastic recoil when the stirring stops. If dispersed in saline, they show non-Newtonian viscosity at low shear rates.

We have attempted to characterize some of these properties by collecting mucus from the snail *Helix pomatia* after stimulating it electrically at 50–100 pulses/min with 20 V. Under these conditions it is possible to collect a "thin" mucus which is opaque, granular and produces a creamy calcareous deposit on standing. A thicker mucus can be collected with glass rods from the sole of the foot (clear mucus) and from the sides of the foot and around the mantle collar (yellow and opaque). All our observations on thick mucus were from mixtures of these types.

Thin mucus was decanted from the sediment and used in a float viscometer rotating in a magnetic field. Samples of distilled water were used as a calibration fluid. It was found that over a range of 0·8 sec/rev to 10 sec/rev the thin mucus was only 23 to 25% more viscous than water.

Thick mucus was tested in a modified Weissenberg rheogoniometer. The samples were held between two parallel plates, one of which was put through a forced sinusoidal oscillation at small amplitude over three decades of frequency. The movement of the second plate was monitored to determine first the ratio of the input to output amplitude of the movable plates and second the phase angle between their sine functions. The data were analysed according to the methods of Walters & Kemp (1968).

The equation of state for a viscoelastic material undergoing forced harmonic oscillation is

$$\sigma = 2\eta^{*}\gamma$$

where σ is shear stress, γ is shear rate and η^{*} is the complex dynamic viscosity. It is usually expressed as real and imaginary parts

$$\eta^{*} = \eta' - i\frac{G'}{\omega}$$

where η' is dynamic viscosity; i is $\sqrt{-1}$ and ω is radians/sec. For a purely Newtonian liquid, η' is constant at all frequencies and thus G' is zero. G' is therefore referred to as the storage modulus since it is a measure of the energy stored and recovered during each cycle of oscillation, i.e. it is a measure of elasticity. The loss modulus

$$G'' = \eta'\omega$$

is a measure of the energy dissipated or lost as heat/cycle. There is therefore a complex modulus (G^*) with the following relationships

$$G^* = G' + iG''.$$

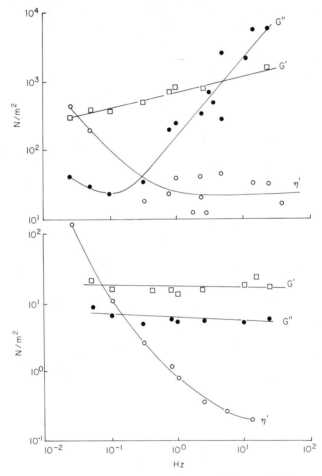

FIG. 9. Dynamic viscoelastic parameters for mucus of the snail *Helix pomatia*. The top graph represents fresh mucus subjected to shearing at various frequencies (Hz). The storage modulus (G') and loss modulus (G'') both increase with the rate of shearing while the dynamic viscosity (η') falls. This fall in viscosity is typical of most mucus secretions but the results shown here are unusual in that the mucus viscosity plateaus at high shear rates, i.e. the mucus then behaves like a Newtonian fluid. Different samples contain different concentrations of mucus and in order to normalize the data they have therefore all been plotted on an arbitrary abscissa scale. The results shown in the bottom graphs are for mucus treated with detergent. Similar results are obtained if the mucus is treated with EDTA or stored for two days and these can again be superimposed on these graphs by using an arbitrary abscissa scale.

The results of such an analysis of snail mucus are shown in Fig. 9. Several features are of interest. The material appears to show shear thinning, i.e. as the shear rate increases the dynamic viscosity falls. At low shear rates the mucus is behaving mainly like as elastic body (i.e. G' is many times greater than G''). As the shear rate increases, however, the mucus becomes more like a viscous fluid (i.e. G'' increases faster than G') and the dynamic viscosity tends to become constant (i.e. Newtonian).

Adding thin mucus or small amounts of water to the thick mucus did not modify its general properties but if kept in the refrigerator for two days or if treated with anionic detergents or EDTA at pH 8 its properties were drastically changed (Fig. 9).

These results should be interpreted with care. The samples which were used were pooled and heterogeneous, and the same material was tested over a considerable range of shear rates so that the breakdown of structure may have been occurring. Other authors have found somewhat similar properties and suggested that molluscan mucus was thixotropic (Ronkin, 1955) and dependent upon calcium ions and pH for its properties (Kwart & Shashoua, 1957). Our results suggest an unusual property, namely the development of Newtonian properties in viscosity at high shear rates.

Much could be gained by more detailed investigations of pure molluscan mucus but it is at least now possible to pose the problems that need to be answered.

(i) Is mucus normally in two forms of different viscosity? If so, (a) is this because of surface effects and evaporation on the outer layer, or (b) is it a thixotropic effect, or (c) is there a thin general tissue exudate (= cuticle?) and a thick mucus secretion?

(ii) Shear rates for ciliary activity have now been estimated in at least some systems. For the mucus in the layer directly affected by the beating of the cilia a shear rate of about 100 to 150 sec^{-1} would be reasonable while a shear rate of 10 sec^{-1} might apply to the overlying mucus sheet (Blake, 1973; Blake & Sleigh, 1974). The data in Fig. 9 should not be applied directly to these estimates because they are affected by concentration effects, material thickness etc. of the samples being tested. One can calculate shear rates from them however, and this suggests that shear thinning would normally occur during ciliary beating. Clearly these problems need further investigation to see if they are important in the mucociliary system and to see if they form the basis of the "mucus blanket" effect.

(iii) The high elasticity of snail mucus at very low shear rates may be of great importance in achieving contact with the substratum. The relationship between this and adhesion should be clarified and both effects must presumably be overcome when the sole is lifted and moved forwards.

The viscoelastic properties of thin layers of molluscan mucus would obviously repay further study, although the techniques required for thin films are only just being developed. Viscoelastic properties are usually due to flexible long chain polymers which are in thermal motion in solution. The chains interact by long-range contour relationships and by more local bond interactions. When stressed, new chain configurations and interactions occur giving rise to the changes in physical properties (Ferry, 1970). A number of attempts have therefore been made to produce models of snail mucus in these terms and Kwart & Shashoua (1957) produced an analogue depending upon two polyacidic fragments linked by calcium ions. The involvement of calcium is an interesting possibility in view of the results discussed in pp. 47–48 which suggest that calcium may be able to pass onto the epidermis. According to Hunt & Jevons (1966) 70% of the protein in *Buccinum* mucus could be destroyed without affecting its viscosity which they therefore attributed to sulphated polysaccharides. The possibility of long chain molecules and even of their interaction with granules which might modify the physical properties of mucus have led a number of workers to study mucus in the electron microscope. Using this technique on hypobranchial mucus from *Buccinum canaliculatum* it was possible to detect elliptical bodies (1·06 by 0·28 μm) and oriented fibres (0·028 μm diameter) in the material (Ronkin, 1952). In a later study (Ronkin, 1955) the viscous properties of mucus were associated with particles 0·1 to 0·4 μm in diameter.

In our experiments we have concentrated on observations of mucus trails of *Helix aspersa* using phase contrast, Nomarski optics and electron microscopy. The main structural elements in the mucus are (i) fine filaments many hundreds of microns long and oriented parallel to the direction of motion (Fig. 10); (ii) birefringent granules either free or attached to filaments (Figs. 10a and 11a); (iii) elongate rodlets about 4·5 μm long and with a length:width ratio of approximately 30:1 (Fig. 12); (d) delicate membranes hundreds of microns in area (Fig. 11a).

The elongate rodlets could also be observed in samples of mucus taken from within the pedal gland. In many cases they appeared, in a normal trail, to be fixed at one end and to fray into 11 or, more commonly, 12 strands at the other. From our observations it is not clear whether they represent fragments of cilia or,

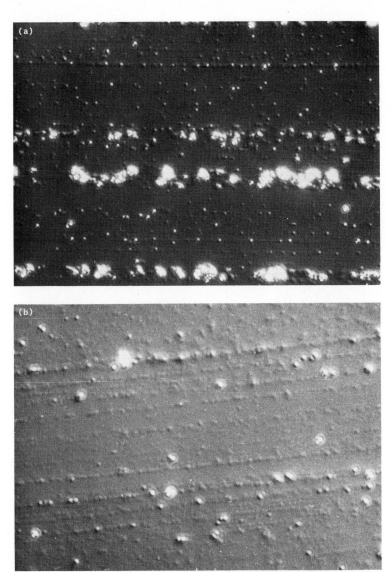

FIG. 10. (a and b) Trail left by *Helix aspersa* when examined by Nomarski optics. Note the orientation of the trail as the animal moved from left to right. The trail contains filaments and small beads with granules (approx. ×900).

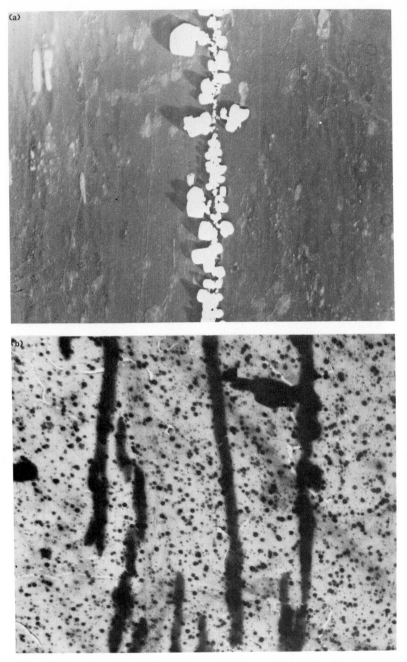

FIG 11. Electron micrograph of part of snail trail. (a) Dense particles apparently associated with a filament cf. Fig. 10a, b. Note membranous material covering entire area. (b) Numerous small particles and elongate strands (approx. ×6400).

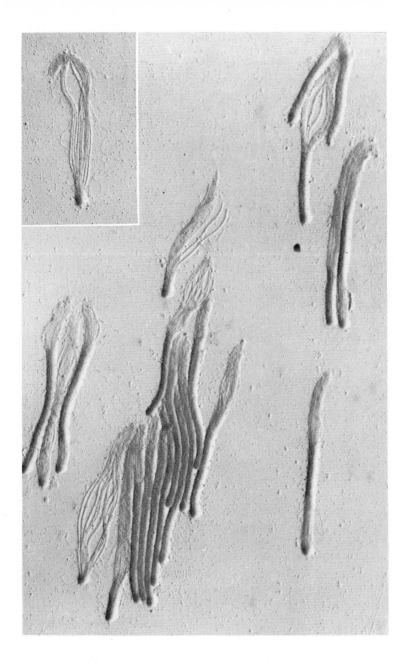

Fig. 12. Elongate rodlets found in electron micrographs of the trail of *Helix aspersa*. Note how they are all oriented in the direction of motion and all fray from one end (approx. ×10 500).

more likely, whether they are a normal component of snail mucus. It is obvious from our observations that snail mucus is highly heterogeneous, containing membranous material as well as granules and an array of filaments that are aligned along the direction of movement. Some of these components are possibly self assembled although the action of the cilia on the foot and the extrusion of mucus from glands will also affect the final structure. As a result of these activities, there is no doubt that considerable order is imposed upon the components of the trail and this will, of course, have to be taken into consideration in interpreting the rheological behaviour of the mucus.

One final set of observations is relevant to the use of mucus in snail locomotion. We have frequently observed that when placed on a new substratum the snail will initially deposit a large mass of mucus but that the amount left in a trail as the animal moves away will vary with the nature of the surface. Trails of various types have been stained with alcian blue to try and quantify this effect but better results are obtained if fluorescein (2 mg in 200 μl saline) was injected into the haemocoel. Under these circumstances fluorescein can be seen to cross the epithelium of the foot rapidly, confirming incidentally that material with a molecular weight of 376 can pass out of the blood onto the epidermis independently of the renal route (pp. 43–44). Snails were allowed to move over wet and dry paper or rough and smooth glass before eluting the mucus and analysing the elutant for protein or fluorescein. The quantity of protein in the trail was not correlated with the fluorescein content and typically dry or rough surfaces received at least twice the fluorescein content as wet or smooth materials. These experiments suggest that the amount of fluorescein passing across the epithelium per unit time is influenced by the nature of the substratum and may be related to the ratio of watery (thin) to viscous (thick) mucus. An alternative explanation would be that on an absorbent substratum the epithelium could not reabsorb mucus so easily. In either case, these experiments indicate a further variable that will have to be considered in relation to the role of mucus in the locomotion of molluscs.

Acknowledgements

We thank Dr J. H. Waite and Dr A. P. Wheeler for helpful discussion of the manuscript. Some of the unpublished studies reported were supported by the National Institute of Dental

Research, National Institutes of Health, Grant DE-01328-06 and the Office of Naval Research, Oceanic Biology Program, Grant Nonr 1181 (06). We are grateful to Dr J. H. Prentice (NIRD) and Drs M. Sherriff and B. Warburton (School of Pharmacy, London WC1) for the use of their rheogoniometer. One of us (KMW) would like to thank the Research Board, University of Reading, for supporting this work.

REFERENCES

Alexander, R. McN. (1966). Rubber-like properties of the inner hinge-ligament of Pectinidae. *J. exp. Biol.* **44**: 119–130.
Andrewartha, H. G. (1964). How animals can live in dry places. *Proc. Linn. Soc. N.S.W.* **89**: 287–294.
Andrews, E. & Little, C. (1971). Ultrafiltration in the gastropod heart. *Nature, Lond.* **234**: 411–412.
Bamford, D. R. & McCrea, R. (1973). Active absorption of neutral and basic amino acids by the gill of the common cockle *Cerastoderma edule*. *Comp. Biochem. Physiol.* **50A**: 811–817.
Beedham, G. E. (1958). Observations on the non-calcareous component of the shell of Lamellibranchia. *Q. Jl microsc. Sci.* **99**: 341–357.
Bevelander, G. & Nakahara, H. (1966). Correlation of lysosomal activity and ingestion by the mantle epithelium. *Biol. Bull. mar. biol. Lab., Woods Hole* **131**: 78–82.
Bevelander, G. & Nakahara, H. (1967). An electron microscope study of the formation of the periostracum of *Macrocallista maculata*. *Calc. Tiss. Res.* **1**: 55–67.
Bevelander, G. & Nakahara, H. (1970). An electron microscope study of the formation and structure of the periostracum of a gastropod *Littorina littorea*. *Calc. Tiss. Res.* **5**: 1–12.
Blake, J. (1973). A note on mucus shear rates. *Resp. Physiol.* **17**: 394–399.
Blake, J. & Sleigh, M. A. (1974). Mechanics of ciliary locomotion. *Biol. Rev.* **49**:85–125.
Blinn, W. C. (1964). Water in the mantle cavity of land snails. *Physiol. Zool.* **37**: 329–337.
Bøggild, O. B. (1930). The shell structure of the molluscs. *K. dansk. Vidensk. Selsk. Skr.* (a) **2**: 231–325.
van der Borght, O. & Puymbroeck, S. van (1964). Active transport of alkaline earth ions as physiological base of the accumulation of some radionucleide in freshwater molluscs. *Nature, Lond.* **204**: 533–534.
van der Borght, O. & Puymbroeck, S. van (1966). Calcium metabolism in a freshwater mollusc: quantitative importance of water and food as supply for calcium during growth. *Nature, Lond.* **210**: 791–793.
Brown, C. H. (1952). Some structural proteins of *Mytilus edulis*. *Q. Jl microsc. Sci.* **93**: 487–501.
Bubel, A. (1973). An E. M. investigation into the distribution of polyphenols in the periostracum and cells of the inner face of the outer fold of *Mytilus edulis*. *Mar. Biol.* **23**: 2–14.

Bullock, T. H. & Horridge, G. A. (1965). *Structure and function in the nervous systems of invertebrates.* San Francisco: W. H. Freeman.

Burton, R. F. (1965). Relationships between the cation contents of slime and blood in the snail *Helix pomatia. Comp. Biochem. Physiol.* **15**: 339–345.

Campbell, J. W. & Speeg, K. V. (1969). Ammonia and biological deposition ot calcium carbonate. *Nature, Lond.* **224**: 725–726.

Campion, M. (1961). The structure and function of the cutaneous glands in *Helix aspersa. Q. Jl microsc. Sci.* **102**: 195–216.

Chaisemartin, C., Martin, P. N. & Bernard, M. (1968). Homéoionemie chez *Margaritana margaritifera* L. (Unionidés), étudiée à l'aide des radioéléments ^{24}Na et ^{36}Cl. *C.r. hebd. Séanc. Soc. Biol.* **162**: 523–526.

Crenshaw, M. A. (1971). The soluble matrix from *Mercenaria mercenaria* shell. *Biomineralization* **6**: 6–11.

Crenshaw, M. A. (1972). The inorganic composition of molluscan extrapallial fluid. *Biol. Bull. mar. biol. Lab., Woods Hole* **143**: 506–512.

Currey, J. D. (1976). Further studies on the mechanical properties of mollusc shell material. *J. Zool., Lond.* **180**: 445–453.

Currey, J. D. & Taylor, J. D. (1974). The mechanical behaviour of some molluscan hard tissues. *J. Zool., Lond.* **173**: 395–406.

Dohke, K. (1973). Studies on the prephenoloxidase-activating enzyme from the cuticle of the silkworm *Bombyx mori. Arch. Biochem. Biophys.* **157**: 203–211.

Eddy, F. B. (1975). The effect of calcium on gill potentials and on sodium and chloride fluxes in the goldfish *Carassius auratus. J. comp. Physiol.* **96**: 131–142.

Edmonds, M. (1968). Acid secretion in some species of Doridacea (Mollusca Nudibranchia). *Proc. malac. Soc. Lond.* **38**: 121–133.

Eliezer, N. (1974). Viscoelastic properties of mucus. *Biorheology* **11**: 61–68.

Ferry, J. D. (1970). *Viscoelastic properties of polymers.* 2nd edition. London: John Wiley.

Fretter, V. (1941). The genital ducts of some British stenoglossan prosobranchs. *J. mar. Biol. Ass. U.K.* **25**: 173–211.

Frick, W. (1965). Der Kalziumstoffwechsel bei *Helix pomatia* unter dem Einfluss wechselnder Kohlensäureatmosphären. *Mitt. zool. Mus. Berl.* **41**: 95–120.

Gilula, N. B., Branton, D. & Satir, P. (1970). The septate junction: a structural basis for intercellular coupling. *Proc. natl Acad. Sci. (Wash.)* **67**: 213–220.

Graham, A. (1957). The molluscan skin with special reference to Prosobranchs. *Proc. malac. Soc. Lond.* **32**: 135–144.

Greenaway, P. (1970). Sodium regulation in the freshwater mollusc *Limnaea stagnalis. J. exp. Biol.* **53**: 147–163.

Greenaway, P. (1971). Calcium regulation in the freshwater mollusc *Limnaea stagnalis.* II Calcium movements between internal calcium compartments. *J. exp. Biol.* **54**: 609–620.

Heilbrunn, L. V. (1952). *An outline of general physiology.* Philadelphia and London: Saunders.

Hillman, R. E. (1961). Formation of the periostracum in *Mercenaria mercenaria. Science, N.Y.* **134**: 1754–1755.

Hunt, S. & Jevons, F. R. (1963). Characterization of the hypobranchial mucin of the whelk *Buccinum undatum. Biochim. biophys. Acta* **78**: 376–378.

Hunt, S. & Jevons, F. R. (1966). The hypobranchial mucin of the whelk *Buccinum undatum.* The polysaccharide sulphate component. *Biochem. J.* **98**: 522–529.

Istin, M. & Fossat, B. (1972). Étude du profil de potential électrique de la partie centrale du manteau de moule d'eau douce. *C.r. hebd. Séanc. Acad. Sci., Paris* **274D**: 119–121.

Istin, M. & Kirschner, L. B. (1968). On the origin of the bioelectrical potential generated by the freshwater clam mantle. *J. gen. Physiol.* **51**: 478–496.

Istin, M. & Maetz, J. (1964). Perméabilité au calcium du manteau du lamelli-branches d'eau douce étudiés à l'aide des isotopes ^{45}Ca et ^{47}Ca. *Biochim. biophys. Acta* **88**: 225–227.

Jones, H. D. (1973). The mechanism of locomotion of *Agriolimax reticulatus* (Mollusca: Gastropoda). *J. Zool., Lond.* **171**: 489–498.

Jones, H. D. (1975). Locomotion. In *Pulmonates*: **I**: 1–32. Fretter, V. & Peake, J. (eds). London and New York: Academic Press.

Karlson, P. & Liebau, H. (1961). Darstellung, Kristallisation und substratspecifitat der o-Diphenoloxydase aus *Calliphora erythrocephala*. *Z. phys. Chem.* **326**: 135–146.

Kennedy, W. J., Morris, N. J. & Taylor, J. D. (1970). The shell structure, mineralogy and relationships of the Chamacea (Bivalvia). *Paleontology* **13**: 379–413.

Kerkut, G. A. & Cottrell, G. A. (1962). Amino acids in the blood and nervous system of *Helix aspersa*. *Comp. Biochem. Physiol.* **5**: 227–230.

Kirschenbaum, D. M. (1973). A compilation of amino acid analyses of proteins, IV, residues per thousand residues. *Analytical Biochem.* **53**: 223–244.

Kniprath, E. (1972). Formation and structure of the periostracum in *Lymnaea stagnalis*. *Calc. Tiss. Res.* **9**: 260–271.

Krogh, A. (1939). *Osmotic regulation in aquatic animals*. Cambridge: Cambridge University Press.

Kwart, H. & Shashoua, V. E. (1957). The structure and constitution of mucus. *Trans. N.Y. Acad. Sci.* **19**: 595–612.

Lane, N. J. (1963). Microvilli on the external surfaces of gastropod tentacles and body walls. *Q. Jl microsc. Sci.* **104**: 495–504.

Lissmann, H. W. (1945). The mechanism of locomotion in gastropod molluscs. I. Kinematics. *J. exp. Biol.* **21**: 58–69.

Lissmann, H. W. (1946). The mechanism of locomotion in gastropod molluscs. II. Kinetics. *J. exp. Biol.* **22**: 37–50.

Little, C. (1965). The formation of urine by the prosobranch mollusc *Viviparus viviparus* Linn. *J. exp. Biol.* **43**: 39–54.

Little, C. (1972). The evolution of kidney function in the Neritacea (Gastropoda, Prosobranchia). *J. exp. Biol.* **56**: 249–262.

Machin, J. (1964a). The evaporation of water from *Helix aspersa*. I. The nature of the evaporating surface. *J. exp. Biol.* **41**: 759–769.

Machin, J. (1964b). The evaporation of water from *Helix aspersa*. II. Measurement of air flow and the diffusion of water vapour. *J. exp. Biol.* **41**: 771–781.

Machin, J. (1965). Cutaneous regulation of evaporative water loss in the common garden snail *Helix aspersa*. *Naturwissenschaften* **52**: 18.

Machin, J. (1972). Water exchange in the mantle of a terrestrial snail during periods of reduced evaporative loss. *J. exp. Biol.* **57**: 103–111.

Machin, J. (1974). Osmotic gradients across snail epidermis. Evidence for a water barrier. *Science, N.Y.* **183**: 759–760.

Machin, J. (1975). Water relationships. In *Pulmonates*: **1**: 105–163. Fretter, V. & Peake, J. (eds). London and New York: Academic Press.

Martin, A. W., Stewart, D. M. & Harrison, F. M. (1965). Urine formation in a pulmonate land snail *Achatina fulica*. *J. exp. Biol.* **42**: 99–123.

Meenakshi, V. R., Donnay, G., Blackwelder, P. L. & Wilbur, K. M. (1974). The influence of substrata on calcification patterns in molluscan shells. *Calc. Tiss. Res.* **15**: 31–44.

Meenakshi, V. R., Hare, P. E., Watabe, N. & Wilbur, K. M. (1969). The chemical composition of the periostracum of the molluscan shell. *Comp. Biochem. Physiol.* **29**: 611–620.

Meenakshi, V. R., Hare, P. E. & Wilbur, K. M. (1971). Amino acids of the organic matrix of neogastropod shells. *Comp. Biochem. Physiol.* **40B**: 1037–1043.

Mercer, E. C. (1952). Observations on the molecular structure of byssus fibres. *Aust. J. mar. Freshwat. Res.* **3**: 199–205.

Mercer, E. H. (1972). Byssus fibres—Mollusca. In *Chemical zoology*: **7**, Mollusca: 147–154. Florkin, M. & Scheer, B. T. (eds). London and New York: Academic Press.

Munn, E. A. & Bufton, S. F. (1973). Purification and properties of a phenoloxidase from the blow fly *Calliphora erythrocephalia*. *Eur. J. Biochem.* **35**: 3.

Nakahara, H. & Bevelander, G. (1967). Ingestion of particulate matter by the outer surface cells of the mollusc mantle. *J. Morph.* **122**: 139–146.

Neff, J. M. (1972). Ultrastructural studies of periostracum formation in the hard shelled clam *Mercenaria mercenaria*. *Tissue & Cell* **4**: 311–326.

Newell, P. J. (1973). Étude de l'ultrastructure de l'épithélium dorsal et pédieux des limaces *Arion hortensis* et *Agriolimax reticulatus* (Müller). *Haliotis* **3**: 131–141.

Newell, P. F. & Skelding, J. M. (1973). Studies on the permeability of the septate junction in the kidney of *Helix pomatia*. *Malacologia* **14**: 89–91.

Nicol, J. A. C. (1960). *The biology of marine animals*. London: Pitman & Sons.

Parker, G. H. (1911). The mechanism of locomotion in gastropods. *J. Morph.* **22**: 155–170.

Pujol, J. P., Rolland, M., Lasry, S. & Vinet, S. (1970). Comparative study of the amino acid composition of the byssus in some common bivalve molluscs. *Comp. Biochem. Physiol.* **34**: 193–201.

Rogers, D. C. (1971). Surface specializations of the epithelial cells at the tip of the optic tentacle, dorsal surface of the head and ventral surface of the foot in *Helix aspersa*. *Z. Zellforsch. mikrosk. Anat.* **114**: 106–116.

Ronkin, R. R. (1952). Fibrous ultrastructure in the hypobranchial mucus of *Busycon*. *Biol. Bull. mar. biol. Lab., Woods Hole* **103**: 306–307.

Ronkin, R. R. (1955). Some physicochemical properties of mucus. *Archs Biochem. Biophys.* **56**: 76–89.

Rudall, K. M. (1955). The distribution of collagen and chitin in fibrous protein. *Symp. Soc. exp. Biol.* **9**: 49–71.

Runham, N. W., Thornton, P. R., Shaw, D. A. & Wayte, R. C. (1969). The mineralisation and hardness of the radular teeth of the limpet *Patella vulgata* L. *Z. Zellforsch. mikrosk. Anat.* **99**: 608–626.

Sadé, J., Eliezer, N., Silberberg, A. & Nevo, A. C. (1970). The role of mucus in transport by cilia. *Am. Rev. resp. Dis.* **102**: 48–52.

Saleuddin, A. S. M. (1975). An electron microscopic study on the formation of the periostracum in *Helisoma* (Mollusca). *Calc. Tiss. Res.* **18**: 297–310.

Saleuddin, A. S. M. (1976). Ultrastructural studies on the formation of the periostracum in *Helix aspersal* (Mollusca). *Calc. Tiss. Res.* **22**: 49–65.

Satir, P. & Gilula, N. B. (1970). The cell junction in a lamellibranch gill ciliated epithelium. Localization of pyroantimonate precipitate. *J. Cell Biol.* **47**: 468–487.

Sminia, T., Pietersma, K. & Scheeloom, J. E. M. (1973). Histological and ultrastructural observations on wound healing in the freshwater pulmonate *Lymnaea stagnalis*. *Z. Zellforsch. mikrosk. Anat.* **141**: 561–573.

Smyth, J. D. (1954). A technique for the histochemical demonstration of polyphenol oxidase and its application to eggshell formation in helminths. *Q. Jl microsc. Sci.* **95**: 139–152.

Taylor, J. D. (1973). The structural evolution of the bivalve shell. *Paleontology* **16**: 519–534.

Taylor, J. D. & Kennedy, W. J. (1969). The influence of the periostracum on the shell structure of bivalve molluscs. *Calc. Tiss. Res.* **3**: 274–283.

Taylor, J. D., Kennedy, W. J. & Hall, A. (1969). The shell structure and mineralogy of the Bivalvia. Introduction. Nuculacea–Trigonacea. *Bull. Br. Mus. nat. Hist.* suppl. **3**: 5–125.

Taylor, J. D., Kennedy, W. J. & Hall, A. (1973). The shell structure and mineralogy of the Bivalvia. II. Lucinacea–Clavagellacea. Conclusions. *Bull. Br. Mus. nat. Hist.* **22**: 253–294.

Thompson, T. E. (1969). Acid secretion in Pacific ocean gastropods. *Aust. J. Zool.* **17**: 755–764.

Trueman, E. R. (1964). Adaptive morphology in paleoecological interpretation. In *Approaches to paleoecology*: 45–74. Imbrie, J. & Newell, N. (eds). New York: John Wiley & Sons.

de Vlieger, T. A. (1968). An experimental study of the tactile system of *Lymnaea stagnalis*. *Neth. J. Zool.* **18**: 105–154.

Voss-Foucart, M. F., Laurent, C. & Gregoire, C. (1969). Sur les constituants organiques des coquilles d'éthérides. *Archs int. Physiol. Biochim.* **77**: 901–915.

Waite, J. H. & Wilbur, K. M. (1976). Phenoloxidase in the periostracum of marine bivalve *Modiolus demissus* Dillwyn. *J. exp. Zool.* **195**: 359–367.

Walters, K. & Kemp, R. A. (1968). On the use of a rheogoniometer. *Rheol. Acta* **7**: 1–8.

Watabe, N. (1965). Studies on shell formation. XI Crystal-matrix relationships in the inner layers of mollusc shells. *J. Ultrastruct. Res.* **12**: 351–370.

Weil, E. & Pantin, C. F. A. (1931). The adaptation of *Gunda ulvae* to salinity. II The water exchange. *J. exp. Biol.* **8**: 73–81.

Wheeler, A. P. (1975). *Oyster mantle carbonic anhydrase: evidence for plasma membrane-bound activity and for a role in bicarbonate transport*. Duke University: Ph. D. thesis.

Wheeler, A. P., Blackwelder, P. L. & Wilbur, K. M. (1975). Shell growth in the scallop *Argopecten irradians*. I. Isotope incorporation with reference to diurnal growth. *Biol. Bull. mar. biol. Lab., Woods Hole* **148**, 472–482.

Wilbur, K. M. (1972). Shell formation in molluscs. In *Chemical zoology*: **7**: 103–145. Florkin, M. & Scheer, B. T. (eds). London and New York: Academic Press.

Wilbur, K. M. & Jodrey, L. H. (1952). Studies on shell formation I. Measurement of the rate of shell formation using ^{45}Ca. *Biol. Bull. mar. biol. Lab., Woods Hole* **103**: 269–273.

76 K. SIMKISS and K. M. WILBUR

Wilbur, K. M. & Simkiss, K. (1968). Calcified shells. In *Comprehensive biochemistry*: **26A**: 229–295. Florkin, M. & Stotz, E. H. (eds). Amsterdam: Elsevier.

Wondrak, G. (1968). Elektronenoptische untersuchungen der Korperdecke von *Arion rufus*. *Protoplasma* **66**: 151–171.

Wondrak, G. (1969). Electronenoptische untersuchungen der Drusenund Pigmentzellen aus der Korperdecke von *Arion rufus* (L.) (Pulmonata). *Z. mikrosk.-anat. Forsch.* **80**: 17–40.

Zylstra, U. (1972a). Histochemistry and ultrastructure of the epidermis of the subepidermal gland cells of the freshwater snails *Lymnaea stagnalis* and *Biomphalaria pfeifferi*. *Z. Zellforsch. mikrosk. Anat.* **130**: 93–131.

Zylstra, U. (1972b). Uptake of particulate matter by the epidermis of the freshwater snail *Lymnaea stagnalis*. *Neth. J. Zool.* **22**: 299–306.

Zylstra, U. (1972c). Distribution and ultrastructure of epidermal and sensory cells in the freshwater snails *Lymnaea stagnalis* and *Biomphalaria pfeifferi*. *Neth. J. Zool.* **22**: 283–298.

Symp. zool. Soc. Lond. (1977) No. 39, 77–95.

THE MECHANISM OF MELANOGENESIS

P. A. RILEY

Department of Biochemical Pathology,
University College Hospital Medical School,
London, England

SYNOPSIS

The oxidation of tyrosine to give rise to a series of related quinones is a widespread feature of metabolism in plants and animals. The enzyme, tyrosinase, which is responsible for this process is a copper-containing protein frequently found in an aggregated form. Tyrosinase has two activities: it inserts molecular oxygen into monophenolic substrates (cresolase activity) and is also responsible for the dehydration of diphenols (catecholase activity). Binding to oxygen occurs only when the copper in the active centre is in the reduced form. *Ortho*-quinones formed by tyrosine oxidation are highly reactive and take part in many processes including ring formation, polymerization, protein tanning (sclerotization), lipid peroxidation and reactions with sulphydryl compounds. The importance of some of these reactions to various biological systems is discussed.

INTRODUCTION

Quinones

The basic chemical significance of melanogenesis is that it is a process which leads to the generation of *ortho*-quinones.

Quinones possess an electronic structure which endows them with properties that make them useful compounds in biological systems. Probably the most important reaction of quinones as far as biology is concerned is their reversible reduction to the corresponding hydroquinone.

Primary metabolites

The redox reaction of quinones constitutes one of the elements of the electron transport chain found in photosynthesis and respiration. There is little species specificity, and the participation of quinones in cellular chemistry was evidently an early evolutionary development. As Bentley & Campbell (1974) so aptly put it in their review: "The same ubiquinone which powered the muscles of a Caesar's conquering hand provides the lowly alga with its energy needs".

Secondary metabolites

The evolutionary significance of quinones formed as secondary metabolites is perhaps less evident, if only because of the lack of generality in the properties deployed. For example, quinones are found in the defensive secretions of several arthropods such as bombadier beetles (Aneshansley *et al.*, 1969) and millipedes. When roughly handled, the red-legged millipede *Metiche tanganyicense* can propel a quinone-containing secretion a distance of about 40 cm. The spray is irritant to mucous membranes and is effective in preventing predation by the dwarf mongoose (*Helogale parvula*) (Wood *et al.*, 1975). The irritant action of quinones seems to have been discovered by the Chinese in about 2700 B.C., and quinone-containing extracts of plants such as rhubarb and senna have been in use as laxatives for over 4000 years (Giles, 1974). The quinone pigments alizarin and lawsone in the form of madder and henna also have a distinguished history. Henna is believed to be the "Camphire" of *The Song of Solomon* (see Bentley & Campbell, 1974), and there is evidence that the consumption of concoctions of madder (a preparation of the root of *Rubia tinctorum* and other plants) as protection against witchcraft is a custom extending back to the time of the Essenes (Steckoll *et al.*, 1971). Quinones are present in the surface secretions of many small insects (Eisner & Meinwald, 1965; Tschinkel, 1972), presumably with the purpose of discouraging the consumption of their begetters, and it is possible that the quinoid polymers in fungal spores perform the same function (Bu'Lock, 1967), although it seems more probable in the case of sporophores, such as those of *Daldinia*, that the quinoid polymer in the cell wall (Allport & Bu'Lock, 1960) has structural importance.

The polymer-forming capability of quinones results in the production of a complex group of compounds with radiation-absorbing properties collectively known as melanins (for reviews see Nicolaus, 1968; Swan, 1974). As pigments, melanins have importance in the protective colouration of many species. In man melanins are important in reducing the radiation damage to exposed structures, such as the skin and the retina, as well as providing the basis for an unedifying example of human intolerance. It is with the mechanisms of the generation of these *ortho*-quinone polymers that we shall be concerned.

Melanin

Evolutionary aspects

In man, while it is generally accepted that the racial differences in skin pigmentation by melanin have been brought about by a process of natural selection which favours dark skins in tropical climates and light skins in temperate zones, there is no agreement on how such selection may have operated. One possibility is suggested by the diminished vitamin D synthesis in the skin of darkly melanized subjects and their greater susceptibility to rickets in regions where ultraviolet radiation from the sun is low (Loomis,1967)—although this view is not considered to be wholly satisfactory (Cavalli-Sforza & Bodmer, 1971). There is evidence to suggest that skin tumours are less frequent in dark than in lightly pigmented individuals exposed to solar irradiation at the same latitude (see Harrison, 1961) but it has been argued that dark skin has no adaptive value at all (Blum, 1961). Recently Deol (1975) has suggested, on the basis of the evidence of interspecific homology and the pleiotropic effects of the genes which affect pigmentation, that skin colour may have resulted from the action of natural selection on these other functions.

Genetic control of pigmentation

We know remarkably little about the genetic basis of pigmentation in man. It is estimated that about four major loci are involved (Harrison, 1973). A good deal more is known about the genetic control of melanogenesis in the mouse. Altogether about 30 loci with 100 alleles are known to be involved, of which five loci with between five and 14 alleles each are regarded as major loci (see Searle, 1968). Similar loci have been found in other mammals and several are regarded as good examples of interspecific homology (Robinson, 1970).

The majority of the pigmentation loci in the mouse, including the five major ones, are of importance in metabolic pathways unrelated to pigmentation (Searle, 1968). The agouti locus has the allele A^y which is lethal in the homozygote; the brown locus has the allele b that leads to obesity; the colour locus has the albino allele c which causes abnormal visual pathways (Guillery *et al.*, 1973); the dilute locus has the allele d^e that causes myelin degeneration; the pink-eye locus has the allele p^s that causes sterility. In addition there are the loci pallid, muted and mocha which affect the inner ear (Lyon, 1951; Lyon & Meredith, 1969; Lane & Deol, 1974) and the spotting loci (dominant spotting, Steel and White) which have alleles producing microphthalmia, anaemia and sterility (for review see Searle, 1968).

It is clear that the genes which control melanogenesis in mammals have other functions and it is entirely possible that their effects on pigmentation are secondary to other, more profound, effects on which the forces of natural selection can act. The same may be true of pigment genetics in birds (cf. Carver & Brumbaugh, 1974) and insects (see discussion of genetics of melanogenesis by Ziegler, 1961).

MECHANISM OF MELANOGENESIS

Chemical events

The essential steps in melanogenesis consist of enzymatic oxidation of tyrosine and its derivatives linked to spontaneous reduction. The sequence of reaction is outlined in the scheme of equations proposed by Raper (1928).

EQUATION 1. Schematic outline of tyrosine oxidation (after Raper, 1928).

Oxidation

The chemical events which take place during the oxidation of tyrosine begin with the addition of oxygen in the *ortho* position of the aromatic ring. This reaction mechanism probably involves two intermediate stages with a transfer of hydrogen between carbon-3 and carbon-2 of the ring.

EQUATION 2. First stage in the oxidation of tyrosine.

There is no clear confirmation by tritium exchange as in enzymatic oxidation of phenylalanine (for discussion see Evans, 1974). The oxidation product formed, 3, 4-dihydroxyphenylalanine (dopa), undergoes dehydrogenation to give rise to the corresponding quinone.

EQUATION 3. Oxidation of dopa to dopa-quinone.

A similar mechanism accounts for the dehydrogenation of 5, 6-dihydroxyindole. Histochemical studies using the indole substrate in the absence of other intermediates have confirmed that the dehydrogenation of hydroxyindole is catalysed by tyrosinease (Riley, 1967).

The relatively small contribution of the side chain to specificity of substrate binding enables a number of dopa analogues to be oxidized by tyrosinase of which some, such as 4-hydroxyanisole (Riley, 1970), have therapeutic implications. Physiological substrates, such as α-hydroxydopa; 3, 4-dihydroxyphenylacetate; and protochatechuic acid, are important quinone precursors in insects and may possibly be tyrosinase substrates. However, there is evidence that certain substances which are not substrates of tyrosinase, are indirectly oxidized by electron exchanges with dopa-quinone.

Reduction

The reversible oxidation and reduction of *ortho*-quinones has a number of important implications. The reaction can be viewed as a two-stage process with the semi-quinone radical as the intermediate.

EQUATION 4. Oxidation–reduction reactions of *ortho*-quinone.

The significance of these electron exchanges is discussed in pp. 85 *et seq.*

Reductive additions

Apart from redox reactions, probably most of the non-enzymatic reactions in melanogenesis which are of biological interest can be viewed as consequences of the electronic structure of *ortho*-quinones. The molecular orbital scheme for the benzene ring shows that substitution by oxygen results in a delocalization of π electrons from the *ortho* and *para* positions towards the substituent. This makes the quinone oxygen and the *meta* ring carbon susceptible to electrophilic reagents and renders the *ortho* and *para* ring carbons susceptible to nucleophilic attack. In the presence of the side chain (R) and *ortho*-quinone oxygens the majority of reactions which take place are 3, 4 reductive additions of the type described by Michael (1910) (Equation 5).

EQUATION 5. Nucleophilic addition reaction of *ortho*-quinone.

Tyrosinase

Distribution

The starting point for the synthesis of melanin is the amino acid L-tyrosine. The enzyme tyrosinase, which is responsible for its oxidation, is present in both eukaryotic and prokaryotic organisms (Robb, Mapson & Swain, 1963; Lerch & Ettlinger, 1972; Balasingham & Ferdinand, 1970).

It is convenient to classify the copper oxidases which oxidize *ortho*-dihydric phenols (but not ascorbic acid) into two groups distinguished by the added ability of one group to catalyse the *ortho*-hydroxylation of monophenols. This group of enzymes is commonly termed "tyrosinase". Tyrosinases are widespread in nature and those which have been studied appear to be heterogeneous, often occuring in two forms (α, β) and occasionally in larger numbers of isozymes (Bouchillioux, McMahill & Mason, 1963). Some of these multiple forms may be composed of differing aggregates of one or two fundamental units. Modification of the enzyme by reaction with the quinone product has also been suggested. Minor differences in the degree of activity are found but the general properties of the enzyme are broadly identical.

Synthesis and control

In eukaryotic organisms the enzyme is synthesized by specialized cells and the synthesis controlled by hormones. In insects there is evidence that synthesis of tyrosinase is induced (or the activity of the enzyme increased) by ecdysone (see L'Hélias, 1970). In mammals the synthesis of the enzyme is controlled by melanocyte stimulating hormone (MSH) which acts by raising intracellular levels of cyclic adenosine monophosphate in special pigment-producing cells (melanocytes).

In vertebrates tyrosinase is active only in specialized cytoplasmic organelles (melanosomes) but in insects and plants the enzyme is found extracellularly and is presumably secreted by the cells.

Structure and activity

Tyrosinase (E.C. 1.14.18.1)* is a copper-containing enzyme that catalyses the *ortho*-hydroxylation of monophenols to diphenols (cresolase activity) and the subsequent dehydrogenation of *ortho*-diphenols to *ortho*-quinones (catecholase activity).

EQUATION 6. Oxidation of mono and diphenolic substrates.

Both activities require molecular oxygen, the latter reaction involving the complete reduction of oxygen to water. The ubiquitous nature of the enzyme has allowed its characterization with respect to substrate specificity and inhibition but, owing to the wide variations found in the properties of preparations purified from different sources, no clear mechanism has yet been proposed. Some progress has been made recently with studies involving mushroom (Jolley *et al.*, 1974; Duckworth & Coleman, 1970) and *Neurospora crassa* tyrosinase (Gutteridge & Robb, 1975).

Mushroom (*Agoricus bisporus*) tyrosinase exists predominantly as a tetramer of about 130 000 daltons containing four atoms of copper (Kertesz & Zito, 1965). On the basis of the reaction with hydrogen peroxide, Jolley *et al.* (1974) have proposed that there are two copper atoms present at the dimeric active site. A proportion of the copper is thought to exist in the cupric state in which binding with hydrogen peroxide occurs but oxygen can be bound only by the cuprous form of the enzyme. It has been suggested

* This is a recognized abbreviation for Enzyme Commission of the International Union of Biochemistry. The numerals are the code for the particular enzyme.

(Mason, 1956) that the reaction mechanism in monophenol oxidation involves the transfer of two electrons and generates the cupric form of the enzyme.

EQUATION 7. Binding of oxygen to the dimeric active centre of mushroom tyrosinase (after Jolley *et al.*, 1974 and Mason, 1956).

The cupric form of the enzyme is reduced by a reaction with diphenol.

EQUATION 8. Electron donation by diphenol; D: diphenol, Q: quinone.

The tyrosinase purified from *Neurospora* has a molecular weight of 33 000 daltons and contains only one atom of copper per mole of protein (Fling, Horowitz & Heinemann, 1963). Kinetic studies of the catecholase activity indicate the presence of only one binding site (Gutteridge & Robb, 1975). Electron spin resonance data indicate that only about 4% of the copper in the enzyme is in the cupric (oxidized) form and on the basis of spectral absorption at 345 nm about 35% of the enzyme is thought to be complexed with molecular oxygen. Although it has been suggested for prune tyrosinase that the formation of this complex is the first step in the reaction mechanism (Ingraham, 1957), it is now considered that substrate binding occurs as the initial event, as found for the oxidation of L-3,4-dihydroxyphylalanine by tyrosinase from *Streptomyces glaucescens* (Lerch & Ettlinger, 1972) or that the binding sequence is random (Duckworth & Coleman, 1970; Gutteridge & Robb, 1975). A plausible scheme for the reactions is outlined in Equation 9.

The rate-limiting step is probably the initial reduction of oxygen to form the enzyme–oxygen (EO) complex. The subsequent reaction is rapid, irreversible and not inhibited by the quinone product which suggests that the EO complex has an increased affinity for the substrate dependent on the substrate's

EQUATION 9. Reaction scheme for catechol oxidation by monomeric tyrosinase from *Neurospora* (after Gutteridge & Robb, 1975).

reduced state (dopa > tyrosine > quinone). This may well be of importance in relation to the cresolase activity of the enzyme, i.e. the oxidation of monophenolic substrates such as L-tyrosine:

$$EMO_2 \longrightarrow EDO \longrightarrow E+Q+H_2O$$

EQUATION 10. Schematic outline of cresolase activity; M: monophenol.

since the kinetics of this reaction suggest that the binding of a monophenol substrate to the fully oxygenated enzyme is less than that of a diphenol.

Osaki (1963) has shown that the kinetics of the induction or "lag" period in tyrosine oxidation can be explained by competition between the monophenol and the diphenolic product for the active site of the enzyme.

REACTIONS OF TYROSINE OXIDATION PRODUCTS

Endoreactions

Ring formation

The intramolecular reductive addition of amines to quinone has been studied in the case of the formation of adrenochrome (Heacock *et al.*, 1963). A similar reaction leads to the formation of the indolene ring in which, owing to the constraints of the side chain, the addition occurs at the sixth ring carbon (Equation 11) with the formation of the indolene cyclo-dopa.

EQUATION 11. Indole ring formation.

Under appropriate conditions cyclo-dopa becomes rearranged with the loss of carbon dioxide and two hydrogens to give 5,6-dihydroxyindole.

There is some evidence to suggest that the dehydrogenation of the cyclo-dopa is by a redox exchange with dopa-quinone. Occasionally, alternative additive reactions may give rise to oligomers containing cyclo-dopa (Gruhn, Pomeroy & Maurer, 1974) (Equation 12).

EQUATION 12. Oligomer containing cyclo-dopa (after Gruhn *et al.*, 1974).

Polymerization

The process of polymerization to form melanin, which seems to occur with a random assortment of oxidation products of tyrosine, takes place by a series of reductive C-5 additions (Equation 13).

EQUATION 13. Polymerization of tyrosine oxidation products to form melanin.

The resulting product is a highly conjugated system which absorbs radiation throughout the visible spectrum.

Exoreactions

Redox reactions

In addition to their role in ring formation and polymerization reactions of other tyrosine oxidation products, quinones such as dopa-quinone play a part in the oxidation of compounds which cannot be directly oxidized by tyrosinase by virtue either of their composition or their location. One example of this is the oxidation of 3-hydroxykynurenine to form xanthommatin (Equation 14) a reaction which has been studied in *Drosophila* and *Bombyx* (see review by L'Hélias, 1970).

EQUATION 14. Vicarious oxidation of 3-hydroxykynurenine by tyrosinase.

Another possible example is the reaction which gives rise to protein cross-linkage through tyrosyl residues, a phenomenon which is relatively widespread (Andersen, 1964; Labella *et al.*, 1967; Raven, Earland & Little, 1971; Fujimoto, 1975). It is likely that the biphenyl linkage is brought about by the simultaneous dehydrogenation of adjacent tyrosyl residues by a redox reaction involving dopa-quinone (Equation 15).

Reactions with amines

Most external additive reactions of L-3,4-dopa-quinone and indole-5,6-quinone involve the ring carbons adjacent to the oxygen. The addition of aniline to oxidized catechol (Equation 16) is a well established reaction (Kehrmann & Cordone, 1913).

EQUATION 15. Formation of dityrosine by simultaneous dehydrogenation of two molecules of tyrosine by reaction with quinone.

EQUATION 16. Reaction of *ortho*-quinone with aniline.

The less usual reaction which takes place only with sterically hindered quinones (e.g. as in melanin) is an azo-substitution for a quinone oxygen (Equation 17) yielding a bifunctional reagent of the *ortho*-aminophenol type which, under suitable conditions, can undergo condensation with quinones to give phenoxazones which are important insect pigments (Butenandt, Biekert & Neubert, 1957).

EQUATION 17. Azo substitution in hindered quinone.

As in so many fields of biochemistry, the first observations on the reaction between oxidized catechols and amino acids were made by Szent-Györgyi (1925) although, in fact, he wrongly supposed the reactant to be a redox compound which he named "tyrin". It was subsequently found that tyrin was simply a mixture of amino acids. Many studies (see Jackson & Kendal, 1949; Hackman, 1953; Hackman & Todd, 1953) have been made of the reactions of *ortho*-quinones with amines and amino acids. The sequence of events is shown in Equation 18.

EQUATION 18. Sequential addition reactions of substituted *ortho*-benzo-quinone (after Hackman, 1953).

The products are coloured, the reaction with proline giving rise to a purple pigment. In general the colours produced by quinone reactions with amino compounds are found to be more intense where a secondary amino group is present. Oxidation of amino acids such as glycine have been shown to occur with the liberation of ammonia. The reaction of quinones with proteins seems to involve free amino groups such as the ε-amino group of lysine and this reaction provides a means of cross-linking protein chains at points along their length (Equation 19).

EQUATION 19. Quinone tanning of proteins; a possible type of cross-linkage between terminal amino groups projecting from peptide chains.

This seems to be of importance to the hardening and darkening of insect cuticles (Pryor, 1940a,b) since these structures contain very little cysteine, and cross-linkage by disulphide bonds as in keratin cannot occur to any appreciable extent. The absence of sulphydryl groups is perhaps fortuitous since the quinones are produced extracellularly by cuticular tyrosinase which would be inhibited by them. The process of sclerotization (quinone tanning) is reported to be widespread in invertebrates, occuring in the central capsule membrane of *Thalassicola*, the external cortical layer of the cuticle in *Ascaris*, the chaetae of *Aphrodite*, the byssus and periostracum of *Mytilus edule*, the byssus of *Dreissensia polymorpha* and in the egg cases of various selachian fishes (Brown, 1950).

A process which seems to be essentially similar occurs in the formation of melanin granules in mammalian melanocytes. As the melanin precursors form they become attached to the protein stroma of the melanosome, finally obliterating the underlying structure and inactivating the tyrosinase. It is clear that the tanning reaction of quinones is potentially harmful if it is not controlled and confined to regions where essential proteins are not damaged.

There is evidence that some of the quinone precursors of melanin are able to diffuse through the membrane of the melanosome and may take part in intracellular tanning or initiate other damaging reactions such as lipid peroxidation in the melanocytes.

Lipid peroxidation

The importance of this reaction lies in the fact that it is a chain reaction and once set in motion can give rise to a widening zone of pathology within the cell. Lipid peroxidation is a free radical reaction which can be initiated by semi-quinones (Equation 20).

EQUATION 20. Initiation of lipid peroxidation by semi-quinone.

The formation of lipid peroxides in biological membranes is accompanied by an extensive disturbance of their organized structure and loss of many specialized functions. Thus, there is loss of mitochondrial function, liberation of lysosomal enzymes and loss of integrity of the cell membrane (Slater, 1972).

Cellular hazards of pigmentation. Unlike the reactions which occur extracellularly, the internal generation of pigment is clearly a potential hazard to the well-being of the cell. I have argued (Riley, 1974) that the biological importance of melanin as a "photoprotective" agent is that it ensures the destruction of cells which are exposed to radiation which is of sufficient intensity to cause potentially deleterious mutations. This conjecture is supported by experimental evidence (Johnson, Mandel & Daniels, 1972; MacDonald, Snell & Lerner, 1965) and explains the statistical data relating to the incidence of skin cancer (Harrison, 1961).

McGinness and his colleagues (Proctor, McGinness & Corry, 1974) have gone further than this and have suggested that selective destruction of melanin-containing cells is brought about by non-radiative transfer of energy to melanin which acts as an amorphous semiconductor.

It has previously been suggested (Slater & Riley, 1966) that the known radical properties of melanin necessitate encapsulation of the pigment by the melanosomal membrane in order to protect the cells responsible for its synthesis. However, despite this compartmentation and localization of the pigment the possibility exists of undesirable reactions initiated by diffusible intermediate products in the process of melanogenesis, and the need for an active scavenger mechanism for potentially damaging quinones is clear.

Reaction with thiols

Recently, Rorsman and his co-workers (for review see Rorsman, 1974) have shown that in human melanocytes a protective mechanism exists which reduces the potential damage caused by tyrosine

EQUATION 21. Formation of 5-S-cysteinyl dopa from dopa-quinone (after Rorsman, 1974).

oxidation products. Dopa-quinone reacts with glutathione in the cytoplasm to give the reduced C-5 adduct (Equation 21) which is no longer a source of potential damage to the cell.

The 5-*S*-glutathione dopa is modified by peptidases which hydrolyse the peptide linkages to give rise to 5-*S*-cysteinyl dopa which can be detected in melanocytes and in the serum and is excreted in the urine. Using a sensitive fluorimetric method for detecting this metabolite, Rorsman's group have shown that the urinary clearance of cysteinyl dopa is closely related to the extent of melanogenesis.

The importance of this detoxification mechanism to the retention of structural and functional integrity in mammalian melanocytes may be inferred from the selective destruction of melanocytes in experimental animals treated with cysteamine and dimethylcysteamine (Frenk *et al.*, 1968). These substances probably interfere with the formation of glutathione dopa and thus with the elimination of dopa from the cell.

CONCLUSION

Although it may be argued (see pp. 78–80) that many of the modifications of melanogenesis are side effects of genes with more essential functions it is evident that the process of pigment production has itself a number of major side effects. Some of these reactions have been harnessed by different species with selective advantage to themselves. The agent of cuticular hardening in insects has the same origin as the precursor of the obfuscating discharge of the squid. The same melanin protects the moth from predation (Kettlewell & Berry, 1961) and man from radiation.

ACKNOWLEDGEMENTS

Some of the work referred to was performed with the financial assistance of the Medical Research Council.

REFERENCES

Allport, D. C. & Bu'Lock, J. D. (1960). Biosynthetic pathways in *Daldinia concentrica. J. Chem. Soc.* **1960**: 654–662.
Andersen, S. O. (1964). The cross-links in resilin identified as dityrosine and trityrosine. *Biochim. Biophys. Acta* **93**: 213–215.

Aneshansley, D. J., Eisner, T., Widom, J. M. & Widom, B. (1969). Biochemistry at 100°C: Explosive secretory discharge of Bombadier beetles (*Brachinus*). *Science, N.Y.* **165**: 61–63.

Balasingham, K. & Ferdinand, W. (1970). The purification and properties of a ribonucleoenzyme, *o*-diphenol oxidase, from potatoes. *Biochem. J.* **118**: 15–23.

Bentley, R. & Campbell, I. M. (1974). Biological reactions of quinones. In *The chemistry of the quinone compounds*: 683–736. Patai, S. (ed.). London: John Wiley and Sons.

Blum, H. F. (1961). Does the melanin pigment of human skin have adaptive value? *Q. Rev. Biol.* **36**: 50–63.

Bouchillioux, S., McMahill, P. & Mason, H. S. (1963). The multiple forms of mushroom tyrosinase. *J. Biol. Chem.* **238**: 1699–1707.

Brown, C. H. (1950). Quinone tanning in the animal kingdom. *Nature, Lond.* **165**: 275.

Bu'Lock, J. D. (1967). *Essays in biosynthesis and microbial development*. New York: Wiley-Interscience.

Butenandt, A., Biekert, E. & Neubert, G. (1957). Über Ommochrome: IX: Modell-Versuche zur konstitution der Ommochrome. *Ann. Chem.* **602**: 72–80.

Carver, V. H. & Brumbaugh, J. A. (1974). Melanocyte developmental genetics: biphasic control of dopa oxidase activity by the E locus of the fowl. *J. exp. Zool.* **190**: 353–366.

Cavalli-Sforza, L. L. & Bodmer, W. F. (1971). *The genetics of human populations*. San Francisco: W. H. Freeman.

Deol, M. S. (1975). Racial differences in pigmentation and natural selection. *Ann. Hum. Genet. Lond.* **38**: 501-503.

Duckworth, H. W. & Coleman, J. E. (1970). Physiochemical and kinetic properties of mushroom tyrosinase. *J. Biol. Chem.* **245**: 1613–1625.

Eisner, T. & Meinwald, J. (1965). Defensive secretions of Arthropods. *Science, N.Y.* **153**: 1341–1350.

Evans, E. A. (1974). *Tritium and its compounds*. London: Butterworth.

Fling, M., Horowitz, N. H. & Heinemann, S. F. (1963). The isolation and properties of crystalline tyrosinase from *Neurospora*. *J. Biol. Chem.* **238**: 2045–2053.

Frenk, E., Pathak, M. A., Szabo, G. & Fitzpatrick, T. B. (1968). Selective action of mercaptoethylamines on melanocytes in mammalian skin. *J. Invest. Derm.* **18**: 119–125.

Fujimoto, D. (1975). Occurrence of dityrosine in cuticulin, a structural protein from *Ascaris* cuticle. *Comp. Biochem. Physiol.* **51B**: 205–207.

Giles, C. H. (1974). Dyestuffs and pigments. *Encyclopaedia Britannica* **5**: 1105–1107.

Gruhn, W. B., Pomeroy, J. S. & Maurer, L. H. (1974). An oligomeric hydroxyphenylalanine in malignant melanoma: a new type of melanogen. *Biochem. Biophys. Res. Comm.* **61**: 704–709.

Guillery, R. W., Scott, G. I., Cattenach, B. M. & Deol, M. S. (1973). Genetic mechanisms determining the central visual pathways of mice. *Science, N.Y.* **179**: 1014–1016.

Gutteridge, S. & Robb, D. (1975). The catecholase activity of *Neurospora* tyrosinase. *Eur. J. Biochem.* **54**: 107–116.

Hackman, R. H. (1953). Chemistry of insect cuticle: 3. Hardening and darkening of the cuticle. *Biochem. J.* **54**: 371–377.

Hackman, R. H. & Todd, A. R. (1953). Some observations on the reactions of catechol derivatives with amine and amino acids in presence of oxidising agents. *Biochem. J.* **55**: 631–637.

Harrison, G. A. (1961). Pigmentation. In *Genetical variation in human populations*: 99–115. Harrison, G. A. (ed.). Oxford: Pergamon Press.

Harrison, G. A. (1973). Differences in human pigmentation: measurement, geographic variation and causes. *J. Invest. Derm.* **60**: 418; 426.

Heacock, E. A., Hutzinger, O., Scott, B. D., Daly, J. W. & Witkop, B. (1963). Chemistry of catecholamines: Revised structure for the iodoaminochromes. *J. Am. Chem. Soc.* **85**: 1825–1831.

Ingraham, L. L. (1957). *Biochemical mechanisms.* New York: J. Wiley.

Jackson, H. & Kendal, L. P. (1949). The oxidation of catechol and homocatechol by tyrosinase in the presence of amino-acids. *Biochem. J.* **44**: 477–487.

Johnson, B. E., Mandel, G. & Daniels, Jr. F. (1972). Melanin and cellular reactions to ultra violet radiation. *Nature, Lond.* **235**: 147–148.

Jolley, R. L., Evans, L. H., Makino, N. & Mason, H. S. (1974). Oxytyrosinase. *J. Biol. Chem.* **249**: 335–345.

Kehrmann, F. & Cordone, M. (1913). Über Anilino-chinone und Azin-derivative derselben. *Chem. Ber.* **46**: 3009-3014.

Kertesz, D. & Zito, R. (1965). Mushroom polyphenol oxidase 1. Purification and general properties. *Biochem. Biophys. Acta* **96**: 447–462.

Kettlewell, H. B. D. & Berry, R. J. (1961). The study of a cline. *Amathes glareosa* Esp. and its melanic *F. edda* Staud (Lep.) in Shetland. *Heredity* **16**: 403–414.

Labella, F., Keeley, F., Vivian, S. & Thornhill, D. (1967). Evidence for dityrosine in elastin. *Biochem. Biophy. Res. Com.* **26**: 748–753.

Lane, P. W. & Deol, M. S. (1974). Mocha, a new coat colour and behaviour mutation in chromosome 10 of the house mouse. *J. Hered.* **65**: 362–364.

Lerch, K. & Ettlinger, L. (1972). Purification and properties of a tyrosinase from *Streptomyces glaucescens. Pathol. Microbiol. (Basel)* **38**: 23–25.

L'Hélias, C. (1970). Chemical aspects of growth and development in insects. In *Chemical zoology*: 343–393. Florkin, M. & Scheer, B. T. (eds). New York and London: Academic Press.

Loomis, W. F. (1967). Skin pigment regulation of vitamin D biosynthesis in man. *Science, N.Y.* **157**: 501–506.

Lyon, M. F. (1951). Hereditary absence of otoliths in the house mouse. *J. Physiol., Lond.* **114**: 410–418.

Lyon, M. F. & Meredith, R. (1969). Muted, a new mutant affecting coat colour and otoliths of the mouse, and its position in linkage group SIV. *Genet. Res.* **14**: 163–166.

MacDonald, C. J., Snell, R. S. & Lerner, A. B. (1965). The effect of laser radiation on the mammalian epidermal melanocyte. *J. Invest. Derm.* **45**: 110–115.

Mason, H. S. (1956). Structure and functions of the phenolase complex. *Nature, Lond.* **177**: 79–81.

Michael, A. (1910). Über den Mechanismus der Chinonreaktionen. *J. Prakt. Chem.* **82**: 306–321.

Nicolaus, R. A. (1968). *The melanins.* Paris: Herrmann.

Osaki, S. (1963). The mechanism of tyrosine oxidation by mushroom tyrosinase. *Arch. Biochem. Biophys.* **100**: 378–384.

Proctor, P., McGinness, J. & Corry, P. (1974). A hypothesis on the preferential destruction of melanised tissues. *J. Theoret. Biol.* **48**: 19–22.

Pryor, M. G. M. (1940a). On the hardening of the ootheca of *Blatta orientalis*. *Proc. R. Soc.* (B) **128**: 378–393.

Pryor, M. G. M. (1940b). On the hardening of the cuticle of insects. *Proc. R. Soc.* (B) **128**: 393–407.

Raper, H. S. (1928). The aerobic oxidases. *Physiol. Revs* **8**: 245–282.

Raven, D. J., Earland, C. & Little, M. (1971). Occurrence of dityrosine in Tussali silk fibroin and keratin. *Biochim. Biophys. Acta* **251**: 96–99.

Riley, P. A. (1967). Histochemical demonstration of melanocytes by the use of 5, 6 diacetoxyindole as substrate for tyrosinase. *Nature, Lond.* **213**: 190–191.

Riley, P. A. (1970). The mechanism of hydroxyanisole depigmentation. *J. Path.* **101**: 163–171.

Riley, P. A. (1974). Epidermal dendrocytes. In *Physiology and pathophysiology of skin* **3**: 1101–1235. Jarrett, A. (ed.). London and New York: Academic Press.

Robb, D. A., Mapson, L. W. & Swain, T. (1963). On the heterogeneity of the tyrosinase of broad bean (*Vicia faba* L.). *Phytochem.* **4**: 731–740.

Robinson, R. (1970). Homologous mutants in mammalian coat colour variation. *Symp. zool. Soc. Lond.* No. 26: 251–268.

Rorsman, H. (1974). The melanocyte illuminated. *Trans. St. Johns Hosp. Derm. Soc.* **60**: 135–141.

Searle, A. G. (1968). *Comparative genetics of coat colour in mammals.* London and New York: Logos/Academic Press.

Slater, T. F. (1972). *Free radical mechanisms in tissue injury.* London: Pion Ltd.

Slater, T. F. & Riley, P. A. (1966). Photosensitization and lysosomal damage. *Nature, Lond.* **209**: 151–153.

Steckoll, S. M., Goffer, Z., Haas, N. & Nathan, H. (1971). Red stained bones from Qunran. *Nature, Lond.* **231**: 469–470.

Swan, G. A. (1974). Structure, chemistry and biosynthesis of the melanins. *Fortsch. Chem. Org. Naturst.* **31**: 521–582.

Szent–Györgyi, A. (1925). Zellatmung IV Über den oxydations-mechanismus der Kartoffeln. *Biochem. Z.* **162**: 399–412.

Tschinkel, W. R. (1972). 6-Alkyl-1, 4 naphthoquinones from the defensive secretion of the tenebrionid beetle, *Argoporis alutacea*. *J. Insect Physiol.* **18**: 711–722.

Wood, W. F., Shepherd, J., Chong, B. & Meinwald, J. (1975). Ubiquinone-0 in defensive spray of African millipede. *Nature, Lond.* **235**: 625–626.

Ziegler, I. (1961). Genetic aspects of ommochrome and pterin pigments. *Adv. Genet.* **10**: 349–403.

Symp. zool. Soc. Lond. (1977) No. 39, 97–144.

EPIDERMAL ADAPTATIONS OF PARASITIC PLATYHELMINTHS

KATHLEEN M. LYONS

Bryanston School, Blandford Forum, Dorset, England

SYNOPSIS

The sheet of living, syncytial cytoplasm covering parasitic platyhelminths which is in connection with parenchymally situated cell bodies is almost unique amongst invertebrates. The syncytial condition has probably evolved convergently in the major parasitic groups and may have resulted from the characteristic manner of adding to the epidermis from epidermal replacement cells that differentiate in the parenchyma but fail to complete their migration to the surface. The parasite tegument is thought to have evolved from the ciliated, cellular epidermis of a rhabdocoel-like ancestral form. The free-swimming larval stages of the parasitic forms retain a ciliated cellular epidermis but this is shed after host location and is replaced by cytoplasm secreted to the surface via long ducts from epidermal cell bodies lying beneath the basement lamina and integumentary muscle layers. The evolutionary modifications both of the ciliated embryophore of cestodes and of the tegument of post-larvae and adults of the different groups are reviewed. The syncytial tegument is shown not only to be highly differentiated in different body regions but to undergo considerable differentiation throughout the often complex life histories of the various ecto- and endoparasitic types. The functional significance of the various structural changes is discussed in the light of recent findings about the nature and role of the surface coat, surface cytoarchitecture, as well as enzymatic, biochemical and immunological properties of the tegument. The living covering of these parasites is shown to have adhesive, sensory, homeostatic, protective, secretory and, in some cases, immunological roles. Particularly in the case of endoparasites that lack a gut, the tegument may have a digestive–absorptive role either by secretion of intrinsic enzymes or by adsorption of extrinsic host enzymes.

INTRODUCTION

The epidermis of all platyhelminths is a living layer. In the free-living forms (turbellarians) the epidermis is a ciliated, cellular layer similar to that of many other invertebrates, but most stages of the parasitic forms are covered with a continuous syncytial layer of living cytoplasm (i.e. not an inert cuticle) in connection with nucleated "cell body" regions situated beneath the basement lamina and integumentary muscle layers in the parenchyma. The "primitive" cellular ciliated epidermis is retained only by the free-swimming larval stages of the parasitic groups and tends to be replaced by a continuous syncytium fairly early in the life history. The syncytial condition must have arisen convergently because parasitism is thought to have arisen several times in the platyhelminths, probably from ciliated ancestors (Llewellyn, 1965). In fact the body wall of acanthocephalans and the epidermis of certain parasitic nematodes are "syncytial" or at least multinucleate (see Nicholas, 1967; Bonner & Weinstein, 1972 respectively) so this condition is more common in invertebrate epithelia than might be supposed. The gut epithelium of certain digeneans, including *Schistosoma mansoni*, is also syncytial (see Hockley, 1973). The possible advantages and *raison d'être* of this platyhelminth syncytial covering are discussed on p. 134. The living epidermis of platyhelminth parasites obviously constitutes an important boundary layer or interface at which the tissue environments of the host and parasite interact. It must be involved in vital sensory, homeostatic and protective roles including cyst formation, expecially when the host environment is specifically hostile to the parasite. Apart from this, the tegument (the epidermis of these parasites) may be concerned with the absorption of metabolites, digestion of host tissues or host metabolites, and adhesion. The ciliated epidermis of free-swimming larvae is directly concerned with locomotion and tegumental spines and projections of various types may assist this in non-ciliated forms.

Particular groups of platyhelminths have specialized the basic plan of the epidermis to suit their individual life styles and there may also be considerable variation in the nature of the epidermis throughout successive larval and adult stages. The epidermis of these parasites has in fact been accorded a great deal of interest recently and a wide range of representatives from the major groups has now been studied using the electron microscope and with histochemical, cytochemical, biochemical and immunological techniques. Much of this work has already been reviewed by Lee (1966, 1972) in papers on helminth surfaces in general; Erasmus (1972) has reviewed work on the monogeneans and digeneans; Hockley (1973) traces the development and comparative structure and function of the schistosome tegument and Lyons (1973a) has reviewed work on some "rhabdocoel"-like turbellarians, aspidogastreans and, in particular, the monogeneans.

CILIATED LARVAE

Oncomiracidia and miracidia

The plasticity and adaptability of the platyhelminth epidermis is well demonstrated even in the ciliated dispersive larval stages. The fine structure of *Entobdella soleae* oncomiracidium (Monogenea) was studied by Lyons (1973b), that of *Fasciola hepatica* miracidium by Wilson (1969) and Southgate (1970), and the miracidium of *Schistosoma mansoni* by Kinoti (1971), Brooker (in Wright, 1971), Brooker (1972), Wikel (1974), Basch & Di Conza (1974) and Lo

Verde (1975). Both oncomiracidium and miracidium larvae have a partial covering of ciliated cells arranged in tiers. The ciliated cells are large (*c.* 20 μm across in *E. soleae* larva), bear regularly arranged cilia attached by long striated rootlets, contain well developed, multicristate mitochondria and have deposits of triglyceride or glycogen as energy reserves (Fig. 1). The ciliated cells are however unorthodox compared with those of other invertebrate epithelia. In *E. soleae* larva they lack nuclei, these being lost just prior to hatching (Lyons, 1973b). The cells are fully formed at this stage and have only a short life since at the end of the larval free-swimming stage they will be cast off. The ciliated cells of *F. hepatica* are nucleated (Fig. 2) but in *S. mansoni* miracidium the ciliated cells have no superficial nuclei (see, however Wikel, 1974) but there are thin cytoplasmic connections to nucleated regions beneath the basement lamina and muscle layers (Fig. 3) (Brooker, 1972). This condition is similar to that of free-living acoel turbellarians (Dorey, 1965). Factors causing epidermal shedding are not known but this is presumably under nervous control. Changes in the intercellular cement binding the ciliated cells to the underlying basement lamina or in the basal plasma membrane, could be involved in cell release (see Southgate, 1970; Wilson, Pullin & Denison, 1971). The surface of *F. hepatica* larva is covered with alcian blue-staining mucopolysaccharide (Wilson, 1969). This could be osmoregulatory during the free-swimming stage and could protect the invading parasite from its own secretions and from host rejection responses. The source of this material is not known but the ciliated cells are rich in acid mucopolysaccharide which has been shown to have a protective osmotic effect (Wilson *et al.*, 1971). In the oncomiracidium of *E. soleae* the ciliated cells are joined directly by septate desmosomes apically and by tight junctions (which may aid ciliary co-ordination). In miracidia, however, each of the ciliated cells is separated from its neighbour by material called ridge cytoplasm (Figs 2 and 3) but this does not extend completely beneath the ciliated cells. Ridge cell cytoplasm of *S. mansoni* may represent the surface cytoplasm of single "cell bodies". In *F. hepatica* it may form a syncytium which at points joins nucleated "cell body" regions in the parenchyma. When the ciliated cells are shed, ridge cytoplasm spreads out on the surface to cover the post-larva and develops folds and ridges which are presumably absorptive, since the succeeding sporocyst stage lacks a gut, and may play a part in contact recognition with molluscan cells (Southgate, 1970; Wilson *et al.*, 1971; Basch & Di Conza, 1974). The

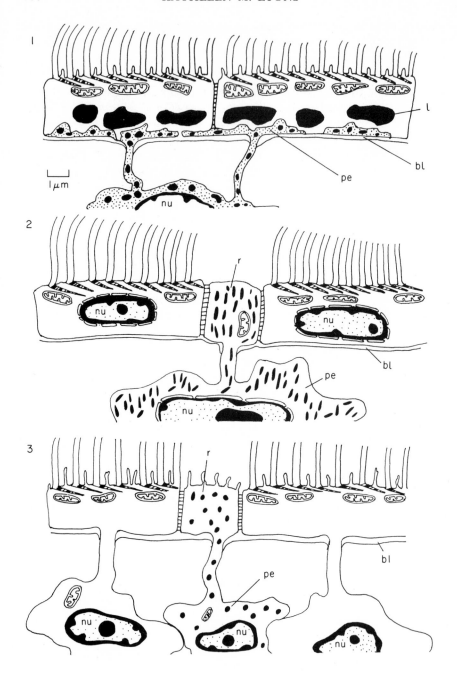

cytoplasm for surface expansion is provided by the ridge "cell bodies". In *E. soleae* oncomiracidium the definitive adult epidermis is formed from discontinuous surface cytoplasm, partially underlying the ciliated cells in connection with parenchymal "cell bodies" (Fig. 1) which spreads out as a syncytium to cover the post-larva when the ciliated cells are shed. The interciliary cytoplasm between the ciliated bands joins with this and contributes to the surface cytoplasm (see Lyons, 1973b).

The apical papilla region of miracidia is ciliated and consists of specialized cytoplasm. In *S. mansoni* this region is covered with folds which may interconnect to form sucker-like cups that assist in attachment to the snail (Brooker, in Wright, 1971; Lo Verde, 1975) and in *F. hepatica* there are less organized surface corrugations (Wilson, 1969; Southgate, 1970). In both types of miracidia the penetration glands (equivalent to accessory glands in *F. hepatica*) pass their contents directly to the exterior, but in *F. hepatica* the apical gland which may secrete enzymes for penetration of snail tissues empties directly into the cytoplasm covering the apical papilla (Wilson *et al.*, 1971).

The types of sensory endings found on monogenean and digenean larvae have been reviewed by Wilson (1970), Brooker (1972), Lyons (1972a, 1973a) and Hockley (1973). Interestingly, sensory endings have not yet been described from coracidia larvae.

Coracidia

Ciliated embryophore

The ciliated embryophore of those cestode coracidia studied so far is unusual in that it appears to be a syncytial, ciliated envelope (Timofeev & Kuperman, 1967; Lumsden, Oaks & Mueller, 1974). This may possibly be associated with the fact that the ciliated larva has to pass into the gut of the first intermediate host before the enclosed hooked oncosphere can escape to penetrate the gut wall; lack of cell boundaries in the embryophore may provide fewer points of attack for host digestive enzymes. In addition, in the ciliated embryophore of *Spirometra mansonoides* coracidium there is

FIGS 1, 2 and 3. Comparison of the epidermis of the ciliated larval stages of: Fig. 1, *Entobdella soleae* (Monogenea); Fig. 2, *Fasciola hepatica* (Digenea) and Fig. 3, *Schistosoma mansoni* (Digenea). The ciliated cells of *E. soleae* oncomiracidium are anucleate, those of *F. hepatica* miracidium have superficial nuclei, whilst those of *S. mansoni* miracidium have connections to a nucleated parenchymal portion. The syncytial presumptive adult epidermis partially underlies the ciliated layer and later replaces it. Abbreviations: bl, basement lamina; l, lipid; pe, presumptive adult epidermis; nu, nucleus; r, ridge cytoplasm.

a band of dense, possibly proteinaceous, filaments near the basal plasma membrane which may be protective during infection. The embryophore nuclei lie between this layer and the basal plasma membrane. A dense outer zone is present in the embryophore of *Diphyllobothrium dendriticum* coracidium (Grammeltvedt, 1973) (Fig. 4). Beneath the (complete) ciliated layer is again a syncytial layer of discontinuous cytoplasm which becomes the oncospheral epidermis after loss of the embryophore (Fig. 4). This was not observed in *Triaenophorus nodulosus* by Timofeev & Kuperman (1967), however.

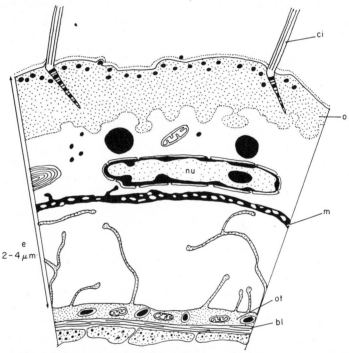

FIG. 4. Diagram of the ciliated embryophore of the coracidium of *Diphyllobothrium dendriticum* which is a nucleated syncytium divided horizontally into zones of various electron density. This is underlain by the oncospheral tegument which is deeply folded into the embryophore layer. Abbreviations: bl, basement lamina; ci, cilium; e, embryophore; m, mid dense zone; nu, nucleus; o, outer dense zone; ot, oncospheral tegument. (After Grammeltvedt, 1973.)

Oncospheral epidermis

The oncosphere of *H. diminuta* is covered with a thin layer of syncytial cytoplasm in connection with multinucleate parenchymal "cell body" regions (Rybicka, 1973). The surface cytoplasm is specialized into three thin layers, the outer two of which are protective, being eventually lost, whilst the inner layer only is retained. Membrane-bound lamellate secretions are added to the membranes of the two outer layers in a way similar to that described for vertebrate keratinosomes or membrane coating granules (also lamellate) which are secreted extracellularly and then bound to the outside surfaces of vertebrate epidermal cell membranes to strengthen them (see Rybicka, 1973). Three days after hatching in a beetle the oncospheral covering is thin and has long microvilli. After five days the microvilli are shorter and often have cytolysed host cells sticking to them, suggesting that the parasite is overcoming host encapsulation reactions (Rybicka, 1973). Collin (1969) observed that the surface cytoplasm of *H. citelli* oncospheres was very irregular and had surface folds and ballooning regions. Transformation of *S. mansonoides* coracidium into the plerocercoid has been studied by Lumsden, Oaks & Mueller (1974) who suggest that the whole of the, at first, discontinuous oncospheral covering becomes the tegument of the pro- and plerocercoid stages. A similar study of the progressive development of coracidium into adult has been made on *Diphyllobothrium dendriticum* by Grammeltvedt (1973).

The oncospheral cytoplasmic epidermis must protect the larva from its own hatching and penetration enzymes. It must also resist host digestive enzymes and encapsulation reactions. At the same time it has to remain permeable and able to absorb simple food molecules from the host.

Protective egg membranes: the modified embryophore

The tapeworms with terrestrial life cycles do not produce a free-swimming coracidium larva, and hatching of the oncosphere is delayed until the eggs have been ingested by the first intermediate host. The chief protective covering of the oncosphere is not the egg shell but the modified, non-ciliated embryophore which becomes internally strengthened with structural protein fibres. The nature and arrangement of the structural protein varies. In the embryophore of *Hymenolepis diminuta* there is an amorphous non-keratin layer (Pence, 1970). However, in taeniids (see Nieland, 1968), *Dipylidium caninum* (see Pence, 1967) and *Catenotaenia pusilla* (see Swiderski, 1972) the embryophore contains structured keratin-like protein which in *C. pusilla* gives reactions for both -SH and S-S groups (Swiderski, 1972). Formation of the protein layer in the embryophore has been described by Rybicka (1972), Nieland

(1968) and Swiderski (1972). In taeniids the keratin material is arranged as blocks separated by non-keratinous proteinaceous material. The blocks form by the accumulation of dense granules on the outer membrane of the embryophore (Nieland, 1968). "Tonofibrils" have been observed to be associated with intracellular condensation of keratin-like material in *C. pusilla* embryophore (Swiderski, 1972). This method of laying down keratin-like material differs from that occurring during metacercarial cyst formation in digenean flukes where keratin bâtonettes composed of tightly rolled keratin sheets are secreted extracellularly (see p. 114).

The cement joining the keratin blocks in taeniids is instrumental in hatching since it is digested to a colloid that imbibes water, swells and splits the keratin blocks apart mechanically. It has been suggested that differences in cement composition could lead to specificity in hatching behaviour in different hosts.

ENDOPARASITIC LARVAL STAGES

Sporocysts

Sporocysts commonly occur in either the digestive gland or gonad tissues of molluscs and, as they have no mouth or gut, have to absorb all nutrients from their host over the tegument. This consists of a thin layer of continuous cytoplasm about 0.5 μm thick which usually connects with nucleated "cell bodies" beneath the muscle layers (see Fig. 5) but in the case of *F. hepatica* mother sporocyst no such connections may occur at this stage. All the various types of sporocyst so far studied with the electron microscope have been shown to have an expanded surface of some kind. Typically the surface cytoplasm is thrown up into irregularly arranged microvilli as in mother sporocysts of *S. mansoni* (see Smith & Chernin, 1974). In some forms the microvilli are branched, as in sporocysts of *C. buccini* (see Køie, 1971a, and Figs 5 and 6), *C. buchanani* (see Bils & Martin, 1966), *Acanthatrium oregonense* (see Belton & Belton, 1971), *Diplostomum phoxini* (see Bibby & Rees, 1971a), *Leucochloridium paradoxum* (see Storch & Welsch, 1970) and *Podocotyle staffordi* (see Gibson, 1974). The surface of *F. hepatica* sporocyst is folded (see Wilson *et al.*, 1971), but that of *Bacciger bacciger* is amplified by the presence of tubular infoldings (Matricon-Gondran, 1967, 1969). The structure of the sporocyst tegument may vary considerably during its life in the mollusc, as described by Gibson (1974).

Various phosphatase enzymes, widely believed to be associated with transport phenomena (see however Lumsden, 1975), have

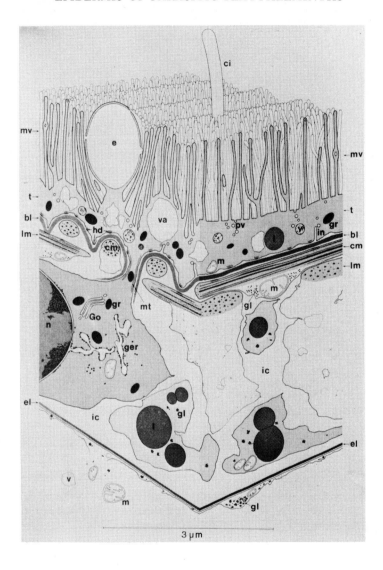

FIG. 5. Diagram of the body wall of the daughter sporocyst of *Cercaria buccini* showing the often branched and presumably absorptive microvilli. A sensory cilium is also shown. Abbreviations: bl, basal lamina; ci, cilium; cm, circular muscle; e, extrusion; el, extracellular layer; ger, granular endoplasmic reticulum; gl, glycogen; Go, Golgi body; gr, granule; hd, half-desmosome; ic, intercellular space; in, basal invagination; l, lipid; lm, longitudinal muscle; m, mitochondrion; mt, microtubule; mv, microvilli; n, nucleus; pv, pinocytotic vesicle; t, tegument; v, vesicles; va, vacuoles. (From Køie, 1971a, by kind permission of the author.)

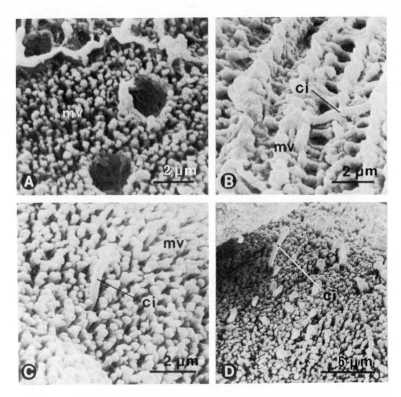

FIG. 6 A, B, C and D. Stereoscan micrographs of the surface of the daughter sporocyst of *Cercaria buccini* showing the densely arranged microvilli, some of which are swollen at the tips and presumed sensory cilia. Abbreviations: ci, cilia; mv, microvilli. (From Køie, 1971a, by kind permission of the author.)

been demonstrated using both histochemical and cytochemical methods in the sporocyst tegument (Dusanic, 1959; Matricon-Gondran, 1967; Dike & Read, 1971; Kinoti, Bird & Barker, 1971; Køie, 1971a; Krupa & Bogitsh, 1972). Histolysis of snail tissue around sporocysts was noted by Køie (1971a) who suggested that extracorporeal digestion occurs followed by absorption. Uptake of labelled sugars and organic acids into sporocysts of *Microphallus similis* has been investigated by McManus & James (1975). Sporocysts migrate actively in mollusc tissues and scanning electron microscope observations by Hansen & Perez-Mendez (1972) and Smith & Chernin (1974) show that there are spines on the anterior of daughter sporocysts of *S. mansoni* which may assist both in gripping and boring through host tissues.

Rediae

The redial tegument is formed anew from the surface of germ balls yet develops a similar structure to the sporocyst covering. The outer syncytial cytoplasm is connected to cell bodies obviously adapted for protein secretion which contain a well developed granular endoplasmic reticulum, Golgi bodies and secretory inclusions. Golgi bodies have also been described from the surface syncytium of *Sphaeridiotrema globulus* redia (Reader, 1972). Dense granules and multivesicular and myelin-like bodies are present in the tegument of several species of redia (see Matricon-Gondran, 1969; Køie, 1971b; Reader, 1972). The former could produce surface mucus or might be zymogen-like; the latter, it has been suggested, might be waste materials or alternatively contribute to surface plasma membrane during growth, replacement, uptake or secretion. The outer tegument bears either irregularly arranged microvilli as in *Acanthopharyphium spinulosum, Cloacitrema narrabeenensis, Parorchis acanthus* and *Sphaeridiotrema globulus* (see Bils & Martin, 1966; Dixon, 1970; Rees, 1966, 1971; Reader, 1972, respectively) or it bears folds. The redia of *Neophasis lageniformis* has an irregularly folded surface (Fig. 7) (Køie, 1971b) but *Cryptocotyle lingua* rediae have thick folds connected by lamellae (Krupa, Bal & Cousineau, 1967; Krupa, Cousineau & Bal, 1968). Although rediae have a pharynx and intestine which are known to be used in feeding (some rediae are predatory and eat other species present in the same snail), some extracorporeal digestion probably occurs so that fluid foods not taken in via the mouth might be absorbed over the expanded tegumental surface (Køie, 1971b). The expanded tegumental surface, large number of mitochondria, presence of pinocytotic vesicles (see below), and internally folded proximal plasma membrane coupled with enzymatic activity in both superficial and "cell body" cytoplasm all point to this layer being extremely active in the metabolism of these rapidly growing and reproducing larvae. There is in fact considerable evidence for tegumental uptake by rediae. Pinocytotic vesicles have been described in the redial teguments of *N. lageniformis* by Køie (1971b) and in hemiurid and echinostome rediae by Matricon-Gondran (1967). Uptake of colloidal thorium by pinocytosis has been demonstrated in the redial tegument of *Cryptocotyle lingua* by Krupa, Cousineau & Inoué (1970), and horseradish peroxidase incorporation has been shown in the redial tegument of *C. narrabeenensis* by Dixon (1970) and *S. globulus* by Reader (1972). Incorporation of radioactive

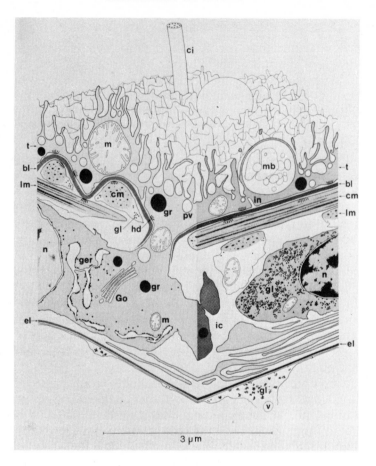

FIG. 7. Diagram of the body wall of the redia of *Neophasis lageniformis* showing the corrugated and greatly folded surface. Membraneous bodies (mb) which may contain waste products are shown, also a sensory cilium. Abbreviations as Fig. 5. (From Køie, 1971b, by kind permission of the author.)

glucose in rediae ligated behind the mouth has been demonstrated in *P. acanthus*, *C. lingua* and *C. narrabeenensis* by McDaniel & Dixon (1967) and Dixon (1970) and in *Himasthla quissetensis* by Hoskin & Cheng (1974). Uptake experiments using ligatures have, however, been criticized by Nollen & Nadakavukaren (1974) as the ligature causes tegumental damage and leakage. Uptake of glucose in these rediae has been correlated with the presence of alkaline phosphatase activity in the tegument. The teguments of various species of rediae have also been shown to contain a variety of hydrolytic enzymes which could be used in direct digestion of host tissues or may be concerned with absorption and transport of nutrients across the body wall (see Køie, 1971b). Snail tissues in contact with the redial surface of *N. lageniformis* become disrupted and the amoebocytes, which constitute part of the snail defence mechanisms, are apparently able to offer little resistance and are destroyed (Køie, 1971b). Whether these cells are damaged directly by local secretions of the tegument or by secretions from the gut is not known.

Sense organs ending in cilia have been found mainly at the anterior end and actually inside the mouth of rediae (see Køie, 1971b). Long cilia on the flanks of *N. lageniformis* may assist circulation of body fluids (Køie, 1971b).

Cercariae and metacercariae

Cercarial tegument

After release from the first intermediate host, cercariae usually have a free-swimming dispersive stage. The succeeding metacercarial or schistosomula stage may either occur outside a host or may be endoparasitic so these larval stages will be considered here for convenience. Early in development the cercarial germ ball is surrounded by a thin, nucleated, cytoplasmic layer termed the "primitive" or "embryonic" epithelium. There is some controversy about whether this layer is formed by sporocyst or redial cells or whether it arises from the surface of the embryo (see Bils & Martin, 1966; James & Bowers, 1967; Belton & Belton, 1971; Cheng & Bier, 1972; Hockley, 1972). As a rule the definitive cercarial tegument forms beneath the primitive epithelium and replaces the latter when this is shed, a process which typically occurs early in development, although the timing is variable in different species. In *Himasthla quissetensis*, for example, a loose "epithelial sac", presumably equivalent to the embryonic epithelium, separates from the underlying cercarial tegument only during encystation in a mussel (Laurie, 1974). This layer does not receive cyst-forming granules directly but prevents loss of cystogenous secretions until the cyst wall has consolidated. The true cercarial tegument developing beneath this embryonic epithelium often arises by fusion of nucleated cells to form a syncytium. Loss of the superficial nuclei then occurs and connections are eventually established with underlying, newly differentiated "subtegumental" cells situated in the parenchyma (see Matricon-Gondran, 1971; Southgate, 1971; Hockley,

1972, 1973). Bils & Martin (1966) differ in their interpretation of the way the cercarial tegument is formed and suggest that the nucleated parts of the surface syncytium migrate *inwards* into the parenchyma to establish "cell bodies". A similar process has been described in *Cloacitrema narrabeenensis* by Dixon (1970). The cercarial tegument of *F. hepatica* may be exceptional in that it seems to develop from the embryonic epithelium which is retained for much longer than usual and actually becomes filled with cystogenous gland material prior to encystation (Dixon & Mercer, 1967). This layer is not actually shed until the cyst wall of the metacercaria is formed. The metacercarial tegument is then formed in a manner similar to that of the definitive cercarial tegument of other digeneans. In this case it is said to arise by cytoplasm from those "subtegumental cells" that had secreted keratin bâtonettes during cyst formation, extruding cytoplasm onto the larval surface. Development of the cercarial tegument of *N. attenuatus* throughout its inception and transformation into a metacercaria was studied by Southgate (1971). He suggests that sequential differentiation of the tegument of *N. attenuatus* occurs by each of four secretory cell types making and then breaking contact with the superficial tegument at the appropriate time (see later). The fully differentiated cercarial tegument is a syncytium containing mitochondria, electron dense materials of various kinds and often vesicles of ruthenium red and alcian blue-staining acid mucopolysaccharide (Belton & Belton, 1971; Southgate, 1971). This outer covering is rarely microvillous but is differentiated and varies in different regions of the body (Belton & Harris, 1967; Gibson, 1974; Hockley, 1968; Rees, 1967, 1971, 1974; Matricon-Gondran, 1971; Southgate, 1971). Gibson (1974) suggests that microvilli around the edges of the oral and ventral sucker of *Podocotyle staffordi* cercaria could be used in feeding; alternatively they could be adhesive. Studies with the scanning electron microscope have been useful in demonstrating surface differences over the cercarial body surface (Hockley, 1968; Rees, 1971; Køie, 1971c, 1973, 1975; Race, Martin, Moore & Larsh, 1971; Robson & Erasmus, 1970; Short & Cartrett, 1973). The nature of seta-like processes on the tail of certain cercariae (see Køie, 1975) and of the hair-like fringe around the mouth of *Allopodocotyle lepomis* (see Lo, Hall, Allender & Klainer, 1975) will not be fully appreciated until these structures are studied using transmission electron microscopy. The surface tegument of the body, but not of the tail, contains crystalline spines which protrude only slightly from the general level of the tegument and are invested at their tips with plasma membrane (Figs 8 and 9). Basally these backwardly pointing spines rest on the basement lamina. They are composed of protein and may be stabilized by disulphide bonds (see Lyons, 1966). The spines often have flattened ends and may be serrated (see Figs 8 and 9). In *Diplostomum phoxini* spines on the cercaria

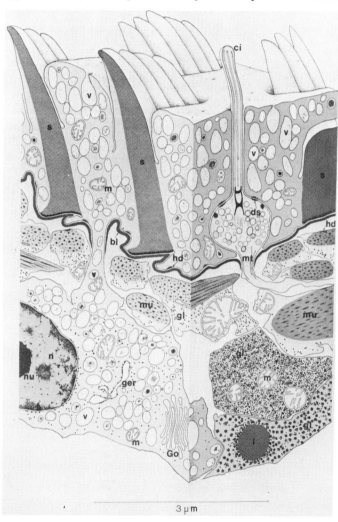

3 µm

FIG. 8. Diagram of the cercarial tegument of *Neophasis lageniformis* showing the ridged spines closely set in syncytial cytoplasm containing much secretory material. A sense ending is shown (ci), also a septate desmosome (ds), muscle layers (mu), nuclei (nu) and spines (s). Other abbreviations as Fig. 5. (From Køie, 1973, by kind permission of the author.)

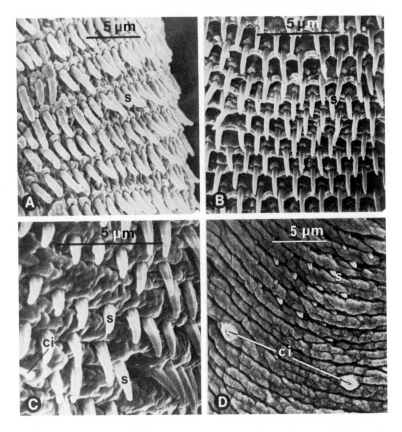

FIG. 9. Stereoscan micrographs of the surface of cercariae in different stages of development. A, Mature cercaria; B and C, almost mature cercariae; D, immature cercaria showing small spins almost hidden in furrows. Sensory papillae with cilia are visible. Abbreviations: ci, cilia; s, spines. (From Køie, 1971c, by kind permission of the author.)

degenerate after penetration of the fish host and new ones are formed in the metacercaria which will be carried through into the adult (Bibby & Rees, 1971a). Cercarial tegumental spines may be used in penetration of snail tissues prior to escape, penetration of the second host and attachment in this host. They are so densely set in some cercaria that they could even fulfil a protective function rather like fish scales when the body of the cercaria is contracted. In addition to cystogenous granular secretions which accumulate in the cercarial tegument, there are often rod-shaped granules and dense-cored spherical vesicles present. The chemical composition of these granules is poorly understood, but they are generally thought to be acidic or neutral mucopolysaccharide. Outside the unit membrane of *S. mansoni* cercaria is a thick (0·5–1 μm) layer of glycoprotein or neutral to slightly acidic mucosubstance. This is periodate-thiocarbohydrazide-osmium method (PATCO) positive, colloidal iron negative at acid pH but appears to contain hidden acidic groups since removal of the superficial layer with 8 mM urea allows the epidermal surface to bind colloidal iron (Stein & Lumsden, 1973). Whether this surface mucus layer is a true surface coat is not yet clear. A "surface coat" is by no means a feature of all free-swimming cercariae. Some cercariae may have a surface coat in the snail and lose it subsequently (reviewed in Hockley, 1973). The "surface coat" of *S. mansoni* cercaria may be involved in permeability control (Morris, 1971) since schistosomula newly penetrated into mouse skin, which have lost some of the surface layer, swell if placed into fresh water, whilst cercariae do not. The "surface coat' is known from immunochemical work to bind serum from an infected animal and to produce the cercarienhüllen reaction (CHR) which may or may not immobilize the cercaria, according to the severity of the reaction (see Hockley, 1973). Thus the surface coat of free-swimming cercariae is like that of cells in general in that it determines surface immunogenicity. This could affect cell–cell interactions with a mouse host during penetration and could assist schistosomula (with only a reduced coat) to avoid host rejection responses until more long term protective measures are adopted, apparently about four days after penetration, by incorporation of host antigenic determinants into the worm's surface (Clegg, 1972, 1974). The negative charge on post-cercarial schistosomes could also possibly assist repulsion of host leucocytes and platelets and so assist in the early establishment of the parasite (Stein & Lumsden, 1973). Other possible functions of the cercarial surface coat are to protect it from its own enzyme secretions during penetration, to act as a lubricant, to bind ions or other particles and to regulate the environment around the cercaria (Stein & Lumsden, 1973). The surface coat of cercariae is unlikely to be involved with adsorption of food molecules prior to incorporation across the tegument since most free-swimming cercariae rely on glycogen reserves in the parenchyma and do not feed. The enzyme histochemistry of the cercarial tegument has been reviewed by Køie (1971c). Acid and alkaline phosphatase activity has been demonstrated in the tegument and subtegument of various cercariae but is not invariably present. Esterases, lipases and aminopeptidases are present only in a few types.

Metacercarial tegument and encystment

Cyst formation has been studied in the cercariae of *F. hepatica* (by Dixon & Mercer, 1967; Mercer & Dixon, 1967), *Ascocotyle leighi* (by Stein & Lumsden, 1971), in *Notocotyle attenuatus* (by Southgate, 1971), *Microphallus opacus* (by Strong & Cable, 1972), *Himasthla quissetensis* (by Laurie, 1974) and in *Allopodocotyle lepomis* (by Lo, Hall, Allender & Klainer, 1975). Formation of the cyst wall of *Parorchis acanthus* and *Philophthalmus megalurus* has been compared by Cable & Shutte (1973). The encysting cercaria typically attaches by the ventral sucker, loses the tail and pours cystogenous secretions around itself via the tegument. These may be moulded by rotatory body movements and eventually harden. Usually three to four cyst layers are formed from different types of secretion which are produced by cystogenous cell bodies opening into the tegument. The granules are released from the surface of the tegument. In *F. hepatica* the cyst consists of four main layers: (1) a layer of tanned protein not complete ventrally; (2) a layer of carbohydrate-protein material, also incomplete; (3) a separate layer of carbohydrate-protein material extending right round the larva; (4) a keratin-like layer also complete. Each layer is secreted by a different kind of cystogenous gland cell containing typical secretion bodies (see Mercer & Dixon, 1967). The inner cyst layer is particularly interesting because it is secreted by cells that contain rods of keratin material arranged as rolled protein sheets. These keratin bâtonettes give reactions for disulphide groups and in transverse section can be seen to be made up of a tightly spiralled sheet. The keratin layers of the cyst are formed by unwinding of the keratin bâtonettes brought about by rotatory movements of the encysting cercariae. The cyst wall of *Cloacitrema narrabeenensis* was found by the same author to have a similar structure and origin (Dixon, 1975). Although an inner keratin layer is typical of most metacercarial cysts it is absent from *Philophthalmus megalurus* cyst, which has only two layers (Cable & Shutte, 1973). Metacercarial cyst walls are by no means impermeable and there is no major lipid component. Survival of *F. hepatica* metacercariae depends on high relative humidity (70%) when they can survive on herbage for 270 to 340 days. Cysts of the lung fluke *Paragonimus* have been reported to survive in crab meat treated with soya sauce for 30 min and in millet wine (10% alcohol) for 43 h. They normally infect man via undercooked crab meat in the East (quoted in Erasmus, 1972). Most encysted metacercariae enter their definitive hosts via the gut and the specific conditions there that stimulate excystation contribute to host specificity (see Erasmus, 1972). The unencysted metacercariae of *Diplostomum phoxini* in the brain of minnows have been studied by means of scanning and transmission electron microscopy by Bibby & Rees (1971a). The tegument is more folded than in the cercarial stage. It did not incorporate ferritin but uptake of labelled glucose was recorded (Bibby & Rees, 1971b). Whether this occurred by active transport or diffusion is not clear since no control was used to try and inhibit glucose transport.

The transformation of *S. mansoni* cercariae into schistosomulae has been reviewed by Hockley (1973). This involves loss of the tail and considerable reorganization of tegument structure. Transition to the much higher temperatures of the mammalian host must involve far reaching metabolic changes. The tegumental changes observed after either active penetration or inoculation into the final experimental host (Eveland, 1972) are: reduction and eventual loss of the surface coat and loss of the CHR reaction, development of the unit membrane into a seven-layered structure, probably from laminated bodies that appear in the tegument at this time which are secreted by tegumental cells newly joined to the outer tegument (Hockley, 1973). The tegument gradually thickens, the mitochondria reduce in number, the basal plasma membrane becomes more folded and the surface area is also increased by means of folds and pits. Ferritin was not incorporated by the tegument of a 14-day schistosomula (Hockley, 1973).

Endoparasitic cestode larvae
Transformation of oncosphere to procercoid and plerocercoid

The oncospheral surface cytoplasm develops microvilli rapidly after reaching the haemocoel of the first intermediate host; in 12–24 h in *S. mansonoides* oncosphere in a copepod according to Lumsden, Oaks & Mueller (1974). These microvilli are completely replaced by true microtriches which have a thickened, spine-like tip and arise flat on the surface of the epidermis. The dense tip of the microthrix is formed from disc-like granules and oval bodies with a multilaminate membrane present in the outer layer. Formation commences in the procercoid and pyramidal protrusions mark the start of microthrix development. The dense terminal cap is formed from the dense granules whilst the multilaminate bodies are deposited along the sides of the microthrix shaft and form the less opaque region proximal to the cap. Both types of secretion contribute to the membrane baseplate and surface plasma membrane (Lumsden, Oaks & Mueller, 1974). The tegument of

S. mansonoides plerocercoid in mice has two types of microthrix, (1) a conoid type typical of the procercoid tegument, (2) an elongate digitiform type characteristic of adults. Well developed microtriches with thick terminal spines have also been described from the surface of *Diphyllobothrium latum* pro- and plerocercoids (Bråten, 1968a,b) and from those of *Triaenophorus nodulosus* (by Timofeev & Kuperman, 1967). Variation in microthrix type has been recorded in three different species of *Diphyllobothrium* by Andersen (1975). It has been suggested that microtriches, in addition to giving grip during locomotion and assisting in adhesion, could almost form a protective covering during penetration into the gut wall of the second intermediate host since the spine tips are set so close together that they overlap. The larva of *Bothrimonus* in the hæmocoel of *Gammarus* is covered by a mucous-like sheath which may prevent encapsulation (Burt & Sandeman, 1974). Plerocercoids of other species have a similar tegument covered with larval microtriches which are rather squat at the base (0·25–0·50 µm long) compared with the long tip (up to 5 µm) (see Morris & Finnegan, 1969). Bråten (1968b), studying the transformation of plerocercoids to adults, noted the sixfold increase in the number of microtriches per unit area and the four- to sevenfold increase in the length of the shaft region of the microtriches. In addition to the squat plerocercoid microtriches, which would appear to be mainly protective or locomotory rather than absorptive, Charles & Orr (1968) have also observed thin finger-like projections from the surface which could be absorptive or secretory. The "pit organelles" described on the anterior of *Spirometra erinacei* may also be secretory and possibly involved in the digestion of host gut tissue (Kwa, 1972). The metacestode larva of *Tylocephalum* sp. encysted in the oyster has a very specialized tegument. The surface microvilli are long and branched and have a tip that is not thickened but vesicular. These may be secretory and help to resist host encapsulation mechanisms. If contactile they might circulate host tissue fluids (Rifkin, Cheng & Hohl, 1970).

The cysticercoid tegument

The outer cyst wall of fully formed cysticercoids is a protective structure which may develop collagen fibres and myelin-like material internally. The covering syncytium of the outer cyst wall is densely microvillous and the microvilli may be branched (Caley, 1973; Rees, 1973).

The fine structure of the complex cysticercoid *Tatria octacantha* was studied by Rees (1973). In this larva from the haemocoel of a damsel fly, the scolex and young strobila are enclosed in an inner and outer cyst, both covered with a modified tegument which originally developed from the oncosphere and was once continuous throughout the larva. As the cysticercoid develops these various structures become cut off from one another and differentiate to fulfil different functions. The outer cyst is absorptive and protects against the action of host haemocytes. It is covered with syncytial cytoplasm bearing branched microvilli. The tegument of the inner cyst wall protects the enclosed scolex and strobila during passage through the gut of the definitive bird host and is covered with a remarkably thick glycocalyx and bears flat, dense plates. Only the tegument of the scolex and young strobila bear microtriches characteristic of adult cestodes, and indeed only these regions produce the adult, the outer and inner cysts being discarded during infection of the bird host. The cysticercoid of *T. octacantha* is similar to the simpler cysticercoid of *Raillietina* described by Baron (1971) where the outer cyst wall and scolex remain in continuity throughout. Again some surface differentiation is present but it is not as marked as in *T. octacantha*.

The cysticercus tegument

The nature of the surface of various bladder worms has been reviewed by Lee (1972), Šlais (1973) and Voge (1973). The syncytial tegument of the bladder wall bears microvilli which lack a thickened tip but which are peculiarly attenuated. The cysticercus of *T. solium* is actually situated in lymph spaces, which is convenient for the absorption of soluble food materials but must produce problems of an immunological nature. Absorption of amino acids by the cysticercus of *T. crassiceps* was demonstrated by Haynes (1970) and Haynes & Taylor (1968). Esch & Kuhn (1971) have demonstrated uptake of [14]C-*Chlorella* protein by *T. crassiceps* larvae. The scolex tegument may bear true microtriches with a thickened tip (Baron, 1968; Featherston, 1972).

Scolex hook formation

Mount (1970) stated that the scolex hooks arise around fused microtriches on which hook protein is deposited. Bilquees & Freeman (1969), however, state that the hooks of *T. crassiceps* larvae arise *de novo*. Baron (1968) described the scolex hooks as small cones at first, the base being added secondarily. The shaft of the scolex hooks contains "keratin".

118   KATHLEEN M. LYONS

The surface of the syncytial cytoplasmic covering of adult flukes is specialized in a characteristic fashion in each of the major groups of parasites. This characteristic cytomorphology is remarkably constant even in members of a group parasitizing unusual host sites.

Monogeneans

Most monogeneans are typically ectoparasitic on the gills and skin of fish. A range of skin and gill parasitic forms has now been investigated with the electron microscope and the dorsal epidermis of most of these bears short, scattered microvilli (reviewed in Lyons, 1973a) (Fig. 10). This is also true of juvenile *Amphibdella flavolineata* which is most unusual in parasitizing the blood system of an electric ray before adopting an ectoparasitic existence on the gills of its host (Lyons, 1971, 1973a). The length of these simple microvilli varies throughout the group. They are very long in *Entobdella soleae* and *Acanthocotyle elegans* (see Lyons, 1970a) and

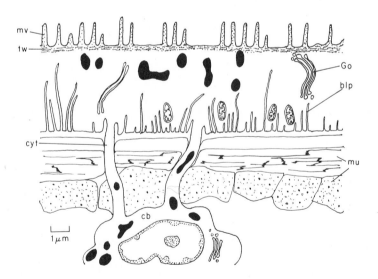

FIG. 10. Diagram of the syncytial epidermis of the polyopisthocotylinean monogenean gill parasite *Plectanocotyle gurnardi* showing the small scattered microvilli and thickened outer cytoplasm resembling a terminal web. The basal plasma membrane sends long folds into the epidermal cytoplasm. Abbreviations: blp, basal plasma membrane; cb, epidermal cell body; cyt, cytoplasmic connection with outer epidermis; Go, Golgi body; mu, integumentary muscles; mv, microvilli; tw, terminal web.

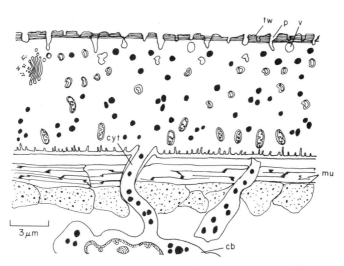

FIG. 11. Diagram of the epidermis of the polyopisthocotylinean gill parasite *Rajon-chocotyle emarginata* showing the absence of microvilli and the pitted surface similar to that described for *Polystoma integerrimum* by Bresciani (1972). A very thick terminal web is present and may be contractile. Abbreviations: cb, epidermal cell body; cyt, cytoplasmic connection with outer epidermis; mu, integumentary muscles; p, surface pits; tw, terminal web; v, secretory vesicles.

short in *Gyrodactylus* (see Lyons, 1970b). Only the dorsal surface may be microvillous, the ventral surface and sucker linings may be smooth-surfaced. The functions of these microvilli are not clear; they resemble those found generally on epithelia of a wide variety of vertebrates and invertebrates. Monogeneans have a gut and as they are mostly ectoparasitic it would seem unlikely that the epidermis plays a significant role in nutrient uptake, except perhaps in regions around the pharynx or adhesive organs. It has not however been demonstrated convincingly whether monogeneans incorporate labelled nutrients across the epidermis, this being partly due to difficulties of leakage caused by damaging the epidermis by ligaturing the gut (Halton & Arme, 1971). Colloidal-ferritin and thorium dioxide were not taken up by pinocytosis into the epidermis of those monogeneans tested (see Lyons, 1973a). Few acidic groups have been demonstrated in the surface coat of *Entobdella soleae* compared with, for example, tapeworms and this may also indicate that ion or amino acid binding associated with uptake is less important in these ectoparasites (see, however, Lumsden, 1975). Three groups of monogeneans have an atypical epidermis. The viviparous gyrodactylids (i.e. *Gyrodactylus* sp.) appear to be covered with an anucleate syncytium with no connection to cell bodies as adults (Lyons, 1970b). The single representatives of the gill parasitic hexabothriids (see Lyons, 1972b) and bladder parasitic polystomatids (see Bresciani, 1972) studied so far have an avillous epidermis containing shallow pores, rather like that of digeneans, and interestingly there is a much more obvious terminal web present than in other monogeneans (Fig. 11). There is increasing evidence that the terminal web microfilaments of vertebrates may be actin-like since they bond with heavy meromyosin (Ishikawa, Bischoff & Holtzer, 1969). If this were true also of the terminal webs found in the epidermis of parasitic platyhelminths, surface contractility could facilitate discharge of surface secretions or assist in flushing the parasites' surface (see Lyons, 1972b, 1973a).

Aspidogastreans

Work on the adult and larval epidermis of this group of endoparasites has been reviewed in detail by Rohde (1972), and see Lyons (1973a). All the adults studied so far have small knob-like projections, the microtubercles, regularly arranged on the surface (Fig. 12). These measure $0.08–0.1\,\mu$m in *Aspidogaster conchicola*, described by Bailey & Tompkins (1971) and Halton & Lyness

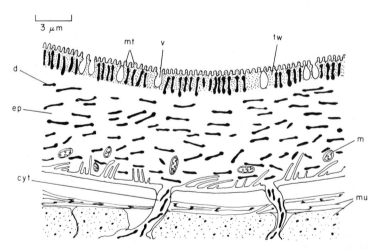

FIG. 12. Diagram of the tegument of the aspidogastrean *Taeniocotyle* sp. from *Hydrolagus colliei* Friday Harbour USA showing the regular surface microtubercles and disc-shaped inclusions. (From unpublished work by Laurie & Lyons.) Abbreviations: cyt, cytoplasmic connection; d, disc-shaped inclusions; ep, epidermis=tegument; m, mitochondria; mt, microtubercles; mu, integumentary muscle layers; tw, terminal web; v, secretory vesicle.

(1971). It has been suggested that the adult microtubercles of *Multicotyle purvisi* may represent the thickened bases of very fine (12–18 nm thick) processes, or microfila present in the larva, which may be flotation devices and break off at the end of larval life (Rohde, 1972). It is not, however, known whether microfila occur on other aspidogastrean larvae.

Digeneans

General tegument stucture and function

All adult digeneans so far described have basically the same type of tegument (reviewed in Lee, 1966, 1972; Hockley, 1973). This is quite different in surface specialization from the microvillous epidermis of monogeneans, the microtubercle-covered tegument of aspidogastreans and the microthrix-bearing tegument of cestodes, though all have the same basic syncytial plan (Fig. 13). The epidermal surface of digeneans is typically avillous and is infolded into a series of pits or tortuous channels. These presumably increase the surface available for metabolic exchanges into and out of the worms. The pits have been investigated in surface view using the scanning electron microscope as well as in section (see Hockley,

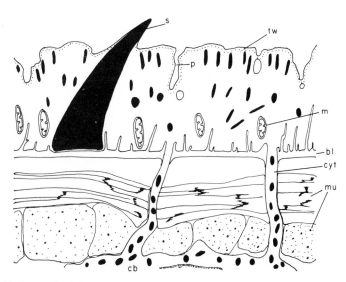

FIG. 13. Generalized diagram of the tegument of an adult digenean showing the absence of surface microvilli (although the tegument may be folded) and the presence of spines. Abbreviations: bl, basement lamina; cb, cell body; cyt, cytoplasmic connection; m, mitochondrion; mu, muscle; p, surface pits; s, spine of crystalline protein; tw, slightly developed terminal web region.

1973). Despite this characteristic surface the tegument of digeneans is regionally differentiated.

Complex folding may occur on the adhesive organ surface of
strigeoids and this may be elaborately pitted and chambered (see
Erasmus, 1969). These specializations probably assist the
adhesive/digestive functions of this surface. Surface differentiation
is also particularly evident in schistosomes which are unusual in
having separate sexes. Many of the surface specializations appear
to be related to attachment to the host and to the way in which the
female worm is grasped in the gynecophoric canal of the male.
Male schistosomes have been shown by the scanning electron
microscope (Morris & Threadgold, 1968; Smith, Reynolds & von
Lichtenberg, 1969; Silk, Spence & Buch, 1970; Race et al., 1971;
Miller, Tulloch & Kuntz, 1972) to be covered with blunt tubercles
or bosses most numerous dorsally bearing spine clusters. These are
absent from females and probably assist in attachment inside host
blood vessels. At the edges of the gynecophoric canal are spines
which interlock across the middle to hold the females in position
and the lining is ridged and contains backwardly pointing spines to
grip the female. The spines in the female, which occur only
posteriorly, are directed anteriorly so may interlock with those of
the male. The surfaces of the oral suckers of both sexes bear small
spines directed inwardly towards the mouth. These body spines,
like those of all digeneans, are secreted within the tegument and
have a characteristic crystalline structure.

The thickness of the tegument depends upon the age and
species concerned. In young worms it may be as little as $0.25\ \mu$m, in
adults 3.5 to 15–$20\ \mu$m (in F. hepatica, an unusually large fluke,
Threadgold, 1963). The surface of the tegument is covered with a
"surface coat" usually consisting of acidic PAS positive material. In
Schistosoma mansoni there is evidence that the glycocalyx consists of
sialic acid-containing glycoprotein (see Hockley, 1973; Stein &
Lumsden, 1973). It has been suggested that this coat could either
mask the parasite's own antigens, or could bind host antigens and
so form a protective coat preventing rejection of worms by host
immune mechanisms (Smithers, Terry & Hockley, 1969) (Fig. 14).
The bound host antigens have been shown, using immunological
methods, to be likely to be glycolipids from host red blood cells
(Clegg, 1972, 1974; McLaren, Clegg & Smithers, 1975) (Fig. 14).

The surface coat of S. mansoni may derive from laminated
bodies in the tegument which may be secreted to the surface and
contribute new membrane and attached glycocalyx at the same

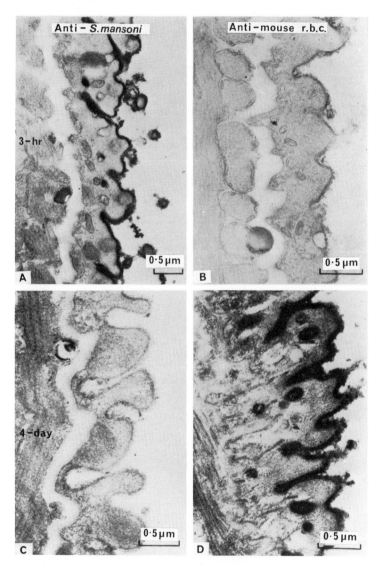

FIG. 14. Immunological properties of the surface of schistosomulae of *S. mansoni* of different ages shown using an antibody enzyme bridge technique. A, Electron micrograph of a transverse section of a 3-h schistosomula after culture for 24 h in hyperimmune monkey serum then stained to show the accumulation of monkey antibodies at the surface of the tegument. B, Electron micrograph of a 3-h schistosomula after culture in non-immune serum showing absence of mouse red cell antigens from the surface (no stain). C, Electron micrograph of a transverse section of a 4-day schistosomula from mouse lung subsequently incubated in immune monkey serum. No monkey antibody has been bound to the surface. D, Similar preparation of a 4-day schistosomula treated to demonstrate the presence of mouse red blood cell antigens which have bound to the surface whilst the schistosome was in the tissues of its host. These will disguise the worm against recognition by host antibodies. Obviously protective antigen binding must occur somewhere between days 1–4 in the host.

time. The surface membrane of adult *S. mansoni* is most unusual in being 11 to 15 layers thick compared with the usual trilaminate structure, and undergoes rapid recycling (see Hockley, 1973; Wilson & Barnes, 1974). The function of rod-shaped secretory granules found in the tegument of *S. mansoni* and other digeneans is not certain; they could contribute to surface mucus, form glycocalyx or contribute to the tegument itself if dispersed internally (see Bogitsh, 1968). Both types of inclusion are secreted by Golgi bodies present usually in the cell body regions, but also occasionally in the outer tegumental layer (Bogitsh, 1971, 1972). Gut parasites may rely upon the surface coat for protection against host digestive enzymes, in the same way that the vertebrate epithelium is itself protected. In tissue sites the glycocalyx could mediate in cell–cell interactions as already outlined. A terminal web-like structure is present just under the plasma membrane in many flukes (Threadgold, 1963; Burton, 1966; Threadgold, 1968; Hockley, 1973) (see p. 120). Except in *Gorgoderina*, a bladder fluke, the tegument contains few mitochondria with few cristae. Those of *S. mansoni* are reported to be even more poorly developed than most, suggesting that transport of materials across the tegument may be minimal and require little energy. The basal membrane of the tegument is an ordinary unit membrane infolded to form finger-like processes that penetrate the tegument. In most cases these infoldings are not closely associated with mitochondria and there is no evidence that they are involved in ion regulatory processes. They may be skeletal. The underlying connective tissue basement lamina is thickest in the suckers where it is obviously developed for muscle attachment. The tegumental cell bodies are secretory, as described. More than one type of cell may be joined to the tegument at any one time and each cell may have several processes linking it with the upper tegument. The sub-tegumental cells may make close contact with neighbouring parenchyma cells by means of junctional complex and doubtless exchanges occur between the two.

Uptake across the tegument of digeneans

Adult digeneans take up most of their food material over the caecal epithelium via the mouth, but there is considerable evidence that the tegument may also be involved in the uptake of small food molecules (reviewed in Lee, 1966, 1972; Erasmus, 1972). *In vitro* experiments with *S. mansoni* have demonstrated the uptake of labelled glucose and amino acids across the tegument (Mansour,

1959; Uglem & Read, 1975). Glucose uptake has been located in the main body region rather than in the oral sucker region of *S. mansoni* by Rogers & Bueding (1975). Uglem & Read (1975) have found that glucose, galactose and glucosamine enter by both mediated transport and diffusion, whereas fructose enters only by diffusion. The transport mechanism involved is Na^+ dependent and is thought to be similar to sugar uptake mechanisms of both tapeworms and vertebrates. The tegument of *F. hepatica* has been shown by Knox (1965) to be permeable to both glucose and various amino acids using both ligated and non-ligated worms. Uptake has also been investigated by Isseroff & Read (1969) and Isseroff & Walczak (1971). Insulin may have an effect on glycogen levels in *F. hepatica* but there is controversy about the nature of the effect (see Pantelouris, 1964; Hines, 1969). Nollen (1968) demonstrated that in *Philophthalmus megalurus* some metabolites are absorbed preferentially via the tegument and others via the gut (see also Pappas, 1971).

Uptake of labelled glucose in *H. medioplexus* and *Gorgoderina* was compared by Parkening & Johnson (1969) who found that tegumental glucose incorporation was far less in *Gorgoderina* (a bladder fluke) than in *H. medioplexus* (a lung fluke). The amino acids adenine and thymidine can be absorbed across the tegument of *G. attenuata in vitro*, however, and were taken up in equal amounts by ligated and non-ligated flukes, but this probably occurs little *in vivo* since the flukes probably feed mainly on bladder tissue (Nollen, Restaino & Alberico, 1973). The validity of the methods used in these experiments has recently been questioned by Nollen & Nadakavukaren (1974). These authors have demonstrated, using the scanning electron microscope, that tegumental damage and therefore leakage is caused by ligatures. Similar findings were reported for *Diclidophora*, a monogenean, by Halton & Arme (1971). Uptake of high molecular weight substances, such as ferritin and thorium dioxide, across the tegument, is controversial. Dike (1969) described incorporation of ferritin by pinocytosis via the gut and tegument of various digeneans, however, the ferritin being in membrane bound vesicles. Knox (1965) was unable to demonstrate tegumental uptake of labelled albumen, insulin or labelled algal protein in *F. hepatica*. In *S. mansoni*, horseradish peroxidase was incorporated in vesicles only in the dorsal tegument of the male (Smith *et al.*, 1969). Iron is said to be absorbed by diffusion, in simple ionic form across the tegument of *H. medioplexus* (see Shannon & Bogitsh, 1969).

Tegumental alkaline phosphatase activity has been demonstrated in several adult digeneans. In *S. mansoni*, for example, there are probably several different kinds of alkaline phosphatases present superficially (Bogitsh & Krupa, 1971). Specific nucleoside di- and triphosphatases have been located in *H. medioplexus* tegument (Bogitsh & Krupa, 1971). The presence of alkaline phosphatase activity in epithelia is usually correlated with membrane transport and particularly with monosaccharide uptake although the evidence for this is somewhat slender (see Lumsden, 1975). These enzymes may be involved in phosphate group transfer during ATP cleavage or hydrolysis of sugar phosphates prior to uptake (see Dike & Read, 1971). Acid phosphatase activity occurs in the general tegument of *F. hepatica* and *Paragonimus westermani* but is confined to the tegument of lappets and adhesive glands in strigeoids (see Erasmus, 1972). Non-specific esterase occurs in the tegument of some schistosomes, and Halton (1967) demonstrated the presence of cholinesterases in *F. hepatica* tegument.

Apart from being involved in the digestion of host tissue (e.g. the strigeioid adhesive organ), possible absorption of nutrients, adsorption of host antigens and disguise (in *S. mansoni*) and adhesion, the tegument also serves as a sense organ having numerous sensory bulbs embedded in it, and doubtless serves protective ion and osmoregulatory roles as well as being an excretory surface. Little is known at present about the regenerative capacity of this highly specialized surface.

Cestodes, "cestodarians" and cestoideans

"Cestodarians" and cestoideans

Both the externally unstrobilated gyrocotylideans, amphilideans and caryophyllideans and the strobilated tapeworms lack a gut at all stages in their development, and this is reflected in the highly specialized nature of their tegument which is amplified by "microvilli" presumably to facilitate the uptake of food molecules. These are regularly arranged and superficially resemble those on the surface of the vertebrate intestinal cells, with which the parasite surface itself competes. The microvilli of the so-called "cestodarians" *Gyrocotyle* and *Amphilina* (Fig. 15) are relatively unspecialized (Lyons, 1969; J. S. Laurie, pers. comm.) whilst those of true cestodes have thickened, spine-like tips and are properly referred to as microtriches (singular: microthrix). The amphilideans have only short, stubby, unspined microvilli (J. S. Laurie,

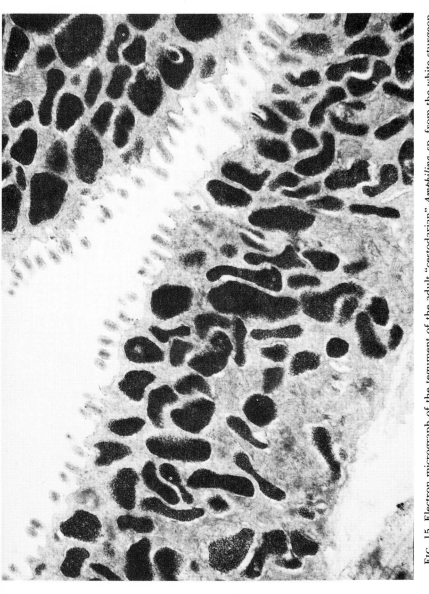

FIG. 15. Electron micrograph of the tegument of the adult "cestodarian" *Amphilina* sp. from the white sturgeon *Acipenser transmontanus* caught in Friday Harbour USA. The tegument has the same basic plan as in cestodes but has shorter scattered microvilli with no terminal spines. (From unpublished work by J. S. Laurie.) ×27 000.

pers. comm.) (Fig. 15). This group has been said to represent an arrested neotenous plerocercoid stage; if this is true the tegument is less developed than that of cestode plerocercoids which already have well developed spines on the microtriches (see p. 116). The microvilli of *Gyrocotyle urna* are much longer than those of *Amphilina* (*c.* 1 μm in length) (Lyons, 1969) and terminate in a fine unthickened spike 0·2 μm long. Those microvilli on the attachment rosette may be bifurcate. The cestoidean *Hunterella nodulosa* (Caryophyllidea) has three types of surface processes. Spined microtriches occur only anteriorly for adhesion, in the middle of the body is an intermediate zone bearing microvilli with short spined endings resembling those of *Gyrocotyle*, and posteriorly are unarmed, sometimes branching, microvilli which are presumably mainly absorptive (Hayunga & Mackiewicz, 1975).

Cestodes

Microtriches with a thickened terminal spine are characteristic of cestodes. They are approximately 0·8–2·0 μm long and divided into a shaft and thickened tip separated by a cap of membrane (Figs 16 and 17). The shaft may contain terminal web microfilaments. There is a cylinder of dense material situated just inside the plasma membrane which is continuous with the tip (Fig. 17). The plasma membrane of the shaft region may be of double thickness (Jha & Smyth, 1969; Grammeltvedt, 1973; Smyth, 1972). Lumsden (1972) found that the surface membrane and coat of the shaft and tip may be associated with different ionic groups capable of binding different kinds of charged molecules. Carrier molecules too probably have a highly patterned arrangement in the tegument plasma membrane. There may be considerable variation in the structure and density of the microtriches in various regions of the tapeworm's body. The scolex spines of *Echinococcus granulosus*, for instance, are better developed than those on the body, and the barbed, curved and hooked tips doubtless aid adhesion (Jha & Smyth, 1969). Conversely the rostellar microvilli of *Raillietina cesticillus* lack spines and may be absorptive whilst the remainder of the scolex has strengthened microtriches (Blitz & Smyth, 1973).

Scanning and transmission electron microscope studies have demonstrated that the density of microtriches varies in different regions of the worms (Berger & Mettrick, 1971; Featherston, 1972; Ubelaker, Allison & Specian, 1973). The increase in surface area produced by the microtriches does not seem to be as great as that produced by microvilli on the host gut epithelium. Densities range from 49/μm^2 on the rostellum, 65/μm^2 on the suckers, 56/μm^2 on the scolex and 48/μm^2 on the mature proglottids of *H. diminuta* (Ubelaker *et al.*, 1973). Besides increasing the surface area for absorption of food, the microtriches offer an expanded surface for either surface digestion or membrane contact digestion or both

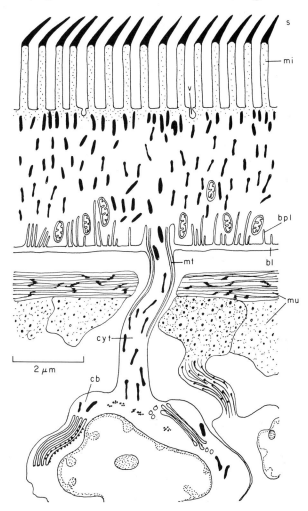

Fig. 16. Diagrammatic representation of the tegument of a cestode. The surface is covered with microtriches each ending in a thickened, spine-like cap. As is usual the epidermal cell bodies are secretory and produce amongst other things surface coat material. Abbreviations: bl, basement lamina; bpl, basal plasma membrane; cb, epidermal cell body; cyt, cytoplasmic connection; mi, microtriches; mt, microtubules; mu, muscle layers; s, microthrix spine; v, vesicle.

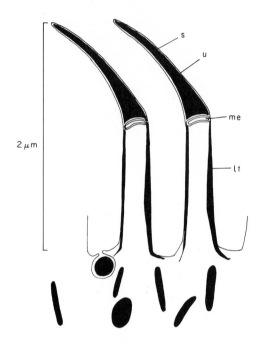

FIG. 17. Diagram of cestode microtriches showing the terminal dense spine separated from the main shaft by a membrane sac. Most authors describe a unit membrane covering the microthrix. Microfilaments continuous with a terminal web may be present. Abbreviations: lt, lateral thickening; me, membrane sac; s, dense terminal spine; u, unit membrane covered by glycocalyx.

(see below). Their thickened recurved tips would seem to facilitate attachment and they might also give leverage during locomotion, since it has been shown that *Hymenolepis diminuta*, at any rate, may perform diurnal migrations within the gut of its rat host and is not permanently anchored to one spot. Fixation of tetraphyllidean tapeworms *in situ* shows that host intestinal microvilli and tapeworm microtriches do not interdigitate to any great extent (McVicar, 1972). It is possible that tapeworm microtriches might be contractile since the shaft contains terminal web microfilaments found to be actin-like in vertebrates (Ishikawa *et al.*, 1969). This could assist in detachment of the microthrix tips and also possibly circulate nutrient-containing fluids at the tapeworm's surface or alternatively aid spreading of protective secretions.

The surface membrane of the tegument is covered with what is termed a surface coat, believed to be mucopolysaccharide or mucoprotein (see Lumsden, 1975, for review). Oaks & Lumsden

(1971) found that the surface coat is renewed every 6–8 h from Golgi secretions. Polyanionic groups of sialic acid in the surface coat have an imputed importance in adsorption of cationic colloids (Lumsden, Oaks & Alworth, 1970; Lumsden, Oaks & Dike, 1970; Lumsden, 1972, 1973). The glycocalyx may bind cations critical to the function of surface enzymes so may play an important part in surface digestion. Lumsden & Berger (1974) have shown that surface phosphohydrolase activity depends on Ca^{2+} activity, and Lumsden (1973) previously showed that this ion was bound by the surface coat. The glycocalyx may also bind host enzymes and assist in membrane contact digestion. The idea of surface digestion involving adsorption of intrinsic amylase to the microvilli of the vertebrate gut itself was first proposed by Ugolev and then investigated for cestodes by Taylor & Thomas (1968) and Read (1973). The latter suggested that extrinsic (i.e. host) amylase is bound to the surface of *H. diminuta* to digest oligosaccharides such as maltose prior to uptake. The theory has, however, been questioned by Mead & Roberts (1972).

It has frequently been speculated that cestodes inhibit the action of host proteolytic enzymes and avoid digestion. There is no known inhibitor of amylase or lipase but trypsin inhibitors are widely distributed. Pappas & Read (1972a,b) suggest that the glycocalyx is the site of interaction for inhibitors that complex with trypsin, the inactivated complex then detaching from the surface. Pancreatic lipase is also said to be inhibited by an adsorption phenomenon. Enzyme deactivation could also be produced by manipulation of local pH and cestodes are known to acidify the gut lumen *in vivo* by absorbing bicarbonate and secreting H^+ ions to maintain internal neutrality. The increase in local acidity may also stimulate Na^+ uptake into the worms. Most of this work applies solely to *H. diminuta* and is reviewed in Mettrick & Podesta (1974).

Small vesicles are present between the microtriches but it is not known whether these are secretory or pinocytotic. Lumsden, Threadgold, Oaks & Arme (1970) have shown that *H. diminuta* does not take up colloids by transmembranosis or incorporate thorium dioxide, ferritin, carbon particles or ^{14}C-labelled *Chlorella* protein in vesicles. The fish tapeworm *Bothriocephalus scorpii* has however been shown to be able to take up denatured proteins *in vitro* and it has been suggested that proteolytic enzymes are present in the tegument to digest these (Dubovskaya, 1971). Thus a picture is being built up of the tegument as a digestive–absorptive surface (see Smyth, 1972). In the vertebrate gut epithelium with which a tapeworm is in competition, some digested proteins may be absorbed as peptides; this may also occur in tapeworms but has not yet been investigated (quoted in Mettrick & Podesta, 1974). The active transport, mediated transport and diffusion of various substances across the cestode tegument have been studied by many workers (mainly in *H. diminuta*) and have been reviewed by Pittman & Fisher (1972) and Mettrick & Podesta (1974). In the vertebrate intestine tight junctions between the cells have been implicated as an extracellular shunt pathway for solute transfer into and out of the mucosa. No such junctions of course occur in tapeworms.

The microthrix region of *H. diminuta* has been shown to have phosphohydrolase activity against a wide variety of substrates (Arme & Read, 1970; Dike & Read, 1971; Pappas & Read, 1974). Hydrolysis of the substrate occurs only on the external face of the membrane and phosphatase action is probably associated with hydrolysis of sugar phosphates or nucleotides prior to uptake (see Page & MacInnis, 1975), or with ATP cleavage. Specific carriers have been demonstrated for particular sugars, amino acids, short and long chain fatty acids, thiamine and riboflavin. *Diphyllobothrium latum* competes for vitamin B_{12} with the host gut by secreting a releasing factor that separates vitamin B_{12} from intrinsic factor. The vertebrate gut can absorb B_{12} only as a complex bound to intrinsic factor, but the tapeworm can absorb B_{12} alone. Sense organs of the type typical to platyhelminths occur throughout the tegument but are concentrated on the scolex region. Space does not permit descriptions of these here.

GENERAL SUMMARY

The epidermis of both the ectoparasitic and endoparasitic platyhelminths probably evolved from the cellular, ciliated covering of a "rhabdocoel"-like ancestral form, similar perhaps to the fecampid, *Kronborgia amphipodicola*, described by Bresciani & Køie (1970) and Køie & Bresciani (1973) (Fig. 18), or to the dalyellioid, *Syndesmis echinorum* (see Lyons, 1973a). Both forms are "endoparasites". It is of interest that the cellular covering of ageing female *Kronborgia* is said to become partially syncytial by breaking down of lateral cell boundaries. Another feature of interest is that the epidermis of this worm may grow by addition of replacement cells from the parenchyma (Køie & Bresciani, 1973). Retention of the ciliated coat, typical of free-living forms, in *Kronborgia* is not

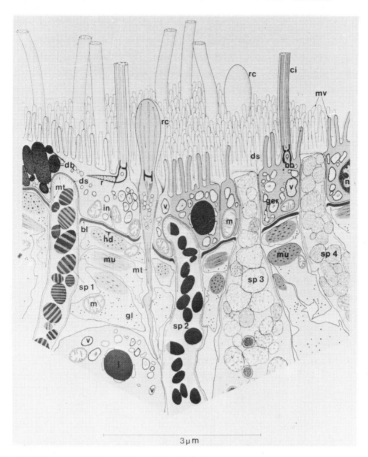

3μm

FIG. 18. Diagram of the cellular, ciliated epidermis of the larva of the neorhabdocoel *Kronborgia amphipodicola* showing the large number of surface microvilli. The surface of the parasitic adult is similar although the microvilli are longer and branch. The syncytial epidermis of the parasitic flukes and tapeworms may have evolved from a similar structure in an ancestral rhabdocoel. Abbreviations: bl, basement lamina; bb, basal body; ci, cilium; db, dense bodies; ds, septate desmosome; ger, granular endoplasmic reticulum; gl, glycogen reserves; hd, half-desmosome; in, basal invagination; l, lipid; m, mitochondrion; mt, microtubules; mu, muscle; mv, microvilli; n, nucleus; r, ciliary rootlet; rc, receptor cilium; sp 1–6, secretory products of different glands; v, vesicle. (From Køie & Bresciani, 1973.)

surprising since the adult female has to escape from the amphipod host to lay eggs. It can be imagined that, as better attachment organs evolved and adult parasites become more closely associated with their hosts, there would be an evolutionary tendency to lose the ciliated coat in the adult and retain this only in a dispersal stage. Ectoparasitic temnocephalan "rhabdocoels" have a non-ciliated epidermis, which is cellular anteriorly but may be partially syncytial, with superficial nuclei (Clark Nichols, 1975). A syncytial condition could be achieved either by cell fusion in a non-ciliated cellular covering [as may have occurred in *Gyrodactylus* sp. (see Lyons, 1973a)] or could be derived by epidermal replacement cells in the parenchyma [these apparently being a feature of turbellarians (see Dorey, 1965; Skaer, 1965)], failing after a time to develop cilia and also failing to migrate completely to the surface. They would then send up cytoplasmic processes to the surface and produce a continuous coat of membrane-bound cytoplasm to cover most of the body. This actually occurs during development of ciliated larvae to adult parasitic forms in monogeneans, digeneans and cestodes, as has been described. This method of forming a syncytium is interesting in that different kinds of cell bodies can apparently make and break connections to the outer layer at different stages in development (see p. 110). Thus the tegument is not a static covering but may receive different secretions and change its surface membrane and associated surface coat as well as remodel its surface architecture in response to the sequential changes in host environment that the parasites, with their complex life histories, undergo. The highly plastic mesenchymal developmental system for producing epidermis in platyhelminths has therefore been put to good use in the parasitic groups. It is far from clear why the parasitic groups have a syncytial rather than cellular epidermis. This has obviously evolved more than once in the various parasitic lines. It may be that the absence of cell boundaries provides fewer points of attack for histolytic host enzymes of other secretions, or it may provide a homogenous procuticle-like zone which can be fortified by internal accumulation of structural proteins (for example). However, invertebrate cuticles probably first made an appearance for skeletal and locomotory reasons rather than to offer physiological protection by sealing the animal off from its environment. That platyhelminth parasites are not "far" from secreting a "cuticle" is shown by the ability of digeneans in particular to form cysts. As has already been pointed out, if the mucus-like material lying between the microvilli on the surface of, for example, monogenean parasites, were to become stabilized, the microvillus permeated cuticle would basically resemble that of annelids, pogonophorans and insects (Lyons, 1973a). In vertebrates the trophoblast of embryos is syncytial; possibly this is connected with its function as an absorptive surface having to maintain contact with tissues of a different immunological character.

Alternatively syncytia in platyhelminths may merely result from the way in which the epidermis is formed in development by fusion of cytoplasm extruded from cell body regions. According to Nicholas (1971) the "syncytial" condition in acanthocephalans may have arisen during the evolution of a small free-living ancestor into a larger form as a result of adopting the parasitic habit. He suggests that a previous evolutionary trend towards miniaturization may have involved restriction of cleavage to an early developmental stage. When the opportunity to increase in size occurred this would be accomplished not by changing determinate development and cleavage patterns but by enlarging each organ which consequently tended to become "syncytial" (or perhaps to be more accurate, "plasmodial"?).

ACKNOWLEDGEMENTS

I should like to thank the Zoology Department, University of London King's College, for photographic assistance, and also the Zoological Society of London for a grant to assist in the preparation of this paper.

REFERENCES

Andersen, K. (1975). Comparison of surface topography of three species of *Diphyllobothrium* (Cestoda, Pseudophyllidea) by scanning electron microscopy. *Int. J. Parasit.* **5**: 293–300.

Arme, C. & Read, C. P. (1970). A surface enzyme in *Hymenolepis diminuta* (Cestoda). *J. Parasit.* **56**: 514–516.

Bailey, H. H. & Tompkins, S. J. (1971). Ultrastructure of the integument of *Aspidogaster conchicola. J. Parasit.* **57**: 848–854.

Baron, P. J. (1968). On the histology and ultrastructure of *Cysticercus longicollis*, the cysticercus of *Taenia crassiceps* Zeder, 1800 (Cestoda, Cyclophyllidea). *Parasitology* **58**: 497–513.

Baron, P. J. (1971). On the histology, histochemistry and ultrastructure of the cysticercoid of *Raillietina cesticillus* (Molin, 1858) Fuhrmann, 1920 (Cestoda, Cyclophyllidea). *Parasitology* **62**: 233–245.

Basch, P. F. & Di Conza, J. (1974). The miracidium-sporocyst transition in *Schistosoma mansoni*: surface changes *in vitro* with ultrastructural correlation. *J. Parasit.* **60**: 935–941.

Belton, J. C. & Belton, C. M. (1971). Freeze-etch and cytochemical studies of the integument of larval *Acanthatrium oregonense* (Trematoda). *J. Parasit.* **57**: 252–260.

Belton, C. M. & Harris, P. J. (1967). Fine structure of the cuticle of the cercaria of *Acanthatrium oregonense* (Macy). *J. Parasit.* **53**: 715–724.

Berger, J. & Mettrick, D. F. (1971). Microtrichial polymorphism among hymenolepidid tapeworms as seen by scanning electron microscopy. *Trans. Am. microsc. Soc.* **90**: 393–403.

Bibby, M. C. & Rees, G. (1971a). The ultrastructure of the epidermis and associated structures in the metacercaria, cercaria and sporocyst of *Diplostomum phoxinii* (Faust, 1918). *Z. ParasitKde* **37**: 169–186.

Bibby, M. C. & Rees, G. (1971b). The uptake of radioactive glucose *in vivo* and *in vitro* by the metacercaria of *Diplostomum phoxinii* (Faust) and its conversion to glycogen. *Z. ParasitKde* **37**: 187–197.

Bilquees, F. M. & Freeman, R. S. (1969). Histogenesis of the rostellum of *Taenia crassiceps* (Zeder, 1800) (Cestoda), with special reference to hook development. *Can. J. Zool.* **47**: 251–261.

Bils, R. F. & Martin, W. E. (1966). Fine structure and development of the trematode tegument. *Trans. Am. microsc. Soc.* **85**: 78–88.

Blitz, N. M. & Smyth, J. D. (1973). Tegumental ultrastructure of *Raillietina cesticillus* during the larval–adult transformation, with emphasis on the rostellum. *Int. J. Parasit.* **3**: 561–570.

Bogitsh, B. J. (1968). Cytochemical and ultrastructural observations on the tegument of the trematode *Megalodiscus temperatus. Trans. Am. microsc. Soc.* **87**: 477–486.

Bogitsh, B. J. (1971). Golgi complexes in the tegument of *Haematoloechus medioplexus. J. Parasit.* **57**: 1373–1374.

Bogitsh, B. J. (1972). Additional cytochemical and morphological observations on the tegument of *Haematoloechus medioplexus. Trans. Am. microsc. Soc.* **91**: 47–55.

Bogitsh, B. J. & Krupa, P. L. (1971). *Schistosoma mansoni* and *Haematoloechus medioplexus*: nucleoside-diphosphatase localization in tegument. *Expl Parasit.* **30**: 418–425.

Bonner, T. P. & Weinstein, P. P. (1972). Ultrastructure of the hypodermis during cuticle formation in the third moult of the nematode *Nippostrongylus brasiliensis. Z. Zellforsch. mikrosk. Anat.* **126**: 17–24.

Bråten, T. (1968a). An electron microscope study of the tegument and associated structures of the procercoid of *Diphyllobothrium latum* (L.). *Z. ParasitKde* **30**: 95–103.

Bråten, T. (1968b). The fine structure of the tegument of *Diphyllobothrium latum* (L.). A comparison of the plerocercoid and adult stages. *Z. ParasitKde* **30**: 104–112.

Bresciani, J. (1972). The ultrastructure of the integument of the monogenean *Polystoma integerrimum* (Frölich 1791). *K. Veterinaer-og Landbohojsk. Arsskr.* **1973**: 14–27.

Bresciani, J. & Køie, M. (1970). On the ultrastructure of the adult female of *Kronborgia amphipodicola* Christensen & Kanneworf, 1964 (Turbellaria, Neorhabdocoela). *Ophelia* **8**: 209–230.

Brooker, B. E. (1972). Sense organs in trematode miracidia. In *Behavioural aspects of parasite transmission*: 171–180. Canning, E. U. & Wright, C. A. (eds). London and New York: Academic Press.

Burt, M. D. B. & Sandeman, I. M. (1974). The biology of *Bothrimonus* (= *Diplocotyle*) (Pseudophyllidea: Cestoda): detailed morphology and fine structure. *J. Fish. Res. Bd Can.* **31**: 147–153.

Burton, P. R. (1966). The ultrastructure of the integument of the frog bladder fluke *Gorgoderina* sp. *J. Parasit.* **52**: 926–934.

Cable, R. M. & Shutte, M. H. (1973). Comparative fine structure and origin of the metacercarial cyst in two philophthalmid trematodes, *Parorchis acanthus*

(Nicoll, 1906) and *Philophthalmus megalunis* (Cort, 1914). *J. Parasit.* **59**: 1031–1040.

Caley, J. (1973). The functional significance of scolex retraction and subsequent cyst formation in the cysticercoid larva of *Hymenolepis microstoma*. *Parasitology* **68**: 207–227.

Charles, G. H. & Orr, T. S. C. (1968). Comparative fine structure of outer tegument of *Ligula intestinalis* and *Schistocephalus solidus*. *Expl Parasit.* **22**: 137–149.

Cheng, T. C. & Bier, J. W. (1972). Studies on molluscan schistosomiasis: an analysis of the development of the cercaria of *Schistosoma mansoni*. *Parasitology* **64**: 129–141.

Clark Nichols, K. (1975). Observations on lesser-known flatworms: Temnocephala. *Int. J. Parasit.* **5**: 245–252.

Clegg, J. A. (1972). The schistosome surface in relation to parasitism. *Symp. Br. Soc. Parasit.* **10**: 23–40.

Clegg, J. A. (1974). Host antigens and the immune response in schistosomiasis. In *Parasites in the immunized host: mechanisms of survival*: 161–183. Porter, R. & Knight, J. (eds). Ciba Foundation Symposium, **25** (new series) Amsterdam: Associated Scientific Publishers.

Collin, W. K. (1969). The cellular organization of the hatched oncospheres of *Hymenolepis citelli* (Cestoda: Cyclophyllidea). *J. Parasit.* **55**: 149–166.

Dike, S. C. (1969). Acid phosphatase activity and ferritin incorporation in the ceca of digenetic trematodes. *J. Parasit.* **55**: 111–123.

Dike, S. C. & Read, C. P. (1971). Relation of tegumentary phosphohydrolase and sugar transport in *Hymenolepis diminuta*. *J. Parasit.* **57**: 1251–1255.

Dixon, K. E. (1970). Absorption by developing cercariae of *Cloacitrema narrabeenensis* (*Philophthalmidae*). *J. Parasit.* **56** (No. 4 Sect. II): 416–417.

Dixon, K. E. (1975). The structure and composition of the cyst wall of the metacercaria of *Cloacitrema narrabeenensis* (Howell & Bearup, 1967) (Digenea: Philophthalmidae). *Int. J. Parasit.* **5**: 113–118.

Dixon, K. E. & Mercer, E. M. (1967). The formation of the cyst wall of the metacercaria of *Fasciola hepatica* L. *Z. Zellforsch. mikrosk. Anat.* **77**: 345–360.

Dorey, A. E. (1965). The organization and replacement of the epidermis in acoelous turbellarians. *Q. Jl microsc. Sci.* **106**: 147–172.

Dubovskaya, A. Ya. (1971). [Comparative investigation of the consumption of proteins of different biological value by the cestodes *Bothriocephalus scorpii*] *Trud. Vses. Inst. Gel 'mintol.* **17**: 41–43. [In Russian.]

Dusanic, D. G. (1959). Histochemical observations of alkaline phosphatase in *Schistosoma mansoni*. *J. infect. Dis.* **105**: 1–8.

Erasmus, D. A. (1969). Studies on the host-parasite interface of strigeoid trematodes. V. Regional differentiation of the adhesive organ of *Apatemon gracilis minor* Yamaguti 1933. *Parasitology* **59**: 193–201.

Erasmus, D. A. (1972). *The biology of trematodes*. London: Edward Arnold.

Esch, G. W. & Kuhn, R. E. (1971). The uptake of ^{14}C-*Chlorella* protein by larval *Taenia crassiceps* (Cestoda). *Parasitology* **62**: 27–29.

Eveland, L. K. (1972). *Schistosoma mansoni*: conversion of cercariae to schistosomula. *Expl Parasit.* **32**: 261–264.

Featherston, D. W. (1972). *Taenia hydatigena* IV. Ultrastructure study of the tegument. *Z. ParasitKde* **38**: 214–232.

Gibson, D. I. (1974). Aspects of the ultrastructure of the daughter-sporocyst and cercaria of *Podocotyle staffordi* Miller, 1941 (Digenea: Opecoelidae). *Norw. J. Zool.* **22**: 237–252.

Grammeltvedt, A. F. (1973). Differentiation of the tegument and associated structures in *Diphyllobothrium dendriticum* Nitsch (1824) (Cestoda: Pseudophyllidea). An electron microscopical study. *Int. J. Parasit.* **3**: 321–327.

Halton, D. W. (1967). Histochemical studies of carboxylic esterase activity in *Fasciola hepatica*. *J. Parasit.* **53**: 1210–1216.

Halton, D. W. & Arme, C. (1971). *In vitro* technique for detecting tegument damage in *Diclidophora merlangi*: possible screening method for selection of undamaged tissues or organisms prior to physiological investigation. *Expl Parasit.* **30**: 54–57.

Halton, D. W. & Lyness, R. A. W. (1971). Ultrastructure of the tegument and associated structures of *Aspidogaster conchicola* (Trematoda: Aspidogastrea). *J. Parasit.* **57**: 1198–1210.

Hansen, E. & Perez-Mendez, G. (1972). Scanning electron microscopy of *Schistosoma mansoni* daughter sporocysts. *Int. J. Parasit.* **2**: 174.

Haynes, W. D. G. (1970). *Taenia crassiceps*: uptake of basic and aromatic amino acids and amino acids by larvae. *Expl Parasit.* **27**: 256–264.

Haynes, W. D. G. & Taylor, E. R. (1968). Studies on the absorption of amino acids by larval tapeworms (Cyclophyllidea: *Taenia crassiceps*). *Parasitology* **58**: 47–59.

Hayunga, E. G. & Mackiewicz, J. S. (1975). An electron microscope study of the tegument of *Hunterella nodulosa* Mackiewicz and McCrae, 1962 (Cestoidea: Caryophyllidea). *Int. J. Parasit.* **5**: 309–319.

Hines, J. W. (1969). An *in vitro* effect of insulin on glycogen levels in the common liver fluke, *Fasciola hepatica* (Linnaeus, 1758). *Comp. Biochem. Physiol.* **28**: 1443–1447.

Hockley, D. J. (1968). Scanning electron microscopy of *Schistosoma mansoni* cercariae. *J. Parasit.* **54**: 1241–1243.

Hockley, D. J. (1972). *Schistosoma mansoni*: the development of the cercarial tegument. *Parasitology* **64**: 245–252.

Hockley, D. J. (1973). Ultrastructure of the tegument of *Schistosoma*. *Adv. Parasit.* **11**: 233–305.

Hoskin, G. P. & Cheng, T. C. (1974). *Himasthla quissetensis*: uptake and utilization of glucose by rediae as determined by autoradiography and respirometry. *Expl Parasit.* **34**: 61–67.

Ishikawa, H., Bischoff, R. & Holtzer, H. (1969). Formation of arrowhead complexes with heavy meromyosin in a variety of cell types. *J. Cell Biol.* **43**: 312–328.

Isseroff, H. & Read, C. P. (1969). Studies on membrane transport—VI. Absorption of amino acids by fascioliid trematodes. *Comp. Biochem. Physiol.* **30**: 1153–1159.

Isseroff, H. & Walczak, I. M. (1971). Absorption of acetate, pyruvate and certain Krebs cycle intermediates by *Fasciola hepatica*. *Comp. Biochem. Physiol.* **39B**: 1017–1021.

James, B. L. & Bowers, E. A. (1967). Reproduction in the daughter sporocyst of *Cercaria bucephalopsis haimeana* (Lacaze-Duthiers, 1854) (Bucephalidae) and *Cercaria dichotoma* Lebour, 1911 (non Müller) (Gymnophallidae). *Parasitology* **57**: 607–625.

Jha, R. K. & Smyth, J. D. (1969). *Echinococcus granulosus*: ultrastructure of microtriches. *Expl Parasit.* **25**: 232–244.

Kinoti, G. K. (1971). The attachment and penetration apparatus of the miracidium of Schistoma mansoni. J. Helminth. 45: 229–235.

Kinoti, G. K., Bird, R. G. & Barker, M. (1971). Electron microscope and histochemical observations on the daughter sporocyst of Schistosoma mattheii & Schistosoma bovis. J. Helminth. 45: 237–244.

Knox, B. E. (1965). Uptake of nutrients by Fasciola hepatica (Abstract). Parasitology 55: 17–18.

Køie, M. (1971a). On the histochemistry and ultrastructure of the daughter sporocyst of Cercaria buccini Lebour, 1911. Ophelia 9:145–163.

Køie, M. (1971b). On the histochemistry and ultrastructure of the redia of Neophasis lageniformis (Lebour, 1910) (Trematoda; Acanthocolpidae). Ophelia 9: 113–143.

Køie, M. (1971c). On the histochemistry and ultrastructure of the tegument and associated structures of the cercaria of Zoogonoides viviparus in the first intermediate host. Ophelia 9: 165–206.

Køie, M. (1973). The host–parasite interface and associated structures of the cercaria and adult Neophasis lageniformis (Lebour, 1910). Ophelia 12: 205–219.

Køie, M. (1975). On the morphology and life-history of Opechona bacillaris (Molin, 1859) Looss, 1907 (Trematoda, Lepocreadiidae). Ophelia 13: 63–86.

Køie, M. & Bresciani, J. (1973). On the ultrastructure of the larva of Kronborgia amphipodicola Christensen and Kanneworff, 1964 (Turbellaria, Neorhabdocoela). Ophelia 12: 171–203.

Krupa, P. L., Bal, A. K. & Cousineau, G. H. (1967). Ultrastructure of the redia of Cryptocotyle lingua. J. Parasit. 53: 725–734.

Krupa, P. L. & Bogitsh, B. J. (1972). Ultrastructural phosphohydrolase activities in Schistosoma mansoni sporocysts and cercariae. J. Parasit. 58: 495–514.

Krupa, P. L., Cousineau, G. H. & Bal, A. K. (1968). Ultrastructural and histochemical observations on the body wall of Cryptocotyle lingua (Trematoda). J. Parasit. 54: 900–908.

Krupa, P. L., Cousineau, G. H. & Inoué, S. (1970). Uptake of colloidal thorium dioxide by the redia of Cryptocotyle lingua. J. Parasit. 56 (No. 4 sect. II): 194.

Kwa, B. H. (1972). Studies on the sparganum of Spirometra erinacei. III. The fine structure of the tegument in the scolex. Int. J. Parasit. 2: 35–43.

Laurie, J. S. (1974). Himasthla quissetensis: induced in vitro encystment of cercaria and ultrastructure of the cyst. Expl Parasit. 35: 350–362.

Lee, D. L. (1966). The structure and composition of the helminth cuticle. Adv. Parasit. 4: 187–254.

Lee, D. L. (1972). The structure of the helminth cuticle. Adv. Parasit. 10: 347–379.

Llewellyn, J. (1965). Evolution of parasites. Symp. Br. Soc. Parasit. 3: 47–78.

Lo, S. J., Hall, J. E., Allender, P. A. & Klainer, A. S. (1975). Scanning electron microscopy of an opecoelid cercaria and its encystment and encapsulation in an insect host. J. Parasit. 61: 413–417.

Lo Verde, P. T. (1975). Scanning electron microscope observations on the miracidium of Schistosoma. Int. J. Parasit. 5: 95–97.

Lumsden, R. D. (1972). Cytological studies on the absorptive surfaces of cestodes. VI. Cytochemical evaluation of electrostatic charge. J. Parasit. 58: 229–234.

Lumsden, R. D. (1973). Cytological studies on the absorptive surfaces of cestodes. VII. Evidence for the function of tegument glycocalyx in cation binding by Hymenolepis diminuta. J. Parasit. 59: 1021–1030.

Lumsden, R. D. (1975). Surface ultrastructure and cytochemistry of parasitic helminths. *Expl Parasit.* **37**: 267–339.

Lumsden, R. D. & Berger, B. (1974). Cytological studies on the absorptive surfaces of cestodes. VIII. Phosphohydrolase activity and cation adsorption in the tegument brush border of *Hymenolepis diminuta. J. Parasit.* **60**: 744–751.

Lumsden, R. D., Oaks, J. A. & Alworth, W. L. (1970). Cytological studies on the absorptive surfaces of cestodes. IV. Localization and cytochemical properties of membrane-fixed cation binding sites. *J. Parasit.* **56**: 736–747.

Lumsden, R. D., Oaks, J. A. & Dike, S. C. (1970). Cytoarchitectural and cytochemical features of tapeworm surfaces. *J. Parasit.* **56**: section 2, 217.

Lumsden, R. D., Oaks, J. A. & Mueller, J. F. (1974). Brush border development in the tegument of the tapeworm, *Spirometra mansonoides. J. Parasit.* **60**: 209–226.

Lumsden, R. D., Threadgold, L. T., Oaks, J. A. & Arme, C. (1970). On the permeability of cestodes to colloids: an evaluation of the transmembranosis hypothesis. *Parasitology* **60**: 185–193.

Lyons, K. M. (1966). The chemical nature and evolutionary significance of monogenean attachment sclerites. *Parasitology* **56**: 63–100.

Lyons, K. M. (1969). The fine structure of the body wall of *Gyrocotyle urna. Z. ParasitKde* **33**: 95–109.

Lyons, K. M. (1970a). The fine structure and function of the outer epidermis of two skin parasitic monogeneans, *Entobdella soleae* and *Acanthocotyle elegans. Parasitology* **60**: 39–52.

Lyons, K. M. (1970b). Fine structure of the outer epidermis of the viviparous monogenean *Gyrodactylus* sp. from the skin of *Gasterosteus aculeatus. J. Parasit.* **56**: 1110–1117.

Lyons, K. M. (1971). Comparative electron microscope studies on the epidermis of the blood living juvenile and gill living adult stages of *Amphibdella flavolineata* (Monogenea) from the electric ray *Torpedo nobiliana. Parasitology* **63**: 181–190.

Lyons, K. M. (1972a). Sense organs of monogeneans. *J. Linn. Soc. (Zool.).* **51** suppl 1: 181–199.

Lyons, K. M. (1972b). Ultrastructural observations on the epidermis of the polyopisthocotylinean monogeneans, *Rajonchocotyle emarginata* and *Plectanocotyle gurnardi. Z. ParasitKde* **40**: 87–100.

Lyons, K. M. (1973a). The epidermis and sense organs of the Monogenea and some related groups. *Adv. Parasit.* **11**: 193–232.

Lyons, K. M. (1973b). Epidermal fine structure and development in the oncomiracidium larva of *Entobdella soleae* (Monogenea). *Parasitology* **66**: 321–333.

Mansour, T. E. (1959). Studies on the carbohydrate metabolism of the liver fluke, *Fasciola hepatica. Biochem. Biophys. Acta* **34**: 456–464.

Matricon-Gondran, M. (1967). Absorptive structures in trematode rediae and sporocysts. *J. Ultrastruct. Res.* **21**: 166.

Matricon-Gondran, M. (1969). Étude ultrastructurale du syncytium tegumentaire et de son evolution chez des trématodes digénétiques larvaires. *C. r. hebd. Séanc. Acad. Sci., Paris* **269**: 2384–2387.

Matricon-Gondran, M. (1971). Étude ultrastructurale des recépteurs sensoriels tegumentaires des quelques trématodes digénétiques larvaires. *Z. ParasitKde* **35**: 318–333.

McDaniel, J. S. & Dixon, K. E. (1967). Utilization of exogenous glucose by the rediae of *Parorchis acanthus* (Digenea: Philophthalmidae) and *Cryptocotyle lingua* Digenea: Heterophyidae). *Biol. Bull. mar. biol. Lab. Woods Hole* **133**: 591–599.

McLaren, D. J., Clegg, J. A. & Smithers, S. R. (1975). Acquisition of host antigens by young *Schistosoma mansoni* in mice: correlation with failure to bind antibody *in vitro*. *Parasitology* **70**: 67–75.

McManus, D. P. & James, B. L. (1975). The absorption of sugars and organic acids by the daughter sporocysts of *Microphallus similis* (Jäg). *Int. J. Parasit.* **5**: 33–38.

McVicar, A. H. (1972). The ultrastructure of the parasite–host interface of three tetraphyllidean tapeworms of the elasmobranch *Raja naevus*. *Parasitology* **65**: 77–88.

Mead, R. W. & Roberts, L. S. (1972). Intestinal digestion and absorption of starch in the intact rat: effects of cestode (*Hymenolepis diminuta*) infection. *Comp. Biochem. Physiol.* **41**A: 749–760.

Mercer, E. H. & Dixon, K. E. (1967). The fine structure of the cystogenic cells of the cercaria of *Fasciola hepatica* L. *Z. Zellforsch. mikrosk. anat.* **77**: 331–344.

Mettrick, D. F. & Podesta, R. B. (1974). Ecological and physiological aspects of helminth–host interactions in the mammalian gastrointestinal canal. *Adv. Parasit.* **12**: 183–278.

Miller, F. H., Tulloch, G. S. & Kuntz, R. E. (1972). Scanning electron microscopy of integumental surface of *Schistosoma mansoni*. *J. Parasit.* **58**: 693–698.

Morris, G. P. (1971). The fine structure of the tegument and associated structures of the cercaria of *Schistosoma mansoni*. *Z. ParasitKde* **36**: 15–31.

Morris, G. P. & Finnegan, C. V. (1969). Studies of the differentiating plerocercoid cuticle of *Schistocephalus solidus*. II. The ultrastructural examination of cuticle development. *Can. J. Zool.* **47**: 957–964.

Morris, G. P. & Threadgold, L. T. (1968). Ultrastructure of the tegument of adult *Schistosoma mansoni*. *J. Parasit.* **54**: 15–27.

Mount, P. (1970). Histogenesis of the rostellar hooks of *Taenia crassiceps* (Zeder, 1800) (Cestoda). *J. Parasit.* **56**: 947–961.

Nicholas, W. L. (1967). The biology of the Acanthocephala. *Adv. Parasit.* **5**: 204–246.

Nicholas, W. L. (1971). The evolutionary origins of the Acanthocephala. *J. Parasit.* **57**: 84–87.

Nieland, M. L. (1968). Electron microscope observations on the egg of *Taenia taeniaeformis*. *J. Parasit.* **54**: 957–960.

Nollen, P. M. (1968). The uptake and incorporation of glucose, tyrosine, leucine and thymidine by adult *Philophthalamus megalurus* as determined by autoradiography. *J. Parasit.* **54**: 295–304.

Nollen, P. M. & Nadakavukaren, M. J. (1974). Observations on ligated adults of *Philophthalamus megalurus*, *Gorgoderina attenuata* and *Megalodiscus temperatus* by scanning electron microscopy and autoradiography. *J. Parasit.* **60**: 921–924.

Nollen, P. M., Restaino, A. L. & Alberico, R. A. (1973). *Gorgoderina attenuata*: uptake and incorporation of tyrosine, thymidine and adenosine. *Expl Parasit.* **33**: 468–476.

Oaks, J. A. & Lumsden, R. D. (1971). Cytological studies on the absorptive surfaces of cestodes. V. Incorporation of carbohydrate-containing macromolecules into tegument membranes. *J. Parasit.* **57**: 1256–1268.

Page, C. R. & MacInnis, A. J. (1975). Characterization of nucleoside transport in hymenolepidid cestodes. *J. Parasit.* **61**: 281–290.

Pantelouris, E. M. (1964). Localization of glycogen in *Fasciola hepatica* L. and an effect of insulin. *J. Helminth.* **38**: 283–286.

Pappas, P. W. (1971). *Haematoloechus medioplexus*: uptake, localization and fate of tritiated arginine. *Expl Parasit.* **30**: 102–119.

Pappas, P. W. & Read, C. P. (1972a). Trypsin inactivation by intact *Hymenolepis diminuta. J. Parasit.* **58**: 864–871.

Pappas, P. W. & Read, C. P. (1972b). Inactivation of α and β chymotrypsin by intact *Hymenolepis diminuta* (Cestoda). *Biol. Bull. mar. biol. Lab. Woods Hole* **143**: 605–616.

Pappas, P. W. & Read, C. P. (1974). Relation of nucleoside transport and surface phosphohydrolase activity in *Hymenolepis diminuta* (Cestoda). *J. Parasit.* **56**: 514–516.

Parkening, J. A. & Johnson, A. D. (1969). Glucose uptake in *Haematoloechus medioplexus* and *Gorgoderina* trematodes. *Expl Parasit.* **25**: 358–367.

Pence, D. B. (1967). The fine structure and histochemistry of the infective eggs of *Dipylidium caninum. J. Parasit.* **53**: 1041–1054.

Pence, D. B. (1970). Electron microscope and histochemical studies on the eggs of *Hymenolepis diminuta. J. Parasit.* **56**: 84–97.

Pittman, R. G. & Fisher, F. M. (1972). The membrane transport of glycerol by *Hymenolepis diminuta. J. Parasit.* **58**: 742–749.

Race, G. J., Martin, J. H., Moore, D. V. & Larsh, J. E. (1971). Scanning and transmission electron microscopy of *Schistosoma mansoni* eggs, cercariae and adults. *Am. J. trop. Med. Hyg.* **20**: 914–924.

Read, C. P. (1973). Contact digestion in tapeworms. *J. Parasit.* **59**: 672–77.

Reader, T. (1972). Ultrastructural and cytochemical observations on the body wall of the redia of *Sphaeridiotrema globulus.* (Rudolphi, 1819). *Parasitology* **65**: 537–546.

Rees, G. (1966). Light and electron microscope studies of the redia of *Parorchis acanthus* Nicoll. *Parasitology* **56**: 589–602.

Rees, G. (1967). The histochemistry of the cystogeneous gland cells and cyst wall of *Parorchis acanthus* Nicoll and some details of the morphology and fine structure of the cercaria. *Parasitology* **57**: 87–110.

Rees, G. (1971). The ultrastructure of the epidermis of the redia and cercaria of *Parorchis acanthus* Nicoll. A study by scanning and transmission electron microscopy. *Parasitology* **62**: 479–488.

Rees, G. (1973). The ultrastructure of the cysticercoid of *Tatria octacantha* Rees, 1973 (Cyclophyllidea: Amatiliidae) from the haemocoele of the damsel-fly nymphs *Pyrrhosoma nymphula*, Sulz and *Enallagma cyathigerum*, Charp. *Parasitology* **67**: 85–103.

Rees, G. (1974). The ultrastructure of the body wall and associated structures of the cercaria of *Cryptocotyle lingua* (Creplin) (Digenea: Heterophyidae) from *Littorina littorea* (L.). *Z. ParasitKde* **44**: 239–265.

Rifkin, E., Cheng, T. C. & Hohl, H. R. (1970). The fine structure of the tegument of *Tylocephalum* metacestodes; with emphasis on a new type of microvilli. *J. Morph.* **130**: 11–24.

Robson, R. T. & Erasmus, D. A. (1970). The ultrastructure, based on Stereoscan observations, of the oral sucker of *Schistosoma mansoni* with special reference to penetration. *Z. ParasitKde* **35**: 76–86.

Rogers, S. H. & Bueding, E. (1975). Anatomical localization of glucose uptake by *Schistosoma mansoni* adults. *Int. J. Parasit.* **5**: 369–371.

Rohde, K. (1972). The Aspidogastrea, especially *Multicotyle purvisi* Dawes, 1941. *Adv. Parasit.* **10**: 77–151.

Rybicka, K. (1972). Ultrastructure of embryonic envelopes and their differentiation in *Hymenolepis diminuta* (Cestoda). *J. Parasit.* **58**: 849–863.

Rybicka, K. (1973). Ultrastructure of the embryonic syncytial epithelium in a cestode *Hymenolepis diminuta*. *Parasitology* **66**: 9–18.

Shannon, W. A. & Bogitsh, B. J. (1969). Cytochemical and biochemical observations on the digestive tracts of digenetic trematodes. IV. A radioautographic and histochemical study of iron absorption in *Haematoloechus medioplexus*. *Expl Parasit.* **26**:376–383.

Short, R. B. & Cartrett, M. L. (1973). Argentophilic "papillae" of *Schistosoma mansoni* cercariae. *J. Parasit.* **59**: 1041–1059.

Silk, M. H., Spence, I. M. & Buch, B. (1970). Observations of *Schistosoma mansoni* blood flukes in the scanning electron microscope. *S. Afr. J. med. Sci.* **35**: 23–29.

Skaer, R. J. (1965). The origin and continuous replacement of epidermal cells in the planarian *Polycelis tenuis* (Ijima). *J. Embryol. exp. Morph.* **13**: 129–139.

Šlais, J. (1973). Functional morphology of cestode larvae. *Adv. Parasit.* **11**: 395–557.

Smith, J. H. & Chernin, E. (1974). Ultrastructure of young mother and daughter sporocysts of *Schistosoma mansoni*. *J. Parasit.* **60**: 85–89.

Smith, J. H., Reynolds, E. S. & Lichtenberg, F. von (1969). The integument of *Schistosoma mansoni*. *Am. J. trop. Med. Hyg.* **18**: 28–49.

Smithers, S. R., Terry, R. J. & Hockley, D. J. (1969). Host antigens in schistosomiasis. *Proc. R. Soc.* (B.) **171**: 483–494.

Smyth, J. D. (1972). Changes in the digestive absorptive surface of cestodes during larval–adult differentiation. *Symp. Br. Soc. Parasit.* **10**: 41–70.

Southgate, V. R. (1970). Observations on the epidermis of the miracidium and on the formation of the tegument of the sporocyst of *Fasciola hepatica*. *Parasitology* **61**: 177–190.

Southgate, V. R. (1971). Observations on the fine structure of the cercaria of *Notocotyle attenuatus* and formation of the cyst wall of the metacercaria. *Z. Zellforsch. mikrosk. Anat.* **120**: 420–449.

Stein, P. C. & Lumsden, R. D. (1971). The ultrastructure of developing metacercarial cysts of *Ascocotyle leighi* Burton 1956 (Heterophyidae). *Proc. helminth. Soc. Wash.* **38**: 1–10.

Stein, P. C. & Lumsden, R. D. (1973). *Schistosoma mansoni*: topochemical features of cercariae, schistosomulae and adults. *Expl Parasit.* **33**: 499–514.

Storch, V. & Welsch, U. (1970). Der Bau der Körperwand von *Leucochloridium paradoxum*. *Z. ParasitKde* **35**: 67–75.

Strong, P. L. & Cable, R. M. (1972). Fine structure and development of the metacercarial cyst in *Microphallus opacus* (Ward, 1894). *J. Parasit.* **58**: 92–98.

Swiderski, Z. (1972). La structure fine de l'oncosphère, du cestode *Catenotaenia pusilla* (Groeze, 1782) (Cyclophyllidea, Catenotatriidae). *Cellule* **69**:207–237.

Taylor, E. W. & Thomas, J. N. (1968). Membrane (contact) digestion in three species of tapeworm: *Hymenolepis diminuta*, *Hymenolepis microstoma* and *Monezia expansa*. *Parasitology* **58**: 535–546.

Threadgold, L. T. (1963). The tegument and associated structures of *Fasciola hepatica. Q. Jl microsc. Sci.* **104**: 505–512.
Threadgold, L. T. (1968). Electron microscope studies of *Fasciola hepatica.* VI. The ultrastructural localization of phosphatases. *Expl Parasit.* **23**: 264–276.
Timofeev, V. A. & Kuperman, B. I. (1967). Ultrastructure of the external integument of the coracidium of *Triaenophorus nodulosus* (Pall.). *Parazitologiya* **1**: 124–129.
Ubelaker, J. E., Allison, V. F. & Specian, R. D. (1973). Surface topography of *Hymenolepis diminuta* by scanning electron microscopy. *J. Parasit.* **59**: 667–671.
Uglem, G. L. & Read, C. P. (1975). Sugar transport and metabolism in *Schistosoma mansoni. J. Parasit.* **61**: 390–397.
Voge, M. (1973). The post-embryonic developmental stages of cestodes. *Adv. Parasit.* **11**: 707–730.
Wikel, S. K. (1974). *Schistosoma mansoni*: penetration apparatus and epidermis of the miracidium. *Expl Parasit.* **36**: 342–354.
Wilson, R. A. (1969). Fine structure of the tegument of the miracidium of *Fasciola hepatica* L. *J. Parasit.* **55**: 124–133.
Wilson, R. A. (1970). Fine structure of the nervous system and specialized nerve endings in the miracidium of *Fasciola hepatica. Parasitology* **60**: 399–410.
Wilson, R. A. & Barnes, P. E. (1974). The tegument of *Schistosoma mansoni*: observations on the formation, structure and composition of cytoplasmic inclusions in relation to tegument function. *Parasitology* **68**: 239–258.
Wilson, R. A., Pullin, R. & Denison, J. (1971). An investigation of the mechanism of infection by digenetic trematodes: the penetration of the miracidium of *Fasciola hepatica* into its snail host *Lymnaea truncatula. Parasitology* **63**: 491–506.
Wright, C. A. (1971). *Flukes and snails.* London: George Allen and Unwin.

Symp. zool. Soc. Lond. (1977) No. 39, 145–170.

THE NEMATODE EPIDERMIS AND COLLAGENOUS CUTICLE, ITS FORMATION AND ECDYSIS

D. L. LEE

*Department of Pure and Applied Zoology,
University of Leeds, Leeds, England*

SYNOPSIS

The body wall of nematodes consists of a collagenous cuticle, a cellular or syncytial epidermis (hypodermis)* and a layer of longitudinal muscle. There is no circular muscle in the body wall. The cuticle can be a simple or a complex structure which varies from genus to genus and may differ in juveniles and adults of the same species. It is basically a three-layered structure consisting of cortical, median and basal layers, but these may be further sub-divided. Large fibres are present in the cuticle of some nematodes. The basic component of the cuticle is a form of collagen, but other substances such as cuticlin, hyaluronic acid and acid mucopolysaccharides may be present. The cuticle is secreted by the epidermis. Most nematodes moult four times during their development and the epidermis plays an important role in this, but many nematodes continue to grow between moults and several species continue to grow after the final moult. In some species the moulted cuticle is partially resorbed by the nematode whereas in others the cuticle is cast almost whole. Moulting appears to be under hormonal control. Development can be arrested at a particular stage in development and a specific stimulus is required to allow it to continue. This is usually associated with arrestment of the moulting cycle prior to ecdysis and occurs in many parasitic nematodes.

The cuticle plays an important role in the locomotion of nematodes and, together with the hypodermis, it is important in osmotic and ionic regulation, in excretion and in the uptake of oxygen.

INTRODUCTION

The typical nematode is spindle-shaped, unsegmented and bilaterally symmetrical. The body wall is composed of an outer cuticle, a cellular or syncytial epidermis (usually called a hypodermis in the literature), and a layer of longitudinal muscle. There is no circular muscle in the body wall. The body cavity, in which lie the gonads and the various parts of the alimentary tract, is a pseudocoelom. The pseudocoelomic fluid is under pressure and, in some species, this can be very high. For example, that of *Ascaris lumbricoides* can be as high as 225 mmHg (Harris & Crofton, 1957), and this has an important bearing on the structure of nematodes. The pressurized fluid in the pseudocoelom together with the cuticle which surrounds the worm form a highly developed hydrostatic skeleton,

* The term hypodermis is used by parasitologists for the nematode epidermis. In vertebrates hypodermis is the subcutaneous tissue, a quite different meaning.

which not only maintains body shape but also plays an important role in locomotion. Certain constraints are placed on the design of nematodes because of this high pressure hydrostatic skeleton. For example, the pharynx will have to create a higher suction pressure than the pressure in the pseudocoelom if food is to be passed from the external environment into the intestine, and is a very powerful pumping organ; the cuticle will have to withstand the large pressures that are generated during locomotion and, as we shall see later, this has had an important bearing on its structure in different species and on different stages of the life cycle. We also find that the thickness of the cuticle is usually proportional to the diameter of the nematode because the tangential stress in a cylinder subjected to internal pressure is proportional to the diameter of the cylinder (Crofton, 1966). The nematode also relies on dilator muscles rather than sphincter muscles to control orifices as the high hydrostatic pressure will close them, but sphincter muscles do control certain important areas of the alimentary tract [intestinal–rectal junction (Lee, 1975)] and the ovijector of some females.

Nematodes undergo four moults during their life cycle. The juvenile (usually referred to as a larva) is similar to the adult nematode but differs from it in size, sometimes in the nature of the mouth parts, in the lack of gonads and of copulatory structures. The structure of the juvenile cuticle often differs from that of the adult nematode. Some nematodes moult once or twice within the egg before hatching, and some undergo a period of arrested development during which they remain ensheathed in the moulted, but not ecdysed, cuticle of the previous stage. This sheath acts as a protective covering against adverse conditions, as in infective juveniles of several animal-parasitic nematodes and in "dauer" juveniles of some free-living species, such as dung-inhabiting nematodes, which are transported from place to place on the body of insects. This sheath is also important in regulating the rate of drying of some of these ensheathed juveniles when they are entering a cryptobiotic state (Ellenby, 1969).

THE EPIDERMIS

The epidermis of nematodes is usually referred to as the hypodermis. It lies between the cuticle and the muscle of the body wall and projects into the pseudocoelom along the dorsal, ventral and lateral lines to form four ridges or cords. The lateral cords are the largest and the excretory canals of the nematode are closely associated with these cords. The main longitudinal nerves of the nematode lie alongside, and are often embedded in, the dorsal and the ventral cords. The nuclei of the epidermis are found only in the epidermal cords. The epidermis of some nematodes is cellular but in others it is a syncytium. It is separated from the cuticle of the body wall by a cell membrane. The epidermis of *Ascaris lumbricoides* is derived from six longitudinal rows of dorsal, ectodermal blastomeres and these give rise to a cellular epidermis. This cellular epidermis becomes syncytial when the nematode becomes a third-stage, parasitic juvenile. There is rapid development of the nematode once it has become a parasitic third-stage juvenile, and both nuclei and cells multiply rapidly. The median rows of cells in the lateral cords remain cellular but the dorsal and ventral cords become syncytial (Thust, 1968). The epidermis of the adult worm becomes completely syncytial (Watson, 1965b).

The epidermis in the inter-cordal area is often very thin, as in *Euchromadora vulgaris* where it is about 1 μm thick (Watson, 1965a) and *Trichuris myocastoris* where it is about 2·5 μm thick (Wright, 1968a) but still contains a few small mitochondria in the cytoplasm in these regions. Ribosomes, granular endoplasmic reticulum and microtubules occur in the cytoplasm of the epidermis and some of these vary in amount at different stages of the moulting cycle. The epidermis is an important storage tissue and contains large amounts of glycogen and lipid. The epidermal membrane is attached to the cuticle by half-desmosomes and fibres extend from these points of attachment to desmosome-type junctions between the epidermis and the longitudinal muscles. The muscles apparently exert their pull on the cuticle by means of these fibres (tonofilaments) during locomotion (Figs 1 and 2). Haemoglobin is present in the epidermis of some nematodes, for example *Ascaris lumbricoides* (Lee & Smith, 1965), but the role of these haemoglobins in the uptake of oxygen by these nematodes is still controversial.

Some modified cells of the epidermis form gland cells in the tail of some marine nematodes and produce a sticky secretion which hardens when it comes in contact with water and attaches the nematode by its tail to the substratum (Lippens, 1974a). Rows of epidermal glands are also present in the lateral cords of some marine nematodes and open to the exterior through pores in the cuticle. These are merocrine gland cells and each has a dendrite associated with it (Lippens, 1974b). Gland-like cells also occur in rows, called bacillary bands, along the length of the animal-parasitic Trichuroidea (Wright, 1968b). These also open to the

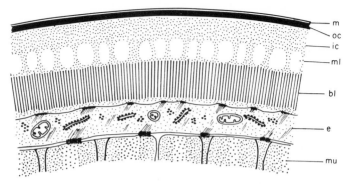

FIG. 1. Diagram of a transverse section through the body wall of a typical juvenile nematode. Some adult nematodes have a similar cuticle. Abbreviations: bl, basal (striated) layer; e, epidermis; ic, inner cortex; m, membrane-like layers; ml, median layer; mu, muscle; oc, outer cortex.

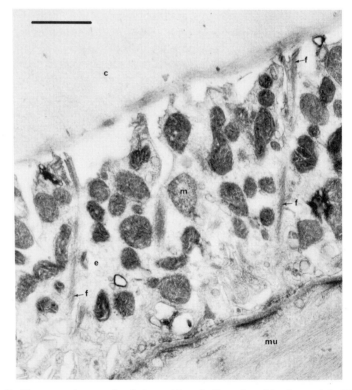

FIG. 2. Electron micrograph of the epidermis (hypodermis) of an adult *Heterakis gallinarum* to show the fibres which traverse the epidermis and, indirectly, link the muscles to the cuticle. Abbreviations: c, cuticle; e, epidermis; f, fibres; m, mitochondria; mu, muscle. The bar respresents 1 μm.

exterior through pores in the cuticle and some have sensory neurones associated with them (Wright & Chan, 1973). The function of these epidermal gland cells is not known, although it has been suggested that they could be involved in the transport of water and ions, the secretion of mucus or the secretion of enzymes.

As well as being one of the most important storage tissues of the body the epidermis plays an important role in the formation and growth of the cuticle (see pp. 157–165).

(see pp. 157–165)

THE CUTICLE

Structure

The cuticle of nematodes can be a relatively simple or a very complex structure which varies from one genus to another and may differ in structure throughout the life cycle of a single species. It is usually superficially annulated and is basically three-layered, consisting of outer cortical, median and inner basal layers (Fig. 1). This three-layered pattern occurs in the juvenile stages of most nematodes and in many free-living adult nematodes, but modifications to the cuticle occur, especially in adult nematodes. The lumen of the buccal cavity, the pharynx, the rectum or cloaca, the vagina, the spicule pouches, the excretory pore, the chemosensory amphids on the head and the sensory phasmids on the tail are lined with cuticle but this has a simpler structure than that of the body wall. The cuticle of the buccal cavity is often shaped and hardened to form small denticles, larger teeth or cutting plates which are used during feeding in some predatory and animal-parasitic nematodes. The mouth stylet of plant-parasitic nematodes and the copulatory spicules of males are also made from toughened cuticle. It is not known how this toughening and hardening is brought about but it is suspected that some tanning or sclerotization occurs.

The cuticle of the body wall is covered by a membrane-like structure which varies in thickness from 25 to 40 μm (Figs 1 and 3). It appears to consist of an outer, triple-layered membrane about 7 μm thick which may be a typical plasma membrane; a middle, osmiophobic layer about 10 to 20 μm thick; and an inner, osmiophilic layer which is about 10 to 20 μm thick (Bird, 1971). There has been considerable controversy about the structure, composition and formation of this layer. Some authors regard it as a layer of lipid (Trim, 1949; Bird, 1957), some as a modified, epidermal membrane (Lee, 1966a,b, 1972) and some as a membrane-like structure deposited as an extracellular secretion on

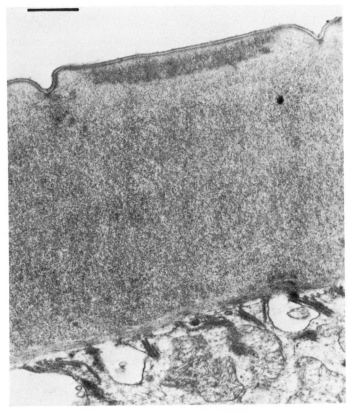

FIG. 3. Electron micrograph of the cuticle of an adult *Heterakis gallinarum* to show the outer, membrane-like layer and the electron dense outer cortex (compare with the cuticlin in Fig. 6). The basal layer is fibrous but is not clearly separated into fibre layers. The bar represents 0·5 μm.

the outside of the cuticle when it is first formed (Bonner & Weinstein, 1972). It has been suggested that this structure may correspond with, and may be similar to, the cuticulin layer found in insects (Locke, in Bird, 1971). The formation of this layer will be discussed later in pp. 157–165.

The main, cortical layer of the cuticle is a single layer in most juveniles and in many free-living adults, and consists of fine fibrils. Inner and outer cortical layers occur in many of the larger, animal-parasitic nematodes. The outer cortex, when present, is more electron dense than the inner cortex and is usually confined to the areas between the grooves which give the cuticle its superficial annulations (Fig. 3). This layer is thought to be tougher than other parts of the body wall cuticle and may strengthen it between the grooves of the annulations, as it will run as a band around each superficial annule of the cuticle. The inner cortical layer varies in thickness in different nematodes. In juveniles it may be about $0.2\ \mu$m thick whereas in some adult, animal-parasitic species it may be $10\ \mu$m thick. It appears to be composed of fine fibrils. The cortical layer of the cuticle of adult female *Mermis nigrescens* is penetrated by canals which extend from the layer just beneath the cortex to the transverse grooves on the surface of the cuticle (Lee, 1970a). The function of these is not known.

The median layer (also called the matrix or homogeneous layer) is relatively structureless and composed of numerous fine fibrils in most nematodes. In some nematodes, especially juvenile stages, this layer is thin relative to the rest of the cuticle (0.1–$0.5\ \mu$m in *Meloidogyne javanica* second-stage juveniles) whereas it forms the major layer in the cuticle of others, especially adult stages (*Nippostrongylus brasiliensis*) (Bird, 1971). In the marine nematode *Acanthonchus duplicatus* the median layer is traversed by dense, skeletal elements and canals extend from it into the epidermis (Wright & Hope, 1968). In adult *Nippostrongylus brasiliensis* this layer is filled with a red fluid containing haemoglobin. It is thought that this haemoglobin plays an important role in the movement of oxygen from the environment (mucosal surface of rat intestine) into the body of the nematode (Lee, 1965). The cuticle of this nematode is longitudinally ridged and the skeletal struts which support these ridges lie in this fluid-filled median layer. Fibres, which exhibit the typical, periodic cross-banding of collagen, connect the basal layer and the cortical layer to these struts and suspend the struts in the median layer (Fig. 4). Other fibres connect the basal layer to the cortical layer. This cuticle seems to operate a form of hydrolastic suspension (apologies to British Leyland Motor Co.) and appears to be ideally suited to the corkscrewing type of locomotion between intestinal villi undertaken by this nematode (Lee, 1965; Lee & Atkinson, 1976). The median layer of pre-parasitic juveniles of *Heterodera rostochiensis* is also thought to contain fluid. It is traversed by thin strands of material which connect the cortical layer to the basal layer (Wisse & Daems, 1968) (Fig. 1).

The basal layer of the cuticle varies in thickness from a very thin layer containing apparently randomly orientated fibrils in some free-living nematodes (*Acanthonchus duplicatus*, Wright & Hope, 1968) to a thick layer containing large fibres which spiral around

152   D. L. LEE

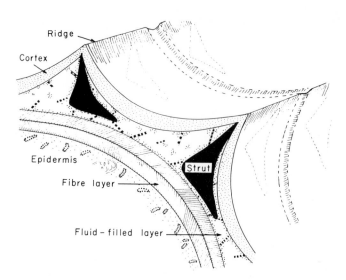

FIG. 4. Diagram of part of the cuticle of an adult *Nippostrongylus brasiliensis* to show the longitudinal ridges, the arrangement of the various layers, the position of the struts, and the fibres of collagen which suspend the struts. Reproduced with permission from Lee (1970b).

the body in some of the larger adult nematodes (*Ascaris lumbricoides, Nippostrongylus brasiliensis*, Harris & Crofton, 1957; Watson, 1965b) (Figs 4 and 5). In juveniles of free-living, plant-parasitic and animal-parasitic nematodes, and in adults of some free-living species, the basal layer contains a material which is regularly striated with a periodicity of about 20 nm (Fig. 1). It is thought that this layer is a tough, almost crystalline, protein which has very close linkages between the molecules. It is probable that this is one of the three natural forms of collagen, the other two being an unstriated form and a striated form with a periodicity of about 64 nm. The layers of the nematode cuticle which contain unstriated fibrils are probably the unstriated form of collagen and the striated fibres which suspend the struts in the cuticle of adult *Nippostrongylus* are probably the striated form of collagen. The striated basal layer shown in Fig. 1 is possibly the main skeletal layer in the cuticle of these nematodes (Lee, 1966a; Wisse & Daems, 1968). It is interesting to note here that many nematodes, including juveniles, possess lateral extensions of the cuticle which run most of the length of the cuticle. These are called lateral alae and may be blunt, ribbon-like extensions or fin-like. In juveniles which possess these alae the basal layer of the cuticle loses the striations in the lateral alae and two fibril layers, which lie at an angle to each other, appear. One must remember that most nematodes move on their sides—that is, on any lateral alae present, and stresses will be set up in the lateral alae when the nematode moves on a solid substratum. It is possible, therefore, that the change from a striated to a fibrous basal layer in this region may be associated with the stresses set up in the lateral alae when the worm is moving.

The basal layer of many larger nematodes is modified to form two or three fibre layers (Figs 4 and 5). There are three fibre layers in *Ascaris lumbricoides* and each fibre in each layer runs in a spiral around the nematode and at about 75° to the longitudinal axis. The middle of the three layers crosses the other two at an angle of 140–150° and the three layers form a lattice which alters its angles as the nematode moves. The success of the hydrostatic skeleton in the larger nematodes depends on these fibres in the cuticle (Harris & Crofton, 1957).

While the cuticles of the juvenile stages and the male of *Heterodera rostochiensis* have the basic, three-layered plan described earlier, the cuticle of gravid females differs significantly from it. It has a cuticle which is more suited to its swollen form, its sedentary habit on the roots of the potato plant, and its eventual role as a protective

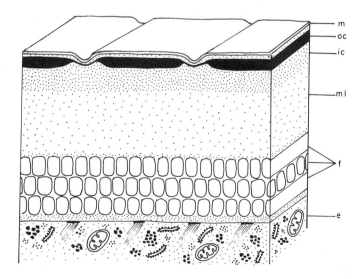

FIG. 5. Diagram of an ascarid-type cuticle in which the basal layer contains large fibres. Note the similarity of the outer cortical layer to the section of cuticlin shown in Fig. 6. Abbreviations: e, epidermis; f, fibre layers; ic, inner cortex; m, membrane-like layer; ml, median layer; oc, outer cortex.

cyst wall for the enclosed eggs when the female dies. The three
basic layers of the juveniles are supplemented by two extra, fibrous
layers in the gravid female. The fibres in the fifth layer are
arranged helicoidally, as in the chitin of insect endocuticle, but they
consist of collagen and not chitin (Shepherd, Clark & Dart, 1972).
Chitin fibres in insect endocuticle lie on a matrix of cross-linked
protein of low modulus and strength. This system has a large
strength to weight ratio, good tensile, flexural and compressive
strength, and is stronger than either of the two components alone.
When fibres of high tensile strength and elasticity are orientated in
a matrix of weak tensile strength and elasticity the strength of the
two-phase system is increased. Mammalian keratins also have a
two-phase structure. A helicoidal arrangement of the fibres gives
an isotropic structure, but once it is formed it can no longer expand
(Weis-Fogh, 1970). The fibres in the innermost layer of *H. rostochiensis* are like this, and such an isotropic layer apparently
favours a spherical structure in response to increased internal
pressure as the female swells (Shepherd *et al.*, 1972).

   Bradynema is an unusual nematode as the adult female has no
cuticle. She lives in the haemocoele of the mushroom fly and the
epidermis has a microvillous surface which forms the outer covering of the nematode. It has no functional alimentary tract and
nutrients are, presumably, taken up across the naked epidermis
(Riding, 1970).

   The cuticle of nematodes has superficial annulations (Figs 3
and 5) which apparently assist in flexure of the worm during
sinusoidal locomotion, but some species also possess longitudinal
or transverse ridges, spines, punctations and inflated areas. Most of
these modifications involve the cortical layer only. The longitudinal ridges of adult *Nippostrongylus* appear to assist coiling of this
nematode. The ridges also abrade the intestinal mucosa of the host
and, in this way, assist in the feeding process (Lee, 1965). Sense
organs at the head end of adult *Nippostrongylus* are so arranged
that distortion of any part of the inflated, cephalic region of the
cuticle will activate the sense organs. This means that the whole of
the head area is sensitive to touch and not just the sense organs
themselves (Wright, 1975).

Composition

Most work on the composition of nematode cuticle has been
carried out on the cuticle of adult *Ascaris lumbricoides*. This is
because most nematodes are less than a millimetre in length and

removal of the cuticle is technically very difficult. The basic component of the cuticle of nematodes is a form of collagen associated with hyaluronic acid, chondroitin sulphate, acid mucopolysaccharide and small amounts of lipid. Chitin is not present. The triple helix of collagen from *Ascaris* cuticle differs from that of vertebrate tropocollagen in that it is formed when subunit polypeptide chains (molar mass 60 000) fold back upon themselves to form a collagen-type triple helix. These subunits are held together by disulphide bonds (Fuchs & Harrington, 1970). Although this collagen exhibits a number of unusual properties, it meets the requirements for inclusion in the "collagen" group. It gives the characteristic wide-angle X-ray diffraction pattern of collagen (Fauré-Fremiét & Garrault, 1944), has high proportions of glycine and imino acids, contains hydroxyproline, and is relatively poor in aromatic acids (Watson & Silvester, 1959; Josse & Harrington, 1964; Fujimoto & Kanaya, 1973). It is also digested by collagenase (Josse & Harrington, 1964; Fujimoto & Adams, 1964). Cuticular collagen of *Ascaris* has a higher molar mass (900 000) than typical vertebrate collagens (300 000) (Josse & Harrington, 1964), and it contains amino acids which differ in their concentrations from vertebrate collagen, elastin, fibroin, resilin and keratin (Table I) (Fujimoto & Kanaya, 1973). Solubilized cuticle collagen is not a suitable substrate for hydroxyproline synthesis by means of a protocollagen proline hydroxylase from chick embryo, but synthesis occurs if the collagen

TABLE I

Comparison of cuticlin from the cuticle of Ascaris *with other structural proteins*

Amino acid	Cuticlin (*Ascaris*)	Collagen (*Ascaris* cuticle)	Elastin (bovine)	Fibroin (*Bombyx*)	Resilin (locust)	Keratin (wool)
		Residues/1000 total amino acids				
Glycine	150	274	330	445	376	85
Small[a]	317	346	441	739	487	146
Imino acids[b]	301	312	221	3	79	85
Basic[c]	36	82	88	9	45	104
Acidic[d]	146	136	117	23	152	173
Half-cystine	24	27	0	0	0	106
Hydroxyproline	0	16	98	0	0	0

[a] Glycine + alanine.   [b] Proline + hydroxyproline.   [c] Lysine + hydroxylysine + histidine + arginine.   [d] Aspartic acid + glutamic acid.

has been denatured by heat. This change in properties may be related to the unusual configuration of the polypeptide chain of the cuticle collagen (Fujimoto & Prokop, 1968). Collagen in the muscles of *Ascaris* contains more hydroxyproline and carbohydrate than collagen from the cuticle (Fujimoto, 1968). Protocollagen proline hydroxylase from *Ascaris* muscle is unusual in that it becomes 50% more active when the oxygen concentration is lowered from 21 to 1%, which suggests that the affinity of the enzyme for oxygen increases when the P_{O_2} decreases (Fujimoto & Prokop, 1969). Maximal hydroxylation of cuticular collagenous proline occurs in the presence of 70% oxygen (Chvapil & Ehrlich, 1970).

Another structural protein, called cuticlin, is present in the cuticle of *Ascaris* and is thought to form the major portion of the outer cortex (Fig. 6). It has high contents of proline and alanine and relatively low amounts of glycine and basic amino acids. It does not give the characteristic X-ray diffraction pattern of collagen nor is it susceptible to collagenase. It is distinct from collagen, fibroin, elastin, resilin and keratin (Table I) (Fujimoto & Kanaya, 1973).

Tanning of the cuticle of nematodes occurs only rarely. The cuticle of gravid female *Heterodera rostochiensis* undergoes polyphenol quinone tanning and this is brought about by the action

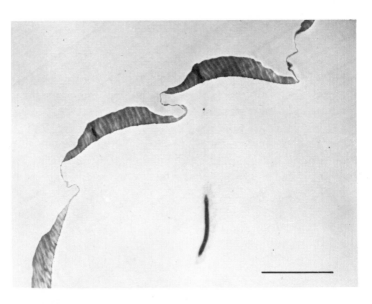

FIG. 6. Electron micrograph of sectioned cuticlin from the cuticle of *Ascaris*. Note the similarity in appearance to the outer cortical layer shown in Figs 3 and 5. The bar represents 5 μm. Reproduced with permission from Fujimoto & Kanaya (1973).

of polyphenol oxidase in the cuticle. This results in the formation of a tough, resistant cyst which encloses, and protects, the eggs after the death of the female (Ellenby, 1946; Ellenby & Smith, 1967).

Formation of the first cuticle

Very little work has been carried out on the ultrastructure of the developing egg, and so little is known about the formation of the first cuticle. The embryo of *Trichinella spiralis* develops in the uterus of the female and is covered by a thin sheet of mucus-like material and a thin, membranous eggshell. Internal to the mucus coat is a thin, dense layer, which was resolved into a three-layered membrane later in development, and a fine homogenous layer. These together make up the early cuticle of the first juvenile stage. The cuticle is attached to crests of the epidermal membrane by half-desmosomes. The epidermis is cellular at this stage of development. In the late-stage juvenile *in utero* the structure of the cuticle is much clearer and consists of an outer, three-layered membrane, an outer cortex and an inner fibril layer. It is thought that during formation of the first cuticle, material is secreted from the epidermis into the troughs between the epidermis and the cuticle, and is retained in position by the previously formed, three-layered membrane (Bruce, 1970).

Lee & Wilkins (in prep.) have studied the formation of the first cuticle in the developing egg of *Heterakis gallinarum*. The embryo, at the tadpole stage, has no cuticle but is coated with a fine filamentous coat, rather like a glycocalyx. Two membranes appear to surround the embryo; one is the epidermal membrane and the other lies external to it. The formation of this outer membrane is still something of an enigma. It could condense from the fine filamentous material which coats the tadpole or it could be an epidermal membrane which has been separated from the epidermis when a second membrane formed beneath it. A similar procedure takes place when the eggshell is being formed in *Ascaris* (Foor, 1967) and in *Heterakis* (Lee & Leštan, 1971). As development of the embryo proceeds, a finely filamentous material begins to appear between these two membranes and separates them. The two membranes move apart as more material passes from the epidermis into this region and gradually it develops into the cuticle of the first juvenile stage. This cuticle has little internal structure. Secretion of the cuticular material takes place over the whole surface of the epidermis and the cuticular material originates from the epidermis.

Moulting and ecdysis

Introduction

Most nematodes moult four times during their development, and
certain stages in the process of moulting and ecdysis are, apparently, controlled by neuroendocrine secretions as in arthropods
(Rogers, 1973).

Moulting seems to occur in four main steps. (1) The stimulus is
received and brings about the discharge of neurosecretory material which initiates step (2), which is separation of the old cuticle
from the epidermis; (3) the new cuticle forms between the epidermis and the old cuticle, with or without the dissolution and absorption of parts of the old cuticle; (4) rupture and ecdysis of the old
cuticle, or the remains, occurs allowing the nematode to escape.
The cuticle which covers the body of the nematode, together with
the cuticular linings of the amphids, phasmids, buccal cavity,
pharynx, excretory pore and the rectum, are shed. In stylet-
bearing nematodes the basal part of the stylet dissolves, the head
becomes disengaged from the anterior part of the old stylet and
this is shed with the old cuticle.

The stimulus

The stimulus which initiates moulting in most nematodes is
unknown. In free-living species it is possible that growth to a
certain size sets off the moulting process or it could be controlled by
a biological clock, such as the gradual loading followed by sudden
discharge of neurosecretory cells. Moulting is initiated in some
parasitic nematodes when the infective juvenile moves from a
free-living to a parasitic existence or when it moves from one
environment to another within the host (for example, migration
from the lungs to the intestine), but this explains the stimulus for
only one moult.

Formation of the new cuticle and ecdysis

The onset of moulting brings about an increase in width and an
increase in the number of ribosomes in the epidermis of
Meloidogyne javanica and of *Phocanema decipiens* (Bird & Rogers,
1965; Kan & Davey, 1968a,b). This does not occur until later in the
moult in *Nippostrongylus brasiliensis* (Lee, 1970b). In *Phocanema*
there is a cycle of RNA synthesis in the epidermis and this is closely
correlated with formation of the cuticle. The onset of moulting in
Hemicycliophora arenaria is preceded by the appearance of globular

"moulting bodies" of unknown function, in the epidermal cords. These moulting bodies disappear when moulting has finished (Johnson, Van Gundy & Thomson, 1970). Leucine aminopeptidase increases in concentration in the epidermis of *Xiphinema index* between moults, reaching a peak just before moulting commences. The concentration of the enzyme falls once moulting begins and, simultaneously, the cuticle becomes loosened from the epidermis. This suggests that the enzyme is involved in the separation of the old cuticle from the epidermal membrane (Roggen, Raski & Jones, 1967).

The epidermal membrane separates from the basal layers of the old cuticle at an early stage in the moult and thus, indirectly, loosens the attachment of the muscles to the cuticle. This explains why some nematodes become immobile prior to, and during, moulting.

The new cuticle is formed in a series of layers which gradually increase in thickness and in complexity. The outer surface of the new cuticle forms at the outer surface of the epidermis as a thin, membrane-like layer. This may be a condensation of new cuticular material, as suggested by Bonner & Weinstein (1972) and by Samoiloff & Pasternak (1969), or it may be the original epidermal membrane which has become underlain by a new epidermal membrane (Lee, 1970b). The cuticle is laid down between the epidermal membrane and the outer membrane.

In *Phocanema* the new cuticle arises as three successive waves of condensation at the outer edge of the epidermis, resulting in a three-layered structure. Ecdysis occurs when the second layer is complete, the third layer being laid down after ecdysis (Kan & Davey, 1968b). During moulting in *Meloidogyne javanica* the newly-formed outer cortex increases in thickness together with the new inner cortical layer and the basal layer (Fig. 7). This new cuticle becomes convoluted and allows for more rapid growth of the nematode after moulting. The inner layers of the old cuticle break down during moulting and are, apparently, resorbed by the nematode, leaving only the outer cortex which becomes broken and dislodged as the nematode increases in size (Bird & Rogers, 1965). Resorption of part of the old cuticle also occurs during the first moult of *Ascaris lumbricoides* (Thust, 1966) and during moulting of *Hemicycliophora arenaria* (Johnson *et al.*, 1970) but does not occur in other nematodes which have been studied, such as *Nippostrongylus brasiliensis* and *Panagrellus silusiae* (Lee, 1970b; Samoiloff & Pasternak, 1969).

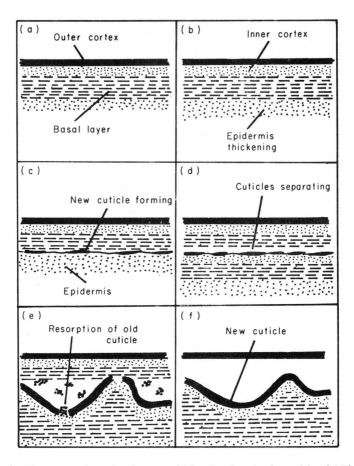

FIG. 7. Diagram to show the changes which take place in the cuticle of *Meloidogyne javanica* during moulting. (a) Normal cuticle; (b) thickening of epidermis; (c) start of formation of new external cortical layer at the surface of the epidermis; (d) new and old cuticle of similar dimensions and starting to separate; (e) inner layers of the old cuticle being resorbed and new cuticle becoming convoluted; (f) completion of moult with only the external cortical layer of the old cuticle remaining. Reproduced with permission from Bird (1971).

The fourth-stage juvenile and the adult of *Nippostrongylus brasiliensis* have a complex cuticle (Fig. 4). At the final moult (Fig. 8) the old cuticle separates from the epidermis, a membrane forms beneath the outer epidermal membrane and cuticular material is laid down between these two membranes. The new cuticle becomes folded into regular annuli, with two to three of these annuli for each single annulus of the old cuticle (Figs 8 and 9).

Extensions of the epidermis extend into these annuli initially and deposit an M-shaped structure which encircles the worm in each annulus. The epidermis then withdraws from the annuli. Material is deposited into the area between the M-shaped girdles and the new epidermal membrane and develops into the two fibre layers of the new cuticle. Once this has formed there is rapid enlargement and deposition of material between the M-shaped girdles and the outer membrane of the cuticle; this becomes oriented to form the cortical layer and, with the deposition of electron dense materials, into the skeletal struts of the cuticle. The M-shaped girdles, which seem to play a role in controlling the formation of the two parts of the cuticle, then flatten out and disappear. Condensation or compaction of the outer part of the cuticle, to form the cortex and the skeletal struts, leaves a fluid-filled space (the median layer) which gradually becomes red as haemoglobin forms within it (Fig. 8). The adult worm emerges from the more or less intact old cuticle when a cap of the old cuticle breaks away at the anterior end. The longitudinal ridges of the new cuticle are formed at an early stage when the epidermis pushes into the space between the epidermis and the old cuticle, deposits new cuticle and then retreats to its original position. There is a rapid increase in the amount of granular endoplasmic reticulum in the epidermis when cuticle formation is actively under way, and this becomes reduced after the moult (Fig. 8). Formation and secretion of the cuticular material is very similar to secretion of collagen precursors by mammalian fibroblasts. It would appear that during moulting in *Nippostrongylus*, amino acids enter the hypodermis from the body fluid, are used to make collagen precursors on the polyribosomes of the granular endoplasmic reticulum, and pass to the outer surface of the epidermis by direct, intermittent communications of the cisternae with the epidermal membrane, or in vesicles which move from the cisternae to fuse with the epidermal membrane, where they release their contents into the new cuticle. Once released into the cuticle the collagen precursors become orientated in the basal fibre layers of the cuticle or pass to the outer layers, where they form the cortex and the skeletal struts (Fig. 10). How these collagen precursors are controlled within the cuticle is not known (Lee, 1970b).

Moulting in several different species of nematode has been described in greater or lesser detail (see Bird, 1957; Lee, 1972; Lee & Atkinson, 1976.

The reasons for differences in the methods of moulting and ecdysis probably lie in the different environments of the different

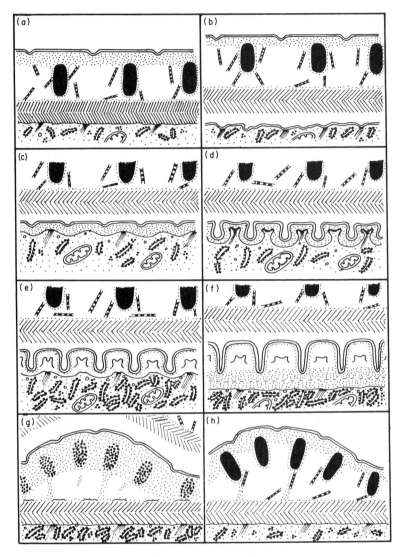

Fig. 8. Diagrams of longitudinal sections to show stages in the loosening of the cuticle of the fourth-stage juvenile and the formation of the adult cuticle in *Nippostrongylus brasiliensis*. (a, b) Loosening of the old cuticle from the hypodermis. (c) Early stage in the formation of the new cuticle. (d) The new cuticle is more extensively folded and thicker than in (c) and the epidermis extends into each fold. (e) The cuticle is thicker and separation into regions has begun. The epidermis retracts from the folds, leaving M-shaped structures in each fold. There is a rapid increase in the amount of granular endoplasmic reticulum in the hypodermis at this stage. (f) A later stage than (e) to show that the fibre layers are almost completely formed before there is any growth of the outer layers of the cuticle. (g) At this stage there is a rapid increase in the size of the outer layers of the cuticle. The M-shaped membrane stays

species. For example, the first-stage juveniles of *Ascaris* and of *Heterodera* moult within the egg, where space and nutrients are at a premium. It is, therefore, to the advantage of the second-stage juvenile to reduce the thickness of the cast cuticle as this will allow it

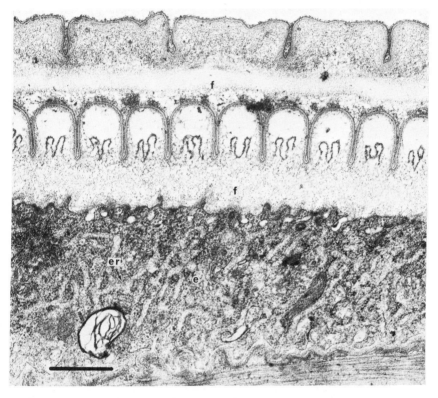

FIG. 9. Electron micrograph of a longitudinal section through the body wall of a moulting, fourth-stage juvenile of *Nippostrongylus brasiliensis* [diagram (f) in Fig. 8] to show the structure of the new cuticle, vesicles passing from the epidermis into the new cuticle, and the build-up of granular endoplasmic reticulum in the epidermis. Abbreviations: e, epidermis; er, granular endoplasmic reticulum; f, fibre layer of old (top) and new (bottom) cuticles. The bar represents 0·5 μm. Reproduced with permission from Lee (1970b).

close to the fibre layers and seems to be important in separating the fibre layers from the rest of the cuticle. The struts are shown at an early stage in their formation and the fluid-filled middle layer is appearing. (h) This diagram shows the adult cuticle shortly after ecdysis. The new cuticle rapidly elongates, causing the folds of the superficial annulations to flatten out. The struts are in the final stages of formation and collagen fibres link them to the cortex and to the basal fibre layer. There is a reduction in the amount of granular endoplasmic reticulum in the epidermis. Reproduced with permission from Lee (1970b).

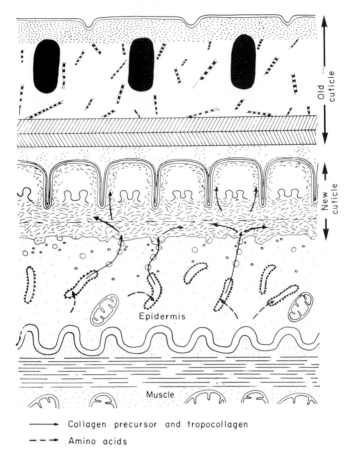

Collagen precursor and tropocollagen

Amino acids

FIG. 10. A diagram to explain how the new cuticle may be formed from amino acids (based on fibroblast production of collagen). Amino acids enter the granular endoplasmic reticulum and are made up into collagen precursors on the polyribosomes. The collagen precursor is then carried to the outer epidermal (hypodermal) membrane in small vesicles and released into the cuticle. In the cuticle the collagen precursors or tropocollagen is orientated in the various layers of the cuticle. Reproduced with permission from Lee (1970b).

more space within the egg and also allow greater freedom of movement within the thinned, first-stage cuticle. The egg is also a closed system, and the developing juvenile relies entirely upon its food reserves until it emerges from the egg. It is, therefore, to the advantage of the juvenile to recycle the proteins obtained from resorption of the old cuticle. Similarly, *Meloidogyne* moults after it has attached itself to the root of the host plant, and reduction in the thickness of the old cuticle will make ecdysis and growth easier for this now semi-sessile nematode. Some nematodes, however, live in more hazardous environments, such as the intestine of other animals, where they are liable to be carried out of the host in a stream of gut contents if they are unable to maintain their position against the mucosa. It is to the advantage of these nematodes to moult as quickly as possible and resorption of the old cuticle may be a hindrance in this respect. Nematodes which live a relatively free existence in the soil can wriggle free from their old cuticle much more easily than those nematodes which live in confined environments. It is, therefore, not surprising to find that some of these nematodes cast their old cuticle intact.

Ecdysis of ensheathed juveniles

The infective stage of many animal-parasitic juveniles is an ensheathed juvenile in which development has been arrested (for example, *Ancylostoma, Trichostrongylus, Haemonchus, Nippostrongylus*). Similarly, many free-living nematodes produce a resistant or dormant "dauer" juvenile when the environment becomes unsuitable for further growth and development. Moulting has occurred in these juveniles but ecdysis has been arrested, resulting in fully-formed juveniles, usually the third-stage juvenile, enclosed by the moulted—but not ecdysed—cuticle of the earlier stage. This sheath affords protection to the juvenile while it awaits entry to a host, or transport to a more suitable habitat if it is a free-living species.

Exsheathment, or ecdysis, seems to require a specific, external stimulus. This stimulus comes from fresh dung in the case of dauer juveniles of nematodes which live in dung (they are carried to it on the surface of insects), or from the alimentary tract of a specific host in the case of infective juveniles of trichostrongyles such as *Haemonchus* and *Trichostrongylus*.

High concentrations of dissolved, gaseous carbon dioxide and/or undissociated carbonic acid at 37°C are the main stimuli which initiate exsheathment of *Haemonchus* and *Trichostrongylus*. The pH and redox potential of the environment are also important in accelerating exsheathment. Digestive enzymes are not responsible for exsheathment of these species (Rogers & Sommerville, 1969), but digestive enzymes assist exsheathment of some other species. Bile and bile salts potentiate exsheathment (Mapes, 1972).

The processes involved in exsheathment are probably not the same as those which initiate moulting. Moulting has already taken place and exsheathment only brings about the release of the juvenile from the cuticle of the previous juvenile stage, that is, ecdysis. These juveniles have apparently lost the ability to initiate ecdysis at the second moult and the stimulus must be supplied by an environment which will be suitable for further growth and development. After these ensheathed juveniles have received the necessary stimulus they secrete an exsheathing fluid, a major constituent of which is leucine aminopeptidase in some species, from the excretory system into the gap between the old and new cuticles. This exsheathing fluid attacks a weak ring in the old cuticle near its anterior end, the inner layer of the sheath dissolves and the outer layer is ruptured by the movements of the activated juvenile. A cap of cuticle becomes detached and the juvenile escapes from the confines of the old cuticle.

Growth

It is not known why nematodes moult, because many nematodes have been shown to increase in size between moults and after the final moult. It has also been shown that the cuticle can increase in thickness after the final moult (Watson, 1965b). The explanation that nematodes moult because they have an inert exoskeleton which must be shed to allow growth to occur appears to be untenable. Crofton (1971) suggested that moulting may not be necessary for gradual changes in size of the nematode to occur, but may be necessary to increase the strength of the cuticle. The tangential forces acting on the walls of a cylinder in which there is an internal pressure (as in nematodes) are proportional to the cross-sectional area of the cylinder. It may be that the growing nematode reaches a stage when it continues to grow but can no longer increase the thickness of the cuticle without decreasing its diameter. Moulting, allowing a rapid change to a larger size followed by gradual thickening of the cuticle as growth continues, may be the answer to this problem (Crofton, 1971). This still does not explain growth of adult *Ascaris*, where the young adult worm can grow to a length of 20–30 cm and also increase the thickness of its cuticle (Watson, 1965b).

Functions of the cuticle

I do not wish to spend much time on this as it is outside the remit of this particular paper. Several excellent reviews have been written on the role of the cuticle in locomotion (Crofton, 1971; Lee & Atkinson, 1976; Clark, 1964; Bird, 1971). In the turgor pressure system of locomotion the muscles are opposed by the hydrostatic pressure of the pseudocoelomic fluid, together with the other contents of the body, and by the elasticity of the cuticle. When the muscles relax these pressures return the muscles to their normal resting length. The success of this system depends on the spiral lattice work of fibres in the basal layer of the cuticle of those nematodes which operate this system, and which allow elongation but not increase in diameter of the worm (Harris & Crofton, 1957; Clark, 1964). Many nematodes do not have a fibre layer in their cuticle and seem to operate a different system. In these nematodes, increase in diameter as the muscles contract and the hydrostatic pressure rises is resisted by the tough, striated basal layer of the cuticle—thus pressure continues to rise in the body cavity and is the returning force which returns the muscles to their resting length when they relax.

Little work has been done on the movement of ions, water and nutrients across the cuticle. Most evidence indicates that the cuticle is unimportant in the uptake of nutrients, except in certain specialized cases such as the mermithids and other insect-parasitic nematodes which live in the body cavity of insects and lack a functional alimentary tract. Water and certain ions move readily across the cuticle of nematodes and presumably play an important role in maintaining the volume of those nematodes which live in euryhaline conditions. Some nematodes can adjust to rapid changes in osmolarity whereas others cannot, and this seems to be partly under the control of the body wall of these nematodes. The marine nematode *Enoplus* has a relatively high overall permeability to water of $4 \cdot 4 \ \mu m^3 H_2O/\mu m^2$ body surface/sec, whereas the soil-inhabiting nematode *Aphelenchus avenae* has a much lower water permeability of $0 \cdot 0005 \ \mu m^3 H_2O/\mu m^2$ body surface/sec. This reduced permeability of the soil-inhabiting species lessens the intensity of the osmoregulatory processes which need to be carried out if the worm is to maintain a normal level of hydration in media of differing osmolarity, as occurs in soil water. This requirement is not necessary for the marine species as it lives in a constant environment and is isomotic with sea-water (D. J. Wright & Newell, 1976).

The cuticle is also important in the protection of the nematode against mechanical and microbial damage.

REFERENCES

Bird, A. F. (1957). Chemical composition of the nematode cuticle. Observations on individual layers and extracts from these layers in *Ascaris lumbricoides* cuticle. *Expl Parasit.* **6**: 383–403.

Bird, A. F. (1971). *The structure of nematodes.* New York and London: Academic Press.

Bird, A. F. & Rogers, G. E. (1965). Ultrastructure of the cuticle and its formation in *Meloidogyne javanica. Nematologica* **22**: 224–230.

Bonner, T. P. & Weinstein, P. P. (1972). Ultrastructure of the hypodermis during cuticle formation in the third molt of the nematode *Nippostrongylus brasiliensis. Z. Zellforsch. mikrosk. Anat.* **126**: 17–24.

Bruce, R. G. (1970). *Trichinella spiralis:* fine structure of body wall with special reference to formation and moulting of cuticle. *Expl Parasit.* **28**: 499–511.

Chvapil, M. & Ehrlich, E. (1970). Effect of increased oxygen on hydroxyproline synthesis in the cuticle and body wall of *Ascaris lumbricoides. Biochem. Biophys. Acta* **208**: 467–474.

Clark, R. B. (1964). *Dynamics of metazoan evolution.* Oxford: Clarendon Press.

Crofton, H. D. (1966). *Nematodes.* London: Hutchinson & Co. Ltd.

Crofton, H. D. (1971). Form, function and behaviour. In *Plant parasitic nematodes.* **1**: 83–113. Zuckerman, B. M., Mai, W. F. & Rhode, R. A. (eds). New York and London: Academic Press.

Ellenby, C. (1946). Nature of the cyst wall of the potato-root eelworm *Heterodera rostochiensis,* Wollenweber, and its permeability to water. *Nature, Lond.* **157**: 302–303.

Ellenby, C. (1969). Dormancy and survival in nematodes. *Symp. Soc. exp. Biol.* **23**: 83–97.

Ellenby, C. & Smith L. (1967). Influence of temperature on polyphenol oxidase activity in three species of *Heterodera. Comp. Biochem. Physiol.* **21**: 51–57.

Fauré-Fremiét, E. & Garrault, H. (1944). Propriétés physiques de l'ascarocollagène. *Bull. Biol. Fr. Belg.* **78**: 206–214.

Foor, E. W. (1967). Ultrastructural aspects of oocyte development and shell formation in *Ascaris lumbricoides. J. Parasit.* **53**: 1245–1261.

Fuchs, S. & Harrington, W. F. (1970). Immunological properties of *Ascaris* cuticle collagen. *Biochim. Biophys. Acta* **221**: 119–124.

Fujimoto, D. (1968). Isolation of collagens of high hydroxyproline, hydroxylysine and carbohydrate content from the muscle layer of *Ascaris lumbricoides* and pig kidney. *Biochem. biophys. Acta* **168**: 537–543.

Fujimoto, D. & Adams, E. (1964). Intraspecies composition differences in collagen from cuticle and body of *Ascaris* and *Lumbricus. Biochem. Biophys. Res. Commun.* **17**: 437–442.

Fujimoto, D. & Kanaya, S. (1973). Cuticlin: a noncollagen structural protein from *Ascaris* cuticle. *Arch. Biochem. Biophys.* **157**: 1–6.

Fujimoto, D. & Prokop, D. J. (1968). Denatured collagen from the cuticle of *Ascaris lumbricoides* as a substrate for protocollagen prolinehydroxylase. *J. Biol. Chem.* **243**: 4138–4142.

Fujimoto, D. & Prokop, D. J. (1969). Protocollagen proline hydroxylase from *Ascaris lumbricoides. J. biol. Chem.* **244**: 205–210.

Harris, J. E. & Crofton, H. D. (1957). Structure and function in the nematodes: internal pressure and cuticular structure in *Ascaris. J. exp. Biol.* **34**: 116–130.

Johnson, P. W., Van Gundy, S. D. & Thomson, W. W. (1970). Cuticle formation in *Hemicycliophora arenaria, Aphelenchus avenae* and *Hirschmaniella gracilis. J. Nematol.* **2**: 59–79.

Josse, J. & Harrington, W. F. (1964). Role of pyrrolidine residues in the structure and stabilization of collagen. *J. Molec. Biol.* **9**: 269–287.

Kan, S. P. & Davey, K. G. (1968a). Molting in a parasitic nematode, *Phocanema decipiens*. II. Histochemical study of the larval and adult cuticle. *Can. J. Zool.* **46**: 235–241.

Kan, S. P. & Davey, K. G. (1968b). Molting in a parasitic nematode, *Phocanema decipiens*. III. The histochemistry of deposition and protein synthesis. *Can. J. Zool.* **46**: 723–727.

Lee, D. L. (1965). The cuticle of adult *Nippostrongylus brasiliensis*. *Parasitology* **55**: 173–181.

Lee, D. L. (1966a). An electron microscope study of the body wall of the third-stage larva of *Nippostrongylus brasiliensis*. *Parasitology* **56**: 127–135.

Lee, D. L. (1966b). The structure and composition of the helminth cuticle. *Adv. Parasit.* **4**: 187–254.

Lee, D. L. (1970a). The ultrastructure of the cuticle of adult female *Mermis nigrescens* (Nematoda). *J. Zool., Lond.* **161**: 513–518.

Lee, D. L. (1970b). Moulting in nematodes: the formation of the adult cuticle during the final moult of *Nippostrongylus brasiliensis*. *Tissue & Cell* **2**: 139–153.

Lee, D. L. (1972). The structure of the helminth cuticle. *Adv. Parasit.* **10**: 347–379.

Lee, D. L. (1975). Structure and function of the intestinal–cloacal junction of the nematode *Heterakis gallinarum*. *Parasitology* **70**: 389–396.

Lee, D. L. & Atkinson, H. A. (1976). *Physiology of nematodes*. 2nd Edn. London: Macmillan.

Lee, D. L. & Leštan, P. (1971). Oogenesis and egg shell formation in *Heterakis gallinarum* (Nematoda). *J. Zool., Lond.* **164**: 189–196.

Lee, D. L. & Smith, M. H. (1965). Hemoglobins of parasitic animals. *Expl Parasit.* **16**: 392–424.

Lee, D. L. & Wilkins, D. (in prep). *Formation of the first cuticle in* Heterakis gallinarum.

Lippens, P. L. (1974a). Ultrastructure of a marine nematode, *Chromadorina germanica* (Buetschli, 1874). I. Anatomy and cytology of the caudal gland apparatus. *Z. Morph. Tiere* **78**: 181–192.

Lippens, P. L. (1974b). Ultrastructure of a marine nematode, *Chromadorina germanica* (Buetschli, 1874). II. Cytology of lateral epidermal glands and associated neurocytes. *Z. Morph. Tiere* **79**: 283–294.

Mapes, C. J. (1972). Bile and bile salts and exsheathment of the intestinal nematodes *Trichostrongylus colubriformis* and *Nematodirus battus*. *Int. J. Parasit.* **2**: 433–438.

Riding, I. L. (1970). Microvilli on the outside of a nematode. *Nature, Lond.* **226**: 179–180.

Rogers, W. P. (1973). Juvenile and moulting hormones from nematodes. *Parasitology* **67**: 105–113.

Rogers, W. P. & Sommerville, R. I. (1969). Chemical aspects of growth and development. In *Chemical zoology* **3**: 465–499. Florkin, M. & Scheer, B. T. (eds). New York and London: Academic Press.

Roggen, D. R., Raski, D. J. & Jones, N. O. (1967). Further electron microscopic observations of *Xiphinema index*. *Nematologica* **13**: 1–16.

Samoiloff, M. R. & Pasternak, J. (1969). Nematode morphogenesis: fine structure of the moulting cycles in *Panagrellus silusiae* (de Man 1913) Goodey 1945. *Can. J. Zool.* **47**: 639–643.

Shepherd, A. M., Clark, S. A. & Dart, P. J. (1972). Cuticle structure in the genus *Heterodera*. *Nematologica* **18**: 1–17.

170   D. L. LEE

Thust, R. (1966). Elektronen mikroskopische Untersuchungen über den Bau des larvalen Integumentes und zur Hautungsmorphologie von *Ascaris lumbricoides*. *Zool. Anz.* **177**: 411–417.

Thust, R. (1968). Submikroskopische Untersuchungen über die Morphogenese des Integumentes von *Ascaris lumbricoides* L. 1758. *Z. wiss. Zool.* **178**: 1–39.

Trim, A. R. (1949). The kinetics of the penetration of some representative anthelmintics and related compounds in *Ascaris lumbricoides* var. *suis*. *Parasitology* **39**: 281–290.

Watson, B. D. (1965a). The fine structure of the body-wall in a free-living nematode, *Euchromadora vulgaris*. *Q. Jl microsc. Sci.* **106**: 75–81.

Watson, B. D. (1965b). The fine structure of the body wall and the growth of the cuticle in the adult nematode *Ascaris lumbricoides*. *Q. Jl microsc. Sci.* **106**: 83–91.

Watson, M. R. & Silvester, N. R. (1959). Studies of invertebrate collagen preparations. *Biochem. J.* **72**: 578–584.

Weis-Fogh, T. (1970). Structure and formation of insect cuticle. *Symp. R. entom. Soc. Lond.* No. 5: 165–185.

Wisse, E. & Daems, W. T. (1968). Electron microscopic observations on second-stage larvae of the potato root eelworm *Heterodera rostochiensis*. *J. Ultrastr. Res.* **24**: 201–231.

Wright, D. J. & Newell, D. R. (1976). Nitrogen excretion, osmotic and ionic regulation in nematodes. In *The organization of nematodes*. Croll, N. A. (ed.). New York and London: Academic Press.

Wright, K. A. (1968a). The fine structure of the cuticle and interchordal hypodermis of the parasitic nematodes, *Capillaria hepatica* and *Trichuris myocastoris*. *Can. J. Zool.* **46**: 173–180.

Wright, K. A. (1968b). Structure of the bacillary band of *Trichuris myocastoris*. *J. Parasit.* **54**: 1106–1110.

Wright, K. A. (1975). Cephalic sense organs of the rat hookworm, *Nippostrongylus brasiliensis*—form and function. *Can. J. Zool.* **53**: 1131–1146.

Wright, K. A. & Chan, J. (1973). Sense receptors in the bacillary band of trichuroid nematodes. *Tissue & Cell* **5**: 373–380.

Wright, K. A. & Hope, W. D. (1968). Elaborations of the cuticle of *Acanthonchus duplicatus* Wieser, 1959 (Nematoda: Cyatholaimidae) as revealed by light and electron-microscopy. *Can. J. Zool.* **46**: 1005–1011.

Symp. zool. Soc. Lond. (1977) No. 39, 171–193.

STRUCTURE AND FUNCTION IN THE OLIGOCHAETE EPIDERMIS (ANNELIDA)

K. SYLVIA RICHARDS

Department of Biology, University of Keele,
Keele, Staffordshire, England

SYNOPSIS

The structure of the lumbricid earthworm cuticle and the three epidermal secretory cell types is briefly reviewed and compared with the epidermis of enchytraeid oligochaetes from terrestrial, freshwater and littoral habitats. The terrestrial species do not possess secretory cells comparable to those of lumbricids.

Detail is centred on the genus *Lumbricillus* in which five species are examined and three secretory cell types identified. Only one type, the small granular cell, equates with a lumbricid type. Of the other two lumbricillid types, the neutral glycoprotein cell is abundant in the large, littoral *L. reynoldsoni* and the uronic acid-containing mucous cell is prominent in the small, littoral *L. georgiensis*, *L. mirabilis* and *L. vancouverensis*. The freshwater *L. rivalis*, of medium size, has the two types almost equally distributed in the epidermis. This acid mucous cell was not recorded in littoral or terrestrial species of other enchytraeid genera and its possible function in *Lumbricillus* is discussed.

Ultrastructurally the secretion of the uronic acid cells is characterized by fingerprint or honeycomb-like patterning established at the mature face of the basally situated Golgi apparatus. An occlusor mechanism in the form of a double sphincter, the inner ring within the gland cell apex and the outer ring within the adjacent supporting cells, exists in *L. georgiensis*, *L. mirabilis* and *L. vancouverensis*. In *L. rivalis* only the inner sphincter occurs and in *L. reynoldsoni* no sphincter mechanism is discernible. All the species possess apical mucous pore microvilli.

The possible interrelationships between the size and habitat of the species, the frequency of this cell type, the nature of the secretion and the degree of occlusor control are discussed.

INTRODUCTION

Oligochaete annelids occur in terrestrial, freshwater and littoral situations. The lumbricid earthworms are terrestrial whereas most of the small, microdrile oligochaetes occupy freshwater habitats. Such ecological diversity has invited studies on the epidermis of a range of oligochaetes and this paper briefly reviews the work on earthworms and presents details of the epidermis of some oligochaetes belonging to the family Enchytraeidae, selected from a variety of habitats including littoral sites.

The lumbricid epidermis consists of an epithelium containing secretory and non-secretory cells overlain by a collagenous cuticle. The products of the secretory cells can provide the lubrication for locomotion and keep the surface moist for respiration. The cuticle contains collagen fibres arranged in layers set at

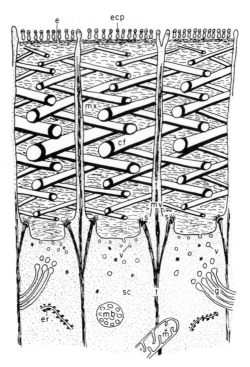

Fig. 1. Diagrammatic representation of oligochaete cuticle structure, showing cross-lamella arrangement of collagen fibres, and ascending microvilli giving rise to the epicuticular projections. Abbreviations: cf, collagen fibre; e, epicuticle; ecp, epicuticular projections; er, endoplasmic reticulum; g, Golgi; m, mitochondrion; mb, multivesicular body; mv, microvillus; mx, cuticle matrix; s, shoulder with attachment microfilaments; sc, supporting cell ; t, tonofilaments; v, vesicles.

right angles to one another and at approximately 45° to the body axis. These lie in a fine fibrillar matrix which extends beyond the fibre zone to form the epicuticle as schematized in Fig. 1. The fibres lack the typical collagen banding because of carbohydrate masking, and Djaczenko & Cimmino (1973) have demonstrated a peripheral periodicity attributable to this carbohydrate component of the fibres. Microvilli, arising from the epithelial surface, have oval bases with paired half-desmosome-like shoulders. The central, ascending portions penetrate the interfibre spaces and terminate at the free edge of the epicuticle where they give rise to the epicuticular projections (Richards, 1974a).

Histochemically the cuticle displays both protein and neutral mucopolysaccharide moieties. The acid mucopolysaccharide hyaluronic acid is also present (Richards, 1975a) and has been recorded in the cuticle of the subtropical megascolecid earthworm *Megascolex mauritii* (Sundara Rajulu & Krishnan, 1967). Its presence might provide a sufficiently viscous matrix for the functioning of the collagen fibres.

Three types of secretory cell occur in the unmodified epidermis of lumbricids. The large granular (orthochromatic) cells secrete a mucopolysaccharide–protein–lipid complex, such a viscous mucus probably serving as a lubricant during locomotion (Richards, 1973). Ultrastructural studies on this cell type reveal electron dense patterns with generic and specific characteristics in the granules in cross-fertilizing species, but not in those forms belonging to parthenogenetic genera (Richards, 1974b). The electron dense configurations are protein sites within the granules and may represent the location of a mating pheromone. The reticulate (metachromatic) cells secrete a predominantly carboxylated acid mucus (Richards, 1974c) considered to be of low viscosity and to provide the permanently present respiratory film trapped by the epicuticular projections. No species differences are apparent at the ultrastructural level, though as a cell ages it produces globules of increased size and different density (Richards, 1975b). The product of the third cell type, the small granular cells, is rich in protein (Richards, 1974d) and might well affect the viscosity of the other secretions, possibly increasing the water retention properties of the acid mucous film. The fine structure of these cells shows no species variation (Richards, 1975c).

The lumbricids studied included species ranging from pasture forms to manure and compost heap worms, yet, apart from the patterning in the orthochromatic cells which was unrelated to ecophysiological factors, the epidermis showed uniformity. However, Rigby & Robinson (1975) have demonstrated that the thermal transition point of the cuticular collagen of the garden and pasture soil-living *Allolobophora caliginosa* and the compost heap-dwelling *Eisenia foetida* is not identical, and that the difference correlates well with their preferred temperature range.

The histochemistry of the epidermal secretions of megascolecid earthworms differs from that of the lumbricids in demonstrating two types of acid mucous cell containing hyaluronic acid (Krishnan & Sundara Rajulu, 1969; Varute & Nalavade, 1970). Since this megadrile family is also terrestrial, it suggests that the epidermal secretions in the oligochaetes may not be prescribed by ecological factors alone.

Enchytraeid oligochaetes differ from the megadrile lumbricids and from other microdrile families in that there are freshwater, terrestrial and littoral species, though no single genus has species occupying all three habitats. Surface problems may be assumed to be of some significance in this family. It seemed appropriate to undertake histochemical and ultrastructural investigations on a range of enchytraeids, and nine species involving four genera were chosen to provide ecological and size comparisons. More detailed studies were made on the genus *Lumbricillus* and are given here. The other genera will be referred to where differences were recorded.

MATERIALS AND METHODS

Enchytraeids were collected from terrestrial sites at the University of Keele, Staffordshire, littoral and sewage filter bed sites in Anglesey, and from Miracle Beach, BC Canada. The species, listed according to ecology and size, were: the terrestrial, small *Fridericia bulbosa, Mesenchytraeus sp.*; the freshwater (sewage), medium sized *Lumbricillus rivalis*; the littoral, large *L. reynoldsoni, Enchytraeus albidus*; the littoral, small *L. georgiensis, L. mirabilis, L. vancouverensis*; the coastal (terrestrial), small *Fridericia callosa*.

Material for the histochemical programme was fixed in Bouin, Zenker or Susa followed by routine processing. The methods undertaken included: periodic acid Schiff (PAS); toluidine blue (TB); azure A (Az.A)–pH extinction 4-5-1·0; alcian blue 8GX (AB) pH 2·5, 1·0; AB–PAS; aldehyde fuchsin (Ald.F); Ald.F–AB; mercuric bromphenol blue (HgBPB); Weigert's commercial resorcin fuchsin (WRF); Sudan black (SB). Chemical blocking/conversion: methylation; saponification; acetylation; deamination; acid hydrolysis–0·1 M HCl at 65°C for 2h, 0·05 M H_2SO_4 at 74°C for 1·25h. Enzymes: diastase, hyaluronidase (ex-ovine testes, Koch Light); β-glucuronidase (BDH).

For electron microscopy, tissue pieces were fixed in 5% glutaraldehyde in 0·1 M phosphate at either pH 6·3 or 7·1, with 1% osmium tetroxide post-fixation in the appropriate buffer. In-block staining with 2% uranyl acetate was performed during acetone dehydration, followed by embedment in Spurr's resin.

RESULTS

Cuticle

The histochemical results for enchytraeid cuticles were broadly similar to those for lumbricids, both protein and mucopolysaccharide moieties being demonstrated, with the neutral mucopolysaccharides predominating in combined techniques. The acid mucopolysaccharide component could not, however, be attributed to hyaluronic acid, since hyaluronidase failed, even after prolonged timings, to abolish TB metachromasia or alcianophilia. Hyaluronic acid, present in the large lumbricids, megascolecids, and nereid polychaetes (Manavalaramanujam & Sundara Rajulu, 1974), would appear to be absent from the cuticle of the considerably smaller enchytraeids.

At the ultrastructural level, the cuticle organization resembles that of lumbricids (Fig. 1) but whereas the number of fibre layers and the depth of the cuticle were proportional to the size of the worm in lumbricids, this is not so in enchytraeids. In the small, terrestrial species thick cuticles, approaching the depth of some lumbricids many times larger in size, are present, the depth being achieved either by an increased number of relatively small diameter fibres (*Mesenchytraeus*) or by fewer layers of thicker fibres as in *Fridericia*. This may account for the stiff movements of *Fridericia* when compared with the littoral lumbricillids of similar size where the cuticle has a large number of small diameter fibres. The microvilli, with their paired shoulders, give rise distally to epicuticular projections in exactly the same way as in lumbricids.

Secretory cells

In the small species of *Lumbricillus* the secretory cells are arranged in transverse rows within each segment (Fig. 2a). This is because of the subdivision of the segmental circular muscle into units and the occurrence of gland cells only in the regions between the units (Fig. 2b). The shallow epidermis overlying the muscle units contains only supporting cells. In the larger species the depth of the epidermis is greater and gland cells are not so restricted in their distribution (Fig. 3).

In the terrestrial *Fridericia* and *Mesenchytraeus* gland cells are infrequent, contrasting sharply with the terrestrial lumbricid earthworms where secretory cells are abundant. Mucous cells are also sparse in *Enchytraeus*, but are prominent in *Lumbricillus* where, at the light microscope level, two types can be recognized histologically and histochemically (Fig. 2a). The one type has distinct granules which give acid mucus reactions and this differs from the earthworm situation where the acid mucous cells are never granular. This type was not observed in the other enchytraeid genera, being exclusive to *Lumbricillus* within this survey. In the second type the secretion is poorly retained in light microscope material,

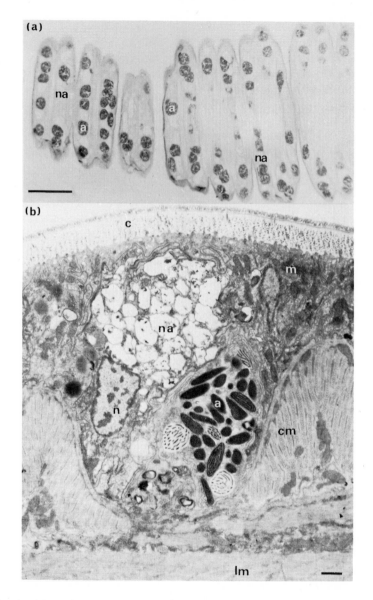

FIG. 2. (a) Superficial L.S. of *Lumbricillus mirabilis* showing transverse rows of secretory cells (Ald.F–AB, green filter). Bar represents 50 μm. Abbreviations: a, granular acid mucous cells; na, non-acid mucous cells.
(b) Epidermis of *L. mirabilis* (L.S.) showing the two secretory cell types positioned between the circular muscle subunits. Bar represents 1 μm. Abbreviations: a, acid mucous cell; c, cuticle; cm, circular muscle; lm, longitudinal muscle; m, mitochondrion; na, non-acid mucous cell; n, nucleus.

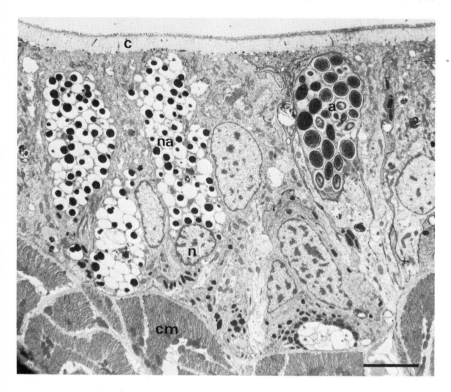

FIG. 3. Epidermis of *L. reynoldsoni* (L.S.). The secretory cells are not restricted in their position. Bar represents 5 μm. Abbreviations: a, acid mucous cell; c, cuticle; cm, circular muscle; na, non-acid mucous cell; n, nucleus.

often appearing reticulate in all but *L. reynoldsoni*. In material fixed for electron microscopy the secretion is in membrane-bound globules (Fig. 2b) which do not lose their integrity as they presumably have done with light microscope fixatives. The secretion of this second type gave negative reactions for acid mucus, again contrasting with the lumbricid condition where the non-acid secretion was always in the form of distinct granules.

The two types of secretory cell differ in their distribution in the lumbricillid species. In the small, littoral *L. georgiensis*, *L. mirabilis* and *L. vancouverensis* the granular cells outnumber the globular ones in all sections examined. In the medium sized *L. rivalis* secretory cells are less common but the two types occur in almost equal numbers, and in the large, littoral *L. reynoldsoni* the granular, acid mucous cells are infrequent, the main type is the globular type showing pronounced condensation of the secretory material within each globule (Fig. 3). A third type was observed only in the ultrastructural study of *Lumbricillus*.

Histochemistry

Granular, acid mucous cells. The significant histochemical results for the granular cells are presented in Table I and detailed arguments for the conclusions can be found in the lumbricid histochemical papers (Richards, 1973, 1974c,d, 1975a). The secretion is primarily a carboxylated acid mucus with identifiable uronic groups susceptible to exposure to testicular hyaluronidase and β-glucuronidase as used by Fullmer (1960). The combined results of these two enzymes suggest that the reactant group in the acid mucus moiety is a glucuronic one and that the staining reactions are due to the presence of hyaluronic acid, the reactant group of

TABLE I

Lumbricillus mirabilis *acid mucous cells: principal histochemical results*

Technique		Result	Conclusion
PAS		$+/++^a$	Periodate reactive material
TB		Metachromatic $++$	Acid mucosubstance present
AB pH 2·5		$++$	⎧Acid mucosubstance present
Methylation–saponification–TB		Metachromatic $++$	⎨Reactive gps re-established, carboxymucin present
Az.A pH extinction		−below pH 3·0	Carboxymucin
Ald.F–AB		AB$++$	Carboxymucin
Hyaluronidase	4h–TB	Metachromatic $++$	⎧Prolonged treatments lessen
	24h–TB	Very pale	⎫and finally abolish meta-
	48h–TB	Extremely pale	⎬chromasia. Uronic-type
	72h–TB	—	⎭groups present
Hyaluronidase	4h–AB	$++$	⎧Alcianophilia decreases
	24h–AB	Pale	⎨with exposure to enzyme
	48h–AB	Extremely pale	⎩Uronic-types gps present
β-Glucuronidase	24h–TB	Metachromatic $+/++$	⎧Metachromasia and alciano-philia negated after 48h enzyme treatment. Glucuronic acid present
	48h–TB	—	
	24h–AB	Pale	
	48h–AB	—	
Acid hydrolysis:			
0·1 M HCl	2h–AB	$++$	
			Sialic acid not present
0·1 M H₂SO₄	1·25h–AB	$++$	

General conclusion:
Carboxylated acid mucus with identifiable uronic groups present.

^{a}+,+/++,++ = degree of staining; ++ = intense colouration.

which is, in fact, the glucuronic acid unit of the repeated disaccharide sequence (Hunt, 1970). The acid mucus therefore differs from that of the lumbricid metachromatic cells (Richards, 1974c) which, although carboxylated, contained neither sialic nor uronic acid groups.

A separate neutral mucopolysaccharide moiety with demonstrable *vic* glycols is presumed to be present, since uronic acid-containing mucosubstances are rarely PAS positive. Low levels of protein appear to be present but bound lipid is absent.

Globular, non-acid mucous cells. All reactions for acid mucus were negative, but positive results for protein and neutral mucopolysaccharides were recorded. The secretion can therefore be classified as a neutral glycoprotein. The limited histochemical techniques applied did not reveal species differences but that is not to say that the secretion is absolutely identical within the lumbricillid genus, or with the secretion from the cells of the other enchytraeid genera studied where similar results were recorded.

Ultrastructure

Granular, acid mucous cells. These cells, only observed in the genus *Lumbricillus*, contain spherical or oval, membrane-bound, secretory inclusions. In all five lumbricillid species the granules are characterized by a distinctive patterning of electron dense strands, 40–50 nm wide, so arranged that fingerprint or honeycomb-like configurations result (Fig. 4). The matrix material between the strands is finely fibrous and in continuity with the peripheral material of each granule. The basally situated endoplasmic reticulum lies in close association with the Golgi apparatus (Fig. 5) from the mature face of which arise the vesicles which coalesce to form the granules. The first manifestation of the electron dense materials appears at the level of the mature Golgi face.

A distinct occlusor mechanism, in addition to the apical ring of pore microvilli (Fig. 6) present in all oligochaete and polychaete epidermal mucous cells, occurs in the granular cells of four of the species of *Lumbricillus*. It is absent in *L. reynoldsoni* and developed to varying degrees within the other species.

In *L. georgiensis*, *L. mirabilis* and *L. vancouverensis* there is a double sphincter of tonofilaments. The inner sphincter ring, consisting of about 50 distinct filaments each 5 nm in diameter, lies within the apical cytoplasmic lining of the mucous cell, just below the pore microvilli and 95 nm below the cell–cuticle interface. The

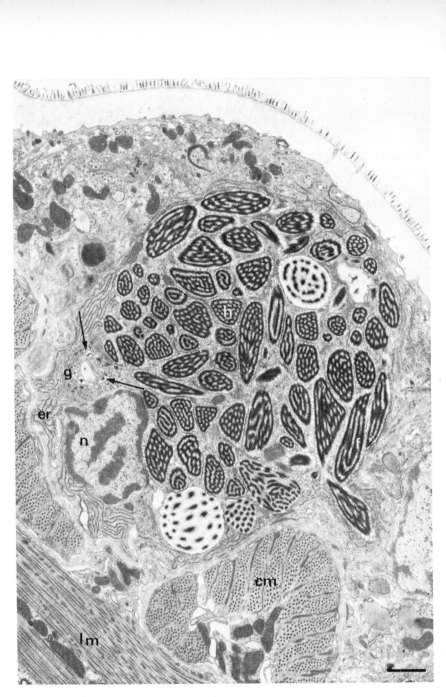

FIG. 4. Acid mucous cell of *L. vancouverensis* showing fingerprint and honeycomb-like secretory granules cut in various planes. The granules show varying degrees of condensation of the secretory material. The electron dense areas are established within the secretory apparatus (arrowed). Bar represents 1 μm. Abbreviations: cm, circular muscle; er, endoplasmic reticulum; f, fingerprint pattern; g, Golgi; h, honeycomb-like pattern; lm, longitudinal muscle; n, nucleus.

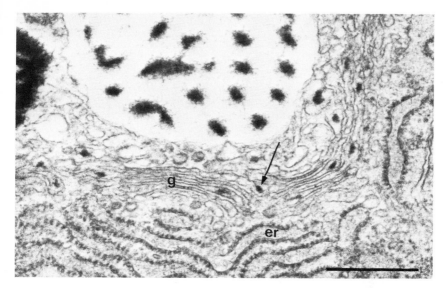

FIG. 5. Base of an acid mucous cell of *L. georgiensis* showing establishment of electron dense areas (arrowed) towards and at the mature face of the Golgi (g). Bar represents 0·5 μm. er, Endoplasmic reticulum.

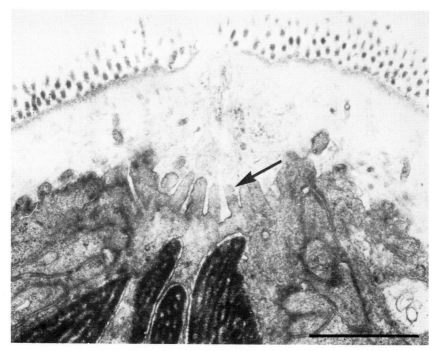

FIG. 6. Apex of an acid mucous cell of *L. georgiensis* (off-centre) showing the ring of mucous pore microvilli (arrowed). Bar represents 1 μm.

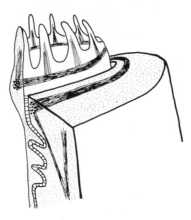

FIG. 7. Diagram of the acid mucous cell occlusor mechanism in *L. mirabilis*. The inner sphincter, within the mucous cell, connects with the tonofilaments of the mucous pore microvilli. The outer sphincter lies within the adjacent supporting cells, the apical region of which is shown as though cut away.

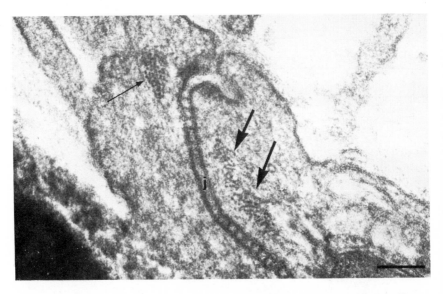

FIG. 8. One side of the occlusor area at the apex of an acid mucous cell and adjacent supporting cell of *L. mirabilis* showing the inner sphincter tonofilaments (thin arrow) and the outer sphincter tonofilaments (thick arrow). Detail of the intercellular junction is also visible. Bar represents 0·1 μm. j, Intercellular junction.

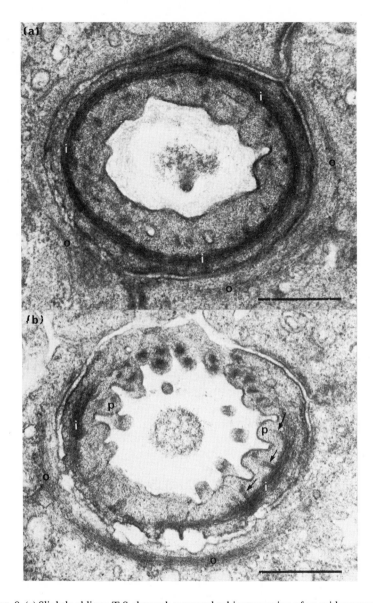

FIG. 9. (a) Slightly oblique T.S. through pore and sphincter region of an acid mucous cell of *L. mirabilis* showing complete inner sphincter (i) within the mucous cell and portions of the outer sphincter (o) within the adjacent supporting cells. Bar represents 0·5 μ m.
(b) A more oblique T.S. through the occlusor area of *L. mirabilis* showing the bases of the mucous pore microvilli on one side. Tonofilament connections between the inner sphincter and the pore microvilli are arrowed. Bar represents 0·5 μm. Abbreviations: i, inner sphincter; o, outer sphincter; p, mucous pore microvillus base.

outer ring lies within the adjacent supporting cells at approximately 180 nm below the cell–cuticle interface. Figure 7 schematizes the sphincter arrangement and Fig. 8 is a median longitudinal section of one side of the pore showing both sphincters in cross-section. Because of the positioning of the two rings, surface sections across this area failed to show both sphincters in their entirety. Figure 9a is an oblique transverse cut through the occlusor region and shows the entire inner ring and traces of the outer sphincter at one side. Figure 9b is a more oblique cut showing portions of both sphincters and revealing that the inner ring filaments are in contact with those that run vertically in the mucous pore microvilli. The outer sphincter is not continuous through the intercellular junctions of the supporting cells involved in the occlusor, but there is evidence that the filaments of this ring are in continuity with the vertically orientated tonofilaments of these supporting cells.

The arrangement is such that contraction of the ring filaments would bring about a closure of the pore in a typical sphincter manner, similar to the contractile ring microfilaments of dividing echinoderm and mammal cells (Schroeder, 1969, 1970). Presumably, however, in the lumbricillids the filaments are also capable of opening the pore by their relaxation, a function not required of those in dividing cells. The association of the mucous pore microvilli filaments and those of the inner sphincter could result in the microvilli altering position depending on the pore aperture and thereby being more effective as a controlling apparatus when the pore is open. The present study has not provided any direct evidence of the control of the sphincter filaments. The epidermal nerve net is well developed in lumbricillids and it is not inconceivable that impulses to the supporting cells could operate on the supporting cell tonofilaments and so affect the outer sphincter. Since there is no structural system of connecting filaments between the two sphincters, and it is presumed that they work synergistically, the state of the outer ring could be relayed to the inner ring by means of pressure changes.

In *L. rivalis* only the inner ring, within the mucous cell, is present and any hypothesis attempting to explain its control must be one involving more general pressure changes. In *L. reynoldsoni* there is no trace of sphincter filaments in either of the positions.

No nerve terminals were observed abutting on to the mucous cells though many of the epidermal nerve fibrils lie close to the bases of the secretory cells.

Globular, non-acid mucous cells. The species of *Lumbricillus* other than *L. reynoldsoni* have globules, approximately 1 μm in diameter, with highly dispersed and flocculated contents in fixed material (Fig. 2b) though near the basally situated secretory apparatus the smaller globules (0·7 μm) have more evenly distributed contents (Fig. 10). In *L. reynoldsoni* the globules are large (1·3–1·6 μm) and the material condensed into a single sphere (Fig. 3). Richards (1975b) has shown the relationship of globule size to the ultrastructural appearance of the contents in lumbricid secretory cells.

In *Fridericia, Mesenchytraeus* and *Enchytraeus* the globular cells show either finely fibrous material distributed uniformly within the small, 0·7 μm diameter globules, or flocculated material in cells with larger, 1·0 μm globules. No cells with both types were seen but it is possible that the differences represent stages in the secretory life of a single cell type. On the limited evidence available, it is likely that the globular cells of these genera equate to those of the lumbricillids.

Small granular cells. Observed in the ultrastructural study of *Lumbricillus*, but not in the light microscope study or in the studies on the other genera, is a cell type containing small, electron dense granules of the same order of size (0·5–0·6 μm) and showing the same range of electron density as the small granular cells of

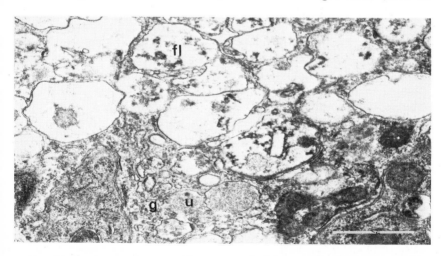

FIG. 10. Basal area of a non-acid mucous cell of *L. mirabilis* showing the smaller, newly-formed globules with uniformly distributed material, and the larger globules housing flocculated material. Bar represents 1 μm. Abbreviations: fl, globule with flocculated material; g, Golgi; u, globule with uniformly distributed material.

lumbricids (Richards, 1975c). They occurred infrequently, as in lumbricids. Speculation that the small granular secretion in lumbricids might affect the viscosity of the acid mucus might also apply in the lumbricillid enchytraeids, since it is only the genus *Lumbricillus* that possesses both acid mucous cells and small granular cells.

Supporting cells

There are numerous mitochondria in the supporting cells of *L. georgiensis*, *L. mirabilis* (Fig. 2b), *L. vancouverensis* and *L. rivalis*. These organelles feature less obviously in *L. reynoldsoni* and *E. albidus*, and in the terrestrial *Fridericia* and *Mesenchytraeus* their numbers approximate to those found in the supporting cells of lumbricids. These findings are subjective; morphometric techniques have not been applied to the micrographs and the tissue blocks were not sampled with this in mind.

There is evidence that a relatively constant mitochondrial/cytoplasm relationship exists in certain mammalian tissue (Berger, 1973). This would appear not to be so in enchytraeids, the small supporting cells of the terrestrial species have appreciably fewer mitochondria than cells of similar size in the small littoral lumbricillids and cells of larger size in *L. rivalis*.

Such observations, although not substantiated statistically, lead to speculation concerning a possible active transport function of the epidermis in the small littoral and the sewage bed species. The association of apparently high mitochondrial numbers and the possession of a hyaluronic acid mucus that might be involved in ion regulation (see Discussion) cannot be ignored. However, active uptake of organic solutes through the epidermis is well documented in polychaetes (Stephens, 1963, 1964; Chapman & Taylor, 1968; Chien, Stephens & Healey, 1972) and the energy demands have been shown not to be excessive (Stephens, 1968). The occurrence of numerous mitochondria in certain lumbricillid species might be linked with such an active uptake but experimental data on these species are not available.

DISCUSSION

The only significant histochemical differences between the cuticle of enchytraeids and that of lumbricids and megascolecids is the absence of hyaluronic acid in the enchytraeids. It may be that within a cuticle housing fibres of small diameter there is less need for a viscous matrix. A similar correlation between cuticle depth, fibre size and the presence or not of hyaluronic acid can be made in leeches where the cuticle is thin (Rutschke, 1970), the fibres are of small diameter, and hyaluronic acid is not present (Damas, 1969). The ultrastructural details of the enchytraeid cuticle are not only similar to those of lumbricids but also to the published descriptions of other microdriles, polychaetes and leeches, reviewed by Richards (in press).

Arising from this present study on the secretory cells are several, perhaps interrelated, points which merit some considera-tion. These are: the possible function of a hyaluronic acid type of mucus; the absence of such a secretion in genera other than *Lumbricillus*; the differences in the distribution of this hyaluronic acid cell type and the degree of development of the occlusor control mechanism within the genus; the habitat differences and the size range of the selected lumbricillids. The pertinent features of the lumbricillids are summarized in Table II.

The possibility that the possession of granular, hyaluronic acid-containing cells is a generic feature must be considered, especially since *L. reynoldsoni* and *E. albidus* are of similar size and occur together at the same littoral sites just above the seaweed drift line. Christensen (1961), for morphological and cytotaxonomic reasons, regards the genus *Lumbricillus* as primitive within the family and suggests that the enchytraeids might have originated in littoral situations. If this were so, then the genus has radiated little, the majority of the present day species being littoral, whereas all the other enchytraeid genera have become more ecologically diverse

TABLE II

Some features of lumbricillid enchytraeids

	L. mirabilis	L. rivalis	L. reynoldsoni
Habitat	Wrack beds	Sewage filter beds	Shingle above weed line
Size (length)	Small (c. 1 cm)	Medium (c.3 cm)	Large (c.4–5 cm)
Hyaluronic acid-containing mucous cells	Numerous	Moderate	Scarce
Mucous pore sphincter	Double	Single	Absent

and have modified the epidermis accordingly. Such a hypothesis links the possession of the granular cells to the problems facing littoral species, yet their absence from the epidermis does not preclude other enchytraeids from this environment as evidenced by *E. albidus*. However, the restriction of *L. reynoldsoni* and *E. albidus* to sites very high up the shore and the preference of *L. reynoldsoni* for low salinities (Tynen, 1969) might be associated with the low frequency of hydraulic acid cells in this species and their absence in *E. albidus*.

The identification of hyaluronic acid in the secretion of the granular cells suggests, from its recorded function at vertebrate and other invertebrate sites, a viscous mucus. The ultrastructural, fingerprint pattern of the granules closely resembles that of the glandulomuscular cells in the basal disc of *Hydra* (Davis, 1973) and, furthermore, this secretion in *Hydra* is very similar histochemically, hyaluronic acid having been identified. Although such close comparisons suggest a chemical nature sufficiently alike as to give, on fixation, similar ultrastructural representations, it must be suspected that other differences, possibly physical ones, exist because in *Hydra* the secretion functions to form an adhering surface and this is not the case in *Lumbricillus*.

Acid mucins are thought to act as selective ion barriers (Kantor & Schubert, 1957) and uronic acid-containing mucosubstances are stated as being hydrophilic (Varute & Nalavade, 1970). The possible functions, in terms of the lumbricillid enchytraeids, would therefore appear to be dehydration prevention, or some involvement in the osmoregulatory mechanism, or both. The former would seem to be unlikely in that the greatest need to limit dehydration must operate in the terrestrial enchytraeids and these do not possess this type of mucous cell. Equally, within the genus *Lumbricillus* the small species living on the wrack beds would receive some protection against water loss by virtue of this habitat and on the sewage filter beds *L. rivalis* is not exposed to desiccation pressures. However, *L. reynoldsoni* is generally found in shingle above the weed line and might well face greater dehydration difficulties than the other species, yet has fewer cells of the hyaluronic acid type.

The littoral species of *Lumbricillus* are exposed to wide extremes of salinity. It is possible that the hyaluronic type of secretion could play some role in the life of the small species (*L. georgiensis, L. mirabilis, L. vancouverensis*) where, because of their size (approximately 1 cm long and 1 mm wide), a relatively large surface area is being permanently exposed to an ever-changing environment. In the much larger *L. reynoldsoni* the surface area relationship is lower and far fewer hyaluronic type cells are found. Although the almost equal numbers of granular and globular cells in the epidermis of the medium sized *L. rivalis* supports the size argument, the environment on primary sewage filter beds is a comparatively constant one. *L. rivalis* is reported from polluted freshwater outlets on the shore but repeated searches for it in these situations were unsuccessful and therefore comparisons of such forms with those collected from sewage beds could not be made. Nevertheless, the filter bed forms must also have osmoregulatory problems which a barrier film of hyaluronic acid mucus might help to alleviate.

However, any such argument linking the acid secretion to the size and environmental demands cannot ignore the fact that *E. albidus* not only occurs together with *L. reynoldsoni* above high-water mark but is also known to occur on sewage filter beds, yet has no secretory cells of the hyaluronic acid type.

The degree of development of the sphincters, hitherto unrecorded in any other annelid mucous cells, lines up well with this size–environment hypothesis. The small species living in wrack beds and exposed to wide environmental fluctuations possess the elaborate double sphincter which could permit a more efficiently controlled mucus flow related to the immediate ambient demands. A suggestion linking mucus flow to environmental salinity is upheld by the situation obtaining in certain migratory fish. The sphincters would enable rapid adjustments to be made in the extrusion rate of this type of mucus. The occlusor mechanism is less well developed in the larger *L. rivalis* and is absent in the even larger *L. reynoldsoni* where the cell frequency is sufficiently low as, perhaps, not to require precise extrusion control.

A more complete understanding of the situation in the lumbricillids must await physiological data concerning the water relations of these forms. This present study can do little more than state the facts and draw attention to the factors, which may or may not be interrelated, operating on these animals.

CONCLUSIONS

Studies on annelid cuticle show its basic structure to be the same in all classes of the phylum irrespective of size or ecology. The features of the cuticle would appear to be related to the annelid level of complexity and the cross-lamella array of collagen fibres might well reflect the locomotory patterns that are so closely linked with the metameric organization. Only in some tubicolous polychaetes is there any modification of this plan (Storch & Welsch, 1970).

Such universality does not hold for the nature of the glandular elements. The secretion forms the interface between the worm and the environment, and since this is different for aquatic and terrestrial annelids in terms of locomotory friction, osmoregulatory and desiccation pressures, it would not be surprising to find the nature of the secretion also differing.

The lumbricid earthworms are all subjected to the same basic environmental pressures and a high degree of uniformity in the secretory cells has been recorded. Ecological preferences for different soil types are not reflected in the structural or histochemical nature of the epidermal secretory cells. The literature indicates that at the histochemical level parallels do not exist between the mucous cells of the megascolecid earthworms and those of the lumbricids, and preliminary electron microscope studies on megascolecid species by the present author show structural differences also, though both families contain large species and are predominantly terrestrial. It would therefore seem that the nature of the epithelium in these two megadrile families cannot solely be related to either size or ecology. The reported differences might be the result of the early divergence of the megadrilid stock, and recent assessments of oligochaete phylogeny (Clark, 1969; Brinkhurst & Jamieson, 1971) stress the separate origins of the Megascolecidae and Lumbricidae.

The origins of the Enchytraeidae are more obscure. Clark (1969) clearly distinguishes them from the rest of the oligochaetes by placing them in a separate order, though Christensen (1961) and Brinkhurst & Jamieson (1971) relate them to the tubificids and naids. As a family they show greater somatic variation and ecological diversity than any of the other oligochaetes. The lack of epidermal uniformity is therefore not altogether unexpected. Within the range of species collected from widely disparate habitats it has not been possible to display firm correlations between the epidermal characteristics and the environment. The terrestrial species do not possess mucous glands comparable to those recorded in terrestrial lumbricids and not all littoral enchytraeids possess the hyaluronic acid gland cells that characterize the genus *Lumbricillus*.

It is possible that the techniques employed in studies of oligochaete skin have not revealed aspects of the secretion which might be linked to the environment and would show similarities between, say, the terrestrial oligochaete forms. It is equally possible that as the various families of oligochaetes adopted the terrestrial habit, they evolved their own type of secretion resulting in the recorded differences in the literature.

ACKNOWLEDGEMENTS

The Biology Department, University of Victoria, Victoria, BC Canada is thanked for facilities which enabled examination of the Canadian lumbricillids, and the assistance of Mr P. M. Webster of Keele University is gratefully acknowledged.

REFERENCES

Berger, E. R. (1973). Two morphologically different mitochondrial populations in the rat hepatocyte as determined by quantitative three-dimensional electron microscopy. *J. Ultrastruct. Res.* **45**: 303–327.

Brinkhurst, R. O. & Jamieson, B. G. M. (1971). *Aquatic Oligochaeta of the world.* Edinburgh: Oliver and Boyd.

Chapman, G. & Taylor, A. G. (1968). Uptake of organic solutes by *Nereis virens. Nature, Lond.* **217**: 763–764.

Chien, P. K., Stephens, G. C. & Healey, P. L. (1972). The role of ultrastructure and physiological differentiation of epithelia in amino acid uptake by the bloodworm *Glycera. Biol. Bull. mar. biol. Lab., Woods Hole* **142**: 219–235.

Christensen, B. (1961). Studies on cyto-taxonomy and reproduction in the Enchytraeidae, with notes on parthenogenesis and polyploidy in the animal kingdom. *Hereditas* **47**: 387–450.

Clark, R. B. (1969). Systematics and phylogeny: Annelida, Echiura, Sipuncula. In *Chemical zoology* **4**: Florkin, M. & Scheer, B. T. (eds). London and New York: Academic Press.

Damas, D. (1969). Données histochimiques sur la cuticule de *Glossiphonia complanata* L. Hirudinée, Rhynchobdelle. *Archs Zool. exp. gén.* **110**: 417–433.

Davis, L. E. (1973). Histological and ultrastructural studies of the basal disk of *Hydra*. 1. The glandulomuscular cell. *Z. Zellforsch. mikrosk. Anat.* **139**: 1–27.

Djaczenko, W. & Cimmino, C. C. (1973). Visualization of polysaccharides in the cuticle of Oligochaeta by the Tris 1-Aziridinyl phosphine oxide method. Demonstration of 62·5 Å and 185 Å periodicities in cuticular fibres. *J. Cell Biol.* **57**: 859–867.

Fullmer, H. M. (1960). Effect of peracetic acid on the enzymatic digestion of various mucopolysaccharides: reversal of the PAS staining reaction in mucins. *J. Histochem. Cytochem.* **8**: 113–121.

Hunt, S. (1970). *Polysaccharide-protein complexes in invertebrates.* London and New York: Academic Press.

Kantor, T. G. & Schubert, M. (1957). The difference in permeability of cartilage to cationic and anionic dyes. *J. Histochem. Cytochem.* **5**: 28–32.

Krishnan, N. & Sundara Rajulu, G. (1969). The integumentary mucous secretions of the earthworm *Megascolex mauritii*. *Z. Naturforsch.* **24b**: 1620–1623.

Manavalaramanujam, R. & Sundara Rajulu, G. (1974). An investigation on the chemical nature of the cuticle of a polychaete *Nereis diversicolor*. *Acta Histochem.* **48**: 69–81.

Richards, K. S. (1973). The histochemistry of the large granular, orthochromatic, mucous cells of some lumbricids (Annelida: Oligochaeta). *Ann. Histochim.* **18**: 289–300.

Richards, K. S. (1974a). The ultrastructure of the cuticle of some British lumbricids (Annelida). *J. Zool., Lond.* **172**: 303–316.

Richards, K. S. (1974b). The ultrastructure of the orthochromatic mucous cells of some British lumbricids (Annelida). *J. Zool., Lond.* **174**: 575–590.

Richards, K. S. (1974c). The histochemistry of the metachromatic mucous cells of some lumbricids (Annelida: Oligochaeta). *Ann. Histochim.* **19**: 187–197.

Richards, K. S. (1974d). The histochemistry of the small granular, proteinaceous cells (albumen cells) of the epidermis of some lumbricids (Annelida: Oligochaeta). *Ann. Histochim.* **19**: 239–251.

Richards, K. S. (1975a). The histochemistry of the cuticle of some lumbricids (Annelida: Oligochaeta). *Ann. Histochim.* **20**: 133–143.

Richards, K. S. (1975b). The ultrastructure of the metachromatic mucous cells of some British lumbricids (Annelida). *J. Zool., Lond.* **177**: 233-246.

Richards, K. S. (1975c). The ultrastructure of the small granular, proteinaceous epidermal cells of some British lumbricids (Annelida) and a reassessment of the identity of the so-called albumen cells. *J. Zool., Lond.* **177**: 517–527.

Richards, K. S. (in press). Epidermis and cuticle. In *Physiology of annelids* Ch. 2. Mill, P. J. (ed.). London and New York: Academic Press.

Rigby, B. J. & Robinson, M. S. (1975). Thermal transitions in collagen and the preferred temperature range of animals. *Nature, Lond.* **253**: 277–279.

Rutschke, E. (1970). Zur Substruktur der Cuticula der Egel (Hirudinea). *Z. Morph. Tiere* **67**: 97–105.

Schroeder, T. E. (1969). The role of "contractile ring" filaments in dividing *Arbacia* eggs. *Biol. Bull. mar. biol. Lab., Woods Hole* **137**: 413–414.

Schroeder, T. E. (1970). The contractile ring. 1. Fine structure of dividing mammalian (HeLa) cells and the effects of cytochalasin B. *Z. Zellforsch. mikrosk. Anat.* **109**: 431–449.

Stephens, G. C. (1963). Uptake of organic material by aquatic invertebrates. II. Accumulation of amino acids by the bamboo worm *Clymenella torquata*. *Comp. Biochem. Physiol.* **10**: 191–202.

Stephens, G. C. (1964). Uptake of organic material by aquatic invertebrates. III. Uptake of glycine by brackish-water annelids. *Biol. Bull. mar. biol. Lab., Woods Hole* **126**: 150–162.

Stephens, G. C. (1968). Dissolved organic matter as a potential source of nutrition for marine organisms. *Am. Zool.* **8**: 95–106.

Storch, V. & Welsch, U. (1970). Über die Feinstruktur der Polychaeten-Epidermis. *Z. Morph. Tiere* **66**: 310–322.

Sundara Rajulu, G. & Krishnan, K. R. (1967). On the possible occurrence of hyaluronic acid in the cuticle of the earthworm *Megascolex mauritii*. *Indian J. exp. Biol.* **5**: 55–56.

Tynen, M. J. (1969). Littoral distribution of *Lumbricillus reynoldsoni* Backlund and other Enchytraeidae (Oligochaeta) in relation to salinity and other factors. *Oikos* **20**: 41–53.

Varute, A. T. & Nalavade, M. N. (1970). Cytochemical study of the mucus and mucus secreting cells in the epidermis of the earthworm *Pheretima elongata*. *Indian J. exp. Biol.* **8**: 225–228.

Symp. zool. Soc. Lond. (1977) No. 39, 195–222.

THE POGONOPHORE EPIDERMIS, ITS STRUCTURE, FUNCTIONS AND AFFINITIES

J. DAVID GEORGE

British Museum (Natural History), London, England

SYNOPSIS

The Pogonophora are a little-known group of worm-like invertebrates living mainly in the deep ocean. They have a long thin body and no digestive tract. The animals dwell within a chitinous tube produced by distinctive glands in the epidermis. A mainly fibrous cuticle, similar to that occurring in annelids, overlays the epidermis and is thickened in various body regions to form the bridle and plaques. The chitinous setae of the girdles and the septate region, whose structure resembles that in several protostomian phyla, are produced in pockets by discrete groups of cells. The epidermal layer also has protein, fat and glycogen-containing cells, mucous glands, ciliary and sensory cells distributed amongst unspecialized cells: all these cell types are common throughout the animal kingdom. The nervous system is intraepidermal, lying between the basal plasma membranes of the epidermal cells and the basal lamina.

The functions of the various epidermal cells and their products are discussed and special reference is made to how the epidermis acts as a nutrient-absorbing surface. Whenever possible, attempts are made to relate the Pogonophora to other animal groups by comparison of epidermal structures.

INTRODUCTION

The pogonophores are a group of benthic marine invertebrates that are little known to the scientific community as a whole, in spite of the fact that they have a worldwide distribution. More than 100 species have been named since the first specimens were described by Caullery in 1914. Over 80% of known species dwell on the continental slopes but some are found in ocean basins and deep trenches (Southward, 1963). They occur rarely in shallow water communities and only where conditions of relatively stable temperature and salinity prevail.

Pogonophores have long worm-like bodies which are enclosed within tightly fitting tubes. The majority of species appear to live with their tubes buried vertically in soft sediments with a short length projecting above the substratum surface (George, 1975), but several species of *Sclerolinum*, for example, have been found with their tubes winding through decaying wood and other vegetable debris lying on the sea bottom (Webb, 1964b; Southward, 1972).

Members of the phylum Pogonophora are unique amongst free-living Eumetazoa in having no mouth, anus or digestive tract at any stage in their life history, and thus must be able to obtain adequate nourishment through their body surface.

In this paper a brief description will be given of the external morphology of pogonophores followed by a review of current knowledge of the structure and function of the epidermis and its derivatives. The phylogenetic position of the group within the Eumetazoa has been a matter of debate ever since the animals were discovered. The structure and function of the epidermis may throw some light on this intriguing question.

EXTERNAL MORPHOLOGY

Pogonophores vary greatly in length according to the species, some being as little as 5 cm long whilst others may reach 30–40 cm and yet have a breadth of less than a millimetre. They form a morphologically discrete group, the bilaterally symmetrical body being divided into a number of recognizable regions regardless of the species examined (Fig. 1). Because of the uncertainty at present surrounding the question of dorsoventral orientation in pogonophores (see George, 1973) the neutral term adneural is used to refer to that side of the body containing the main nerve tract and antineural to the opposite side.

The most anterior region, which is usually conical, bears a crown of long tentacles. The number of tentacles varies from one to several hundred according to the species, but when many tentacles exist they are usually in two bundles or arranged in a spiral (Ivanov, 1963). The tentacles are often highly contractile but sometimes are rigid and held tightly together. In many species the tentacles are provided on one side with rows of filiform extensions known as pinnules.

The frenular region is characterized by a distinct ridge of tissue called the frenulum (or bridle) running obliquely around the body. It shows its greatest development laterally and fails to meet in the mid-line of many species.

A distinct external groove, marking an internal muscular septum, separates the frenular region from the gonadal region. This region forms the bulk of a pogonophore's length and is divided into a pre-annular and post-annular section by annuli (or girdles) composed of setae protruding from ridges. The pre-annular section, which is shorter and sturdier than that following the girdles, is

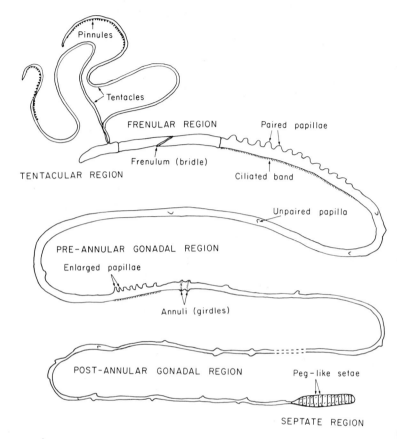

FIG. 1. Diagram of pogonophore (greatly foreshortened posteriorly) showing the body regions and main external features.

characterized anteriorly in all but a few species by pairs of metamerically arranged papillae situated on the antineural side of the body. The papillae usually bear ridges of thickened tissue at their tips (plaques) but in some species of *Siboglinum* the ridges are replaced by glandular openings. More posteriorly the metamerism breaks down, the papillae becoming inconspicuous and seemingly randomly distributed. However, a concentration of enlarged papillae immediately precedes the girdles in all but a few species. A longitudinal ciliated band occurs adneurally but is confined to that part of the pre-annular section bearing the metamerically arranged papillae and the enlarged papillae.

The post-annular gonadal region is very long and fragile and has papillae with plaques, or glandular swellings, scattered along its whole length.

Pogonophores are rarely collected with their rear ends intact due to the frailty of the post-annular body and it was not until 1963 that the first complete specimen was recovered (Webb, 1964a). Since then, with refinement of collecting techniques, the septate regions of several species have been obtained. The region is short and considerably more substantial than that part of the post-annular body immediately preceding it. It is distinctly segmented, each segment bearing several peg-like setae which are aligned with those of other segments to form longitudinal rows.

THE INTEGUMENT AND ITS ASSOCIATED STRUCTURES

Studies on the structure of the main body wall of pogonophores at the light microscope level have shown that it consists of a cuticle overlying a single layer of epidermal cells (Fig. 2). A basal lamina

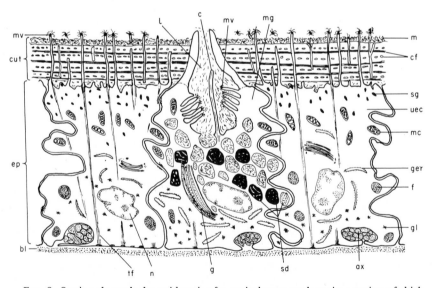

FIG. 2. Section through the epidermis of a typical pogonophore in a region of thick cuticle, showing a generalized mucous gland cell (mg) flanked by two unspecialized cells (uec). Other abbreviations: ax, nerve axons; bl, basal lamina; c, cilium; cf, collagenous fibres; cut, cuticle; ep, epidermis; f, fat globule; g, Golgi complex; ger, granular endoplasmic reticulum; gl, glycogen rosette; l, lumen; m, surface coat of mucus; mc. mitochondrion; mv, microvillus; n, nucleus; sd, secretory droplets of sulphated mucopolysaccharide; sg, "secretory" granule of proteinaceous material; tf, tonofilaments.

separates the epidermal cells from a thin layer of circular muscle and a more strongly developed layer of longitudinal muscles. The nervous system is composed of bundles of axons forming a continuous cylinder of nervous tissue between the epidermal cell membranes and the basal lamina.

This basic arrangement of tissues is maintained throughout the length of the body although the composition and thickness of the layers varies in different regions and from species to species.

Cuticle

The thickness of the cuticle varies considerably along the body. It is at its thickest in the tentacular, frenular and septate regions of the main body, but is very thin over the tentacle pinnules, metameric and non-metameric papillae, over the ciliated bands, and over most of the post-annular gonadal section.

In the frenular region the raised tissue ridge termed the bridle (Fig. 3A) is composed of pigmented and thickened cuticle (Ivanov, 1963; Gupta & Little, 1970) as are variously shaped plaques found on the papillae of many species (Fig. 3B). The function of these cuticular thickenings is not entirely clear but it seems reasonable to suppose that they help the animal to cling to the inside of its tube as it moves up and down. In animals that have a rigid anterior end to their tubes it is possible that the bridle is used to support the animal on the rim of its tube whilst the front end of the body is protruded (Ivanov, 1952). However, the forepart of the tube in the majority of pogonophores is too flimsy to make such a function feasible, as Ivanov (1963) later conceded. Webb (1965) suggested that the bridle is used as a tool for spreading tube-forming glandular secretions over the inside of the tube. George (1975), however, pointed out that although the bridle may well assist in the formation of the anterior end of the tube it is difficult to envisage how it is implicated in the production of the rear end since the animal fits so tightly within the tube that it is unable to reverse its body within it.

The biochemical composition of the cuticle was first investigated by Ivanov (1963) who found that the main part of the cuticle gave a positive periodic acid Schiff reaction indicating that it contained a polysaccharide. More detailed histochemical tests by Southward & Southward (1966) led them to conclude that the cuticle of *Siboglinum atlanticum* is composed of layers of neutral mucopolysaccharide possibly with collagen and some phospholipid. In addition there is a thin coating on the outside of the cuticle which appears to be a sulphated acid mucopolysaccharide.

The fine structure of the cuticle in various body regions in several species of pogonophore has been described by Gupta, Little & Philip (1966), Gupta & Little (1969, 1970) and Southward (1975b). For the most part the cuticle is composed of criss-crossed

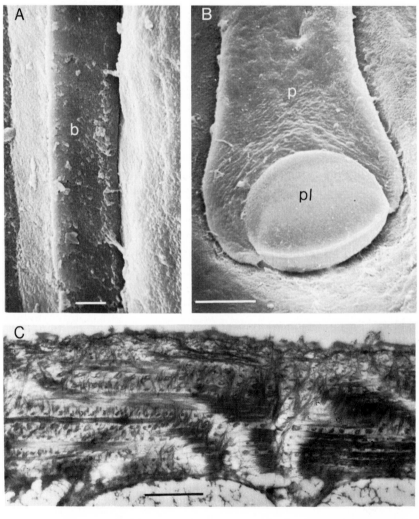

FIG. 3. A. Scanning electron micrograph (SEM) of the bridle (b) of *Polybrachia canadensis*. Scale = 5 μm. B. SEM of a metameric papilla (p) with its terminal plaque (pl) from *Lamellisabella coronata*. Scale = 20 μm. C. Transmission electron micrograph (TEM) of a section through the fibrous cuticle in the frenular region of *Siboglinum fiordicum*. Scale = 2 μm.

layers of parallel bundles of fibres (presumably unstriated collagen fibres), adjacent layers being at an angle of approximately 90° to each other (Figs 2 and 3C). The fibre bundles are embedded in an amorphous or finely fibrillar matrix thought to be a mucopolysaccharide. Microvilli from the underlying epidermal cells penetrate through the fibre lattice, and also through the thin amorphous mucoid layer overlying the meshwork, to the outside. Branching sometimes occurs near the distal ends of the microvilli in *S. fiordicum*, a feature which has also been noted by Gupta *et al.* (1966) in *Siphonobrachia ilyophora*. At high magnification the microvilli are seen to be packed with dense material and numerous fine filaments radiate from them forming a surface fuzz. This surface fuzz probably constitutes the acid mucopolysaccharide layer over the cuticle reported by Southward & Southward (1966). Lumsden (1975) noted the occurrence of "glycocalyces" intimately associated with the tips of the microvilli in several invertebrate groups and Gupta & Little (1969) have pointed out the remarkable similarity between the filament-coated ends of the microvilli in the gastric and intestinal mucosae of vertebrates and those of the pogonophore cuticle. It would seem, therefore, that the fuzz coat may be a universal feature at the exposed tips of microvilli regardless of the animal group.

Both Gupta & Little (1969) and Southward (1975a) have reported the presence of small dark particles (or vesicles) within the surface fuzz, which are probably formed by the pinching off of the tips of the microvilli. Similar vesicles have been seen on the surface of annelid cuticles (Boilly, 1967; Potswald, 1971; Richards, 1974a).

The basic cuticular structure is maintained in the bridle and plaques, although here the amorphous matrix consists of very electron dense material. In areas of the body covered by a very thin cuticle, on the other hand, the fibre bundles are frequently absent, although microvilli still penetrate through the amorphous matrix.

The combination of elasticity and strength afforded by the fibre lattice of the pogonophore cuticle makes it ideally suited for the role of maintaining the body volume constant whilst the animal changes its form during movement.

Evidence favouring the production of the collagenous cuticle in annelids and nematodes from underlying epidermal cells has been produced by Bailey (1968) and Bubel (1973). By comparison it would seem likely that cuticular pogonophore collagens are similarly epidermal derivatives.

Epidermal cells

The epidermal layer covering the body is only a single cell thick and consists largely of unspecialized cells which may be locally differentiated into pinnules, protein, lipid and glycogen-containing cells, absorptive cells and ciliated cells. Unicellular and multicellular glands within the epidermis produce mucus and tube-forming secretions, whilst setae are formed in pouches lined with epidermal cells.

Jägersten (1956) and Ivanov (1963) have provided descriptions of the epidermis at the light microscope level whilst Southward & Southward (1966) have categorized various cell types of the main body on the basis of their histochemistry. More recently the ultrastructure of the epidermal cells of the tentacles and body has been investigated by Nørrevang (1965), Gupta *et al.* (1966), Gupta & Little (1969, 1970).

Unspecialized epidermal cells

The shape and size of these cells varies greatly along the body. On the tentacles and much of the gonadal region they are generally cuboidal or flattened whilst in the tentacular, frenular and septate regions of the main body they are more normally columnar. The cell membranes are interdigitated with the membranes of adjacent cells and the basal plasma membrane often almost surrounds bundles of nerve axons situated beneath the cell. The irregularly contoured nucleus is situated centrally or towards the base of the cell and cisternae of granular endoplasmic reticulum extend up to the apical cell membrane. In regions where the cells are overlain by a well developed cuticle, bundles of tonofilaments are a particularly prominent feature, joining the bases of the microvilli with half-desmosomes on the basal plasma membrane of the cell.

Southward & Southward (1966) were unable to demonstrate histochemically the presence of carbohydrate, lipid or protein in the cytoplasm but electron microscope sections reveal that the apical portion of the cytoplasm contains many electron dense droplets amongst the abundant mitochondria, and that the basal portion contains numerous glycogen and fat droplets. It is possible that the apical droplets contribute to the formation of the collagenous cuticle through a process of exocytosis but no direct evidence is available to confirm this opinion (Gupta & Little, 1970). Certainly these cells are present under thick cuticle where no other cell types exist, and must therefore contribute in some way to the cuticle. Part of the fibrous fuzz coat on the surface of the cuticle is almost certainly contributed by the microvilli.

Pinnule cells

The pinnules of the tentacles are each composed of a single modified epidermal cell (Ivanov, 1963). The cylindrical cell is greatly prolongated distally although the base of the cell remains in contact with the basal lamina of the tentacle and its prominent nucleus remains in the same plane as those of the surrounding unspecialized cells. The cuticle covering the pinnule is exceedingly thin. Inside the cell much of the cytoplasm is occluded by two blood capillaries which unite near the tip of the cell. In some species it has been observed that there are material-filled outgrowths of the capillaries into the cytoplasm which may even link up with the cisternae of smooth endoplasmic reticulum (Gupta *et al.*, 1966). These capillaries are really extracellular in as far as they are invaginations of the basal plasma membrane and of the basal lamina of the cell (Fig. 4). Hama (1960) found that some blood

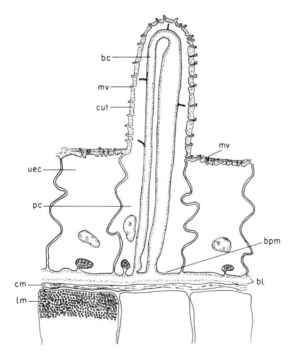

FIG. 4. Longitudinal section through a pinnule cell (pc) of a tentacle. The diagram, which is not drawn to scale, shows how invaginations of the basal plasma membrane (bpm) and of the basal lamina (bl) form the blood capillaries (bc) which connect with the blood space between the epidermal cells and the muscle cells. Other abbreviations: cm, circular muscle; cut, thin non-fibrous cuticle; lm, longitudinal muscle; mv, microvilli; uec, unspecialized epidermal cell.

204 J. DAVID GEORGE

vessels of the earthworm, *Eisenia foetida*, are similarly lined with extracellular basement membrane. The pinnule cell as a whole, however, appears to be a fairly unique cell type in the animal kingdom (Southward, 1975a).

It seems certain that the blood-filled pinnules (and tentacles) have an important respiratory role in pogonophores. Their possible function in the nutrition of the animals will be discussed later (see p. 218).

Protein-containing cells

Three types of protein-containing cells have been recognized within the Pogonophora. These cells do not appear to have the secretory cavity with an opening to the exterior characteristic of gland cells. The cells of the first type ("yellow" protein cells— Southward & Southward, 1966; type I protein cells—Gupta & Little, 1970) lie in strips flanking the ciliated band in the pre-annular gonadal region and where the band of ciliated cells is not present join to form a single strip. The oval protein granules, which have a crystalline structure, fill the cell above the nucleus.

In the second type of protein cell ("white" protein cells— Southward & Southward, 1966; type II protein cells—Gupta & Little, 1970) the granules are larger, more nearly spherical and seen to be packed with a fibrillar material. These cells form a band along the adneural side of the post-annular gonadal region.

The function of the above types of protein-containing cell is unknown. However, the third type of cell, according to Gupta & Little (1970), has features in common with the zymogenic cells of other animals, having an organization typical of those cells engaged in synthesis of secretory protein. The cells correspond to some of the "white" protein cells found by Southward & Southward (1966) in association with the pyriform glands (see p. 209), and are distributed laterally in the frenular and gonadal region and also on the papillae. The cuticle overlying the cells is usually thin and non-fibrous. The "secretory" droplets, which have no apparent substructure, are usually confined to the apical portion of the cell and are sometimes seen being expelled through the apical plasma membrane. The granular endoplasmic reticulum is often arranged in whorls (Fig. 5A).

Cells containing non-collagenous protein granules, in many ways histochemically similar to those described above, have been recorded from the oligochaetes (Richards, 1974b).

Fat-containing cells

These cells, containing much more lipid than unspecialized epidermal cells, are situated on the paired papillae and in the groove between them. The fat is in the form of lipid and phospholipid membrane-bound globules which fill the cell. The cuticle covering the cells is thin and normally lacks the collagenous fibre component. A network of deep invaginations occurs in the apical plasma membrane between the microvilli. According to Gupta & Little (1970) irregular aggregates of a myelin-like structure are frequently found trapped in the invaginations. In contrast the interdigitated form of lateral plasma membranes that normally occurs in unspecialized epidermal cells is replaced by a relatively straight surface. The substructure of the lipid vesicles is very variable but is predominantly of one type in any single cell. Gupta & Little (1970) believe that the fat-containing cells are specialized for the synthesis (and storage?) of fats and phospholipids, and aid this process by absorbing fatty acid precursors from the environment. It is possible, therefore, that the lipoprotein aggregates frequently seen trapped in the apical invaginations are being digested in the subcuticular space, especially as Southward & Southward (1966) have detected enzyme activity in this region.

Glycogen-containing cells

All the epidermal cells of the body, excluding the tube-secreting glands (see p. 209), contain at least some glycogen within the cytoplasm, where it is frequently grouped into rosettes (Fawcett, 1966). However, certain cells are particularly rich in glycogen. Southward (1973) using both histochemical and electron microscope techniques, has found that the cells lining the groove between the paired papillae, the ciliated cells (see p. 206), and the majority of epidermal cells in the very long post-annular gonadal region contain large quantities of glycogen.

In the ciliated cells the glycogen particles are found amongst the ciliary rootlets where they are likely to be acting as an energy reserve for the cilia. Southward (1973) has postulated that the large quantities of glycogen in the epidermis of the post-annular gonadal region could possibly be acting as a reserve for anaerobic respiration. In most species this part of the body is buried deep in the sediment where anaerobic conditions almost certainly prevail.

Absorptive cells

These large cuboidal cells, which are situated in broad bands on either side of protein-containing cells on the adneural side of the post-annular gonadal region, contain no obvious secretory droplets in their extensive cytoplasm. They have an apical cell surface similar to that of the lipid-containing cells and are likewise situated under a thin cuticle. However, they have no extracellular bodies trapped in invaginations of the plasma membrane. The cells have unusually large basally-situated nuclei and contain according to Gupta & Little (1970) numerous "pinocytotic vesicles" which are not found in unspecialized epidermal cells. Although all epidermal cells seem to be well-equipped for an absorptive function they believe that these cells are specialized for absorption.

Ciliated cells

The ciliated cells on the adneural pre-annular gonadal region, and on the tentacles in some species, are composed of cells with bundles of cilia whose rootlets extend deep within the cell (Fig. 5B). The cilia are similar to those occurring in many other animal groups (Sleigh, 1962) and have normal $9+2$ axonemes. The cuticle overlying these cells is very thin and penetrated by microvilli as well as by the cilia. The nucleus is located basally in the cytoplasm which is particularly rich in glycogen granules.

The function of the adneural ciliated bands in adult pogonophores is unknown although my own observations on living specimens of *Siboglinum fiordicum* have revealed that weak water currents are present within the tube as a result of ciliary action. These currents may draw fine particulate organic matter down into the tube or be implicated in removal of waste products from the cuticle surface.

Sensory cells

Very little is known about sensory organs in pogonophores. It is quite conceivable that external stimuli are received all over the body surface and transmitted through the epidermal cells to the nerve net existing between the basal plasma membranes of the cells and the basal lamina. However, the most likely areas for the reception of stimuli are those regions of the body which may on occasions protrude from the tube, namely the tentacular and septate regions. Nørrevang (1974) has recently described in *S. fiordicum* two groups of some 80 cells, situated laterally on either side of the body just in front of the insertion point of the tentacle, which he claims may be acting as photoreceptors. The cells, which lie under a thick fibrous cuticle, are provided with a large vacuole,

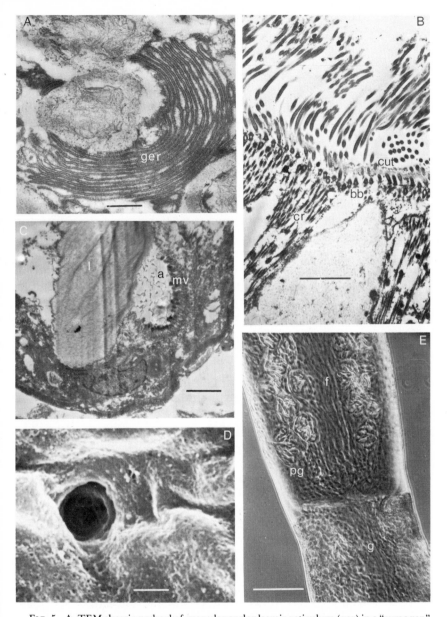

FIG. 5. A. TEM showing whorl of granular endoplasmic reticulum (ger) in a "zymogen" cell of *S. fiordicum*. Scale = 0·5 μm. B. TEM showing cilia of the adneural ciliated band of *P. canadensis*; bb, basal bodies; cr, striated ciliary rootlets; cut, cuticle. Scale = 25 μm. C. TEM through the base of a pyriform gland in *S. fiordicum* revealing an ampulla (a) lined with microvilli (mv) producing material for the lamella (l). Scale = 2 μm. D. SEM of the opening of a pyriform gland on to the body surface in *S. fiordicum*. Scale = 2 μm. E. Phase contrast photomicrograph showing the pyriform glands (pg) protruding into the coelom of the frenular region (f) of *S. fiordicum*; g, gonadal region. Scale = 100 μm.

probably representing an invagination of the apical cell membrane, lined with a mass of projecting microvilli. Axon bundles situated beneath the cell connect directly with the brain mass of the animal. It is claimed that these cells are similar to the visual receptor cells of hirudineans and oligochaetes.

In the detailed study of the septate region of *S. fiordicum* Southward (1975b) located a "sensory" cell in one segment whose apical region penetrated the cuticle and terminated in a bundle of thick straight microvilli and a short cilium. The cell resembles those described on the cirri of the polychaete, *Nereis diversicolor*, by Dorsett & Hyde (1969) and to which a chemosensory function was assigned. Two lateral bulges in the epidermis near the posterior border of each segment contain four types of cells that also may be sensory. The cell types are constructed on a common plan with an apical pit situated beneath the cuticle containing microvilli and/or cilia projecting into the pit. The structure of these cells resembles that found in the epidermal sensory cells of the earthworm, *Lumbricus terrestris*, by Knapp & Mill (1971). The function of these sensory cells remains speculative but they are most likely to be chemoreceptors.

"Mucous" gland cells

The epidermis contains a large number of unicellular glands, resembling the mucous glands in other invertebrates and vertebrates, scattered over the tentacles and body (Jägersten, 1956; Ivanov, 1963). They are characterized by a lumen and have a duct running through the cuticle to the surface. At least three types of these glands have been recognized in pogonophores (Southward & Southward, 1966; Gupta & Little, 1970).

The cells frequently are pear-shaped and the lumen at the distal end is lined by microvilli and has a cilium arising from its base (Fig. 2). The cytoplasm is filled with secretion-packed membrane-bound vesicles whose internal fine structure varies from one vesicle to another.

The glands can be categorized on the basis of their fine structure. The first type are most common in the tentacular, frenular and septate regions of the body, and contain vesicles which are either deeply staining and have a mottled appearance, or are lighter in colour with a distinct fibrillar internal structure. Gupta & Little (1970) believe that the mottled droplets are an intermediate storage form and that the fibrillar contents of the lightly straining vesicles are released into the lumen and form the filamentous coat over the outside of the cuticle. The secretion of the cells is thought to be a sulphated mucopolysaccharide (Southward & Southward, 1966) and may have a different function from the filamentous secretion arising from the epidermal microvilli.

The second type of mucous gland is found on the tentacles of some species, amongst the ciliated and protein-containing cells, and scattered generally over the gonadal and septate regions. The necks of these glands open directly on to the surface of the cuticle whereas those of the first type open above the level of the microvilli of the surrounding epidermal cells (Fig. 2). The secretory granules, at least in the early stage of their formation, have electron dense contents surrounding rods of transparent material (Fig. 2). The mucus produced is a non-sulphated neutral mucopolysaccharide according to Southward & Southward (1966). It is now generally accepted that the Golgi complex is associated with the synthesis of mucopolysaccharides and in this connection it is interesting to note that the cisternae (dictyosomes) of the Golgi complex are particularly abundant and well developed-(Fig. 2).

The third type of gland, which is found in the papillae, although similar in structure to the foregoing is not considered by Gupta & Little (1970) to produce mucus. Rather, it is thought that the homogeneously dense secretory droplets in the cytoplasm are in some way implicated in the phenolic sclerotization of the pogonophore tube (see p. 215).

"Tube-secreting" glands

The importance of the tube to the life processes of pogonophores is probably reflected in the large number of glands producing tube-forming materials.

There are both unicellular and multicellular tube-secreting glands present along the body. The elongated unicellular glands (the swan-neck vesicles of Southward & Southward, 1966) which occur along much of the body have a deep lumen lined with small microvilli, which opens to the surface via a long narrow duct. The septate region has groups of these glands on its antineural side (Southward, 1975b).

The multicellular "pyriform" glands have component units somewhat similar to the unicellular glands. In these glands, however, an individual cell unit has its lumen expanded into an ampulla at the base. The ampulla is lined with distinctive square-ended microvilli with electron dense tips (Fig. 5C). The lumina of the cell units, which are lined with more normal microvilli, open into a common lumen which discharges to the exterior through a short wide duct (Fig. 5D). The duct is lined by thin cuticle and cuboidal cells containing many small dense "secretory" granules above their basally situated nuclei. Histochemical tests by Southward & Southward (1966) have shown that the cytoplasm of the secretory cells surrounding the lumen is filled with granules of polysaccharide, protein and lipid.

Lamellae (flattened in *Siboglinum*) of material with a fibrillar substructure, secreted by the microvilli within the ampullae and individual lumina, project into the common lumen. Histochemically the lamellae consist partly of sulphated acid mucopolysaccharide and partly of chitin. Gupta & Little (1975) have suggested that chitin is secreted by the microvilli of the ampulla and then the Golgi-rich cells surrounding the lumina secrete proteins and other materials. The lamellae appear to be extruded as a continuous thread from the gland openings. It seems likely that the protein-containing "zymogenic" cells surrounding the gland openings contribute to the secretion as it is extruded.

In the frenular and tentacular regions of the body the pyriform glands project into the coelom (Fig. 5E) but in the pre-annular gonadal region they are more usually situated within the metamerically-arranged paired papillae.

Cells of the setal sac

The setae of the annuli and of the septate region are formed within pockets of epidermal cells which have been described in detail by Gupta & Little (1970) and George & Southward (1973). The main body of the seta is produced by a basal cell underlain by a continuation of the basal lamina of the epidermis. Lateral cells lining the pocket support the seta and may contribute material to it. At its distal end the sac is lined by unspecialized epidermal cells and an inpushing of the fibrous cuticle (Fig. 6).

The basal cell is bowl-shaped with microvilli projecting into the bowl. The bulk of the cytoplasmic content of the cell is usually situated to one side of the base of the seta (Fig. 6). Tonofilaments extend from the microvilli to half-desmosomes on the basal plasma membrane. The lateral boundaries of the basal cell are markedly interdigitated with those of the proximal lateral cells. The longitudinally-arranged coalescing cylinders of the shaft of a developing seta (see p. 211) appear to be produced on a template of microvilli which contribute fibrous material consisting of a polysaccharide/protein complex. The polysaccharide is chitin, probably in the β-chitin form (George & Southward, 1973). The lateral cells surrounding the setal shaft are narrow and present a smooth face to the setal wall. Like the basal cell they contain glycogen granules and some larger electron dense droplets. In the material examined the lateral cells of the girdle setae do not appear to contribute to the setal shaft whereas the lateral cells of the setae of the septate region seem to secrete a cortex of amorphous (or finely fibrillar) material around the core of cylinders (Fig. 6).

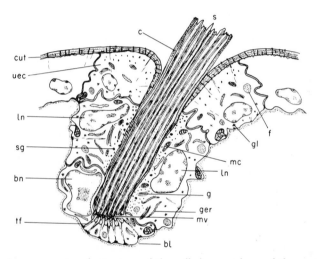

FIG. 6. Arrangement and structure of the cells in a setal sac of the septate region. Abbreviations: bl, basal lamina; bn, nucleus of basal cell; c, cortical material secreted by lateral cells; cut, fibrous cuticle; f, fat globule; g, Golgi complex; ger, granular endoplasmic reticulum; gl, glycogen rosette; ln, nucleus of lateral cell; mc, mitochondrion; mv, microvilli; s, seta; sg, secretory granule; tf, tonofilaments; uec, unspecialized epidermal cell.

Setae

Internal structure

As already mentioned, the shaft of a seta—whether from the girdles or from the septate region—is composed of a number of longitudinally arranged adjoining cylinders which diverge at the distal end to form the teeth of the setal crown. The size of a tooth on the setal head relates to the diameter of the cylinder beneath it, small teeth being formed at the end of small diameter cylinders. The fibrils forming the cylinder walls run in a predominantly

longitudinal direction, the arrangement of microfibres being particularly noticeable towards the setal crown where they are more
electron dense (Fig. 7A). In fully developed setae the cylinders
appear to be empty for most of their length, but in most species so
far examined the heads of the setae are full of electron dense
particulate material associated with the microfibres. The setal
heads, which project above the cuticle, are very hard and often
brown in colour, suggesting that tanning of the proteins has taken
place. In invertebrates tanning of proteins is usually brought about
by quinones but George & Southward (1973) have suggested that
heavy metals may also be implicated in the process. Small, but
significant, quantities of calcium, magnesium and iron have been
found in the setal heads of *Polybrachia canadensis*. Investigations
into the mineralization of radula teeth in a mollusc by Towe &
Lowenstam (1967) showed that iron minerals were precipitated on
a fibrous organic meshwork. Electron dense particles in the teeth of
P. canadensis also seem to be associated with the organic fibres (Fig.
7A). It is possible, therefore, that iron particles are being deposited
in a similar way and may be acting as a cross-linking agent in the
tanning of protein. Iron, chromium or aluminium are certainly
used to promote cross-linking in the industrial tanning of leather.

External morphology

The arrangement of the girdles of setae forming the annuli varies
from species to species but a typical adult has two rings of setae
which are frequently incomplete on the adneural and antineural
sides of the body. The oval-toothed crowns of the setae protrude
only a short distance above the body surface. The crowns are
always orientated with their long axes parallel to that of the body.
The pointed teeth of the setal head are arranged in rows, the teeth
of one row alternating with those of the next. There are usually two
groups of teeth, a large posterior group whose teeth point towards
the anterior of the animal and a smaller anterior group of backward pointing teeth (Fig. 7B).

   The segmentally arranged peg-like setae of the septate region
(Fig. 1) usually only have slightly expanded heads and their teeth
are less well developed. These setae protrude further from the
body than those of the girdles.

Function

Observations on living pogonophores have shown that the annuli
are the structures by which the animal anchors itself firmly in its

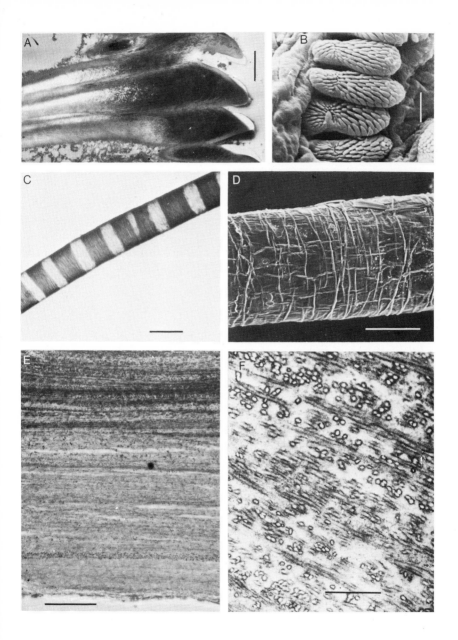

FIG. 7. A. TEM showing a longitudinal section through the head of a seta of *P. canadensis*. Scale = 1 μm. B. SEM showing toothed crowns of the girdle setae of *S. fiordicum*. Scale = 2 μm. C. Photomicrograph of the tube of *S. fiordicum* showing the dark banding that occurs in the buried section of the tube. Scale = 200 μm. D. SEM of the surface of the tube of *S. fiordicum*. Scale = 100 μm. E. TEM through the tube wall of *S. fiordicum* showing its laminated construction. Scale = 2 μm. F. TEM showing the detailed arrangement of fibres in the tube wall of *S. fiordicum*. Scale = 0·5 μm.

tube. When the forepart of the animal is withdrawn or the posterior part of the body is drawn forward, the toothed setal crowns
are pressed into the inner fibrous lining of the tube. As pointed out
by George & Southward (1973) the importance of the withdrawal
movement to the worm is probably reflected in the greater
development of the anterior facing groups of teeth on the setal
heads. It is interesting to note that in several species of *Sclerolinum*
whose tubes wind horizontally through decaying vegetable matter
(see p. 195) the girdles are less well developed.

The setae of the septate region perform a different function
from those of the annuli. Observations by Southward (1971) have
shown that the septate region is used primarily as a burrowing
organ, the peg-like setae serving as anchors in the sediment as the
animal draws itself deeper into the substratum.

Tube

All pogonophores as far as is known live in cylindrical unbranched
tubes secreted by unicellular and multicellular glands in the
epidermis. The detailed architecture of tubes varies considerably
throughout the phylum and has been reviewed by Ivanov (1963)
and more recently by Webb (1971).

The majority of species live in straight tubes of uniform diameter. The most recently formed anterior and posterior parts of the
tube are of a more flimsy nature than the older parts. The flimsi-
ness of the tube protruding from the sediment is not due entirely to
the age of the tube but results from it being formed in contact with
the water instead of with the sediment (George, 1975). Examination of the tubes in transmitted light shows that many of them are
ringed with light and dark bands (Fig. 7C), and in addition often
show annulations at fairly regular intervals. These annulations
may represent pauses between bursts of tube-forming activity.
Most tubes are overlain by filaments (Fig. 7D) which probably
provide the framework on which more homogeneous material is
deposited.

Sections through the tube wall reveal that it is laminated (Fig.
7E). The laminations can be traced through the successive light and
dark bands along the tube. There is a general tendency for the
outer layers to be darker in appearance than the more recently
secreted inner layers. More detailed investigation of a section
through the tube wall shows that it is composed of fine fibres of
material running, according to Gupta & Little (1975), in a helicoidal arrangement (Fig. 7F). In such a design fibres of each lamina

run in parallel and there is a change in fibre angle between one lamina and the next of less than 90°. Such an arrangmenent is not uncommon in biological material (see e.g. Bouligand, 1972; Gubb, 1975). Although there is likely to be a cyclic deposition of material by the glands of the epidermis, the arrangement of fibrillae within the tube wall may arise spontaneously by a natural self-assembly process (Bouligand, 1972; Gupta & Little, 1975) once the secretion has been smeared on the macrofibrous meshwork by the body.

Chemical analysis of the tube of *Siboglinum* sp. by Foucart, Bricteux-Gregoire & Jeuniaux (1965) has shown that it contains amongst other organic materials about 30% chitin and 50% protein. Blackwell, Parker & Rudall (1965) believe that the chitin is present as β-chitin. A more detailed analysis of different tube components of *S. atlanticum* by Southward & Southward (1966) showed that in addition to chitin a considerable amount of sulphated acid mucopolysaccharide is present in the interspaces between the dark rings. They believe that much of the basic protein present in the tube is in the dark rings where it is complexed with chitin. Certainly the rings give every indication of being hardened and tanned. It is not known whether tanning results entirely from quinones derived from mucous-gland cells, as suggested by Gupta & Little (1970), or whether heavy metals present in the sediment may also be implicated. My own preliminary observations using X-ray analysis show that *Siboglinum* tubes from the Norwegian fiords have small quantities of heavy metals incorporated into the parts of the tube buried in the sediment. Those parts of the tube projecting from the sediment rarely seem to be tanned or hardened.

DISCUSSION

The use of collagen as a structural protein is common throughout the animal phyla (Bairati, 1972) but only nematodes, annelids and sipunculans (possibly echiurans—George, prelim. obs.) use it in their cuticles, although it is extensively used in connective tissues. In the deuterostomes (containing echinoderms, hemichordates and chordates), an assemblage of animals to which the pogonophores are believed by some to belong, collagenous tissues are invariably subepidermal (Gupta & Little, 1975). The cuticle of nematodes lacks microvilli and has a differently constructed fibre system (Lee, 1972). The particular combination of microvilli and cuticle that occurs in pogonophores is found elsewhere only in annelids (e.g. Coggeshall, 1966; Moritz & Storch, 1970), sipunculans (Storch & Welsch, 1970) and possibly echiurans (George, prelim. obs.). Furthermore, Southward (1975a) believes that the layer of "surface particles" is confined to oligochaetes and polychaetes. Thus it would seem that on the basis of cuticular structure pogonophores have most in common with annelids. The question remains as to whether this similarity results from convergent evolution or is a manifestation of phylogenetic affinity. However, both nemerteans and the hemichordates have solved the problem of volume control by the development of subepidermal fibre systems.

The presence of possible photoreceptors in S. fiordicum is of interest since this pogonophore is one of the few species which exist in shallow enough water for the presence of receptor organs that could perceive changes in light intensity to be of some advantage in detecting the presence of predators. In this connection it is worth noting that the majority of pogonophores so far examined have one or more giant axons, similar to those existing in many other worm-like tubiculous invertebrates, running from the primitive intraepidermal brain ring in the anterior part of the body as far as the annuli, the major anchoring devices of the body. It seems likely that any "alarm" stimuli received by sense organs at the front of the body would lead to fast transmission of signals along the giant axon and rapid withdrawal of the front end of the animal into the comparative safety of the tube. It must be stated however that experiments so far carried out by myself to test the reaction of S. fiordicum to light stimuli have met with negative results, the animals giving no external sign that they are responding.

The structure, chemical composition and method of formation of the setae in pogonophores is remarkably similar to that in annelids (Bouligand, 1967), echiurans (Orrhage, 1971) and brachiopods (Gustus & Cloney, 1972; Storch & Welsch, 1972; Orrhage, 1973). More recently Brocco, O'Clair & Cloney (1974) have drawn attention to transient epidermal bristles (Kölliker's tufts) found on the surface of juvenile octopods which also seem to have a similar structure and are produced in the same way. The chitinous setae of pogonophores are, therefore, by no means unique in the animal kingdom, although all the phyla in which this type of seta is found belong to the coelomate protostomes (major phyla—annelids, molluscs and arthropods). I have argued (George & Southward, 1973) that the similarity between these setae is more likely to result from a phylogenetic relationship than from convergent evolution due to similarity of function, especially as the setae of brachiopods apparently do not perform any function related to movement of the animal. Various hooks, spines and bristles have evolved to aid movement in soft-bodied invertebrate groups other than those mentioned above (see e.g. Lyons, 1966; Croll, 1970), but these are usually cuticular in origin like the bridle and plaques of pogonophores, and none have the multicylindrical structure characteristic of "annelid-type" setae.

Pogonophores share with annelids the segmental arrangement of setae in the septate region of their body. It has been argued by some that the metamerism of the rear end of pogonophores, unlike that of annelids, is a secondary development. However, the septate region appears as the primary body divisions are forming very early in embryonic development and segments are added from a posterior growth zone as the animal increases in length. This situation closely resembles that in annelids.

The basic similarity between the pyriform gland cells and the cells of the setal sac has not gone unnoticed (Gupta & Little, 1975) and may not be fortuitous, especially as the secretions of both are chemically similar. The metameric arrangement of the pyriform glands in the pre-annular gonadal region is reminiscent of that of the setal sacs in the septate region and of the arrangement of setae in the oligochaetes and polychaetes. The evolution of a chitin/protein-secreting cell in some hypothetical ancestor may have given rise on one hand to the setal sacs of annelids and on the other hand to the tube-secreting cells and setal sacs of the pogonophores.

Jägersten (1956) has drawn attention to the similarity at the light microscope level of the tube-secreting glands in pogonophores to the "bacillary" glands in the epidermis of the archiannelid, *Protodrilus* (Jägersten, 1952). However, I have been unable to find any information on the fine structure of these cells in archiannelids that would corroborate his statement.

The structure and composition of the tubes of pogonophores seem to be unique amongst marine tube-dwelling invertebrates. Membranous and horny tubes are not uncommon amongst tubiculous polychaetes but chitin has not been detected in them (Defretin, 1971; Brown & McGee-Russell, 1971) although it is present in the setae. The tube of the hemichordate, *Rhabdopleura*, which is superficially similar to the tube of a pogonophore, contains keratin-like protein as its structural component (Dilly, 1971).

Besides those of pogonophores only the tubes of phoronids are known to contain chitin (Jeuniaux, 1963).

The tubes of pogonophores have an obvious protective function but in addition probably are involved in the nutrition of these gutless animals. It was originally thought, as a result of superficial comparisons made with tubiculous polychaetes, that the tentacles of pogonophores were extended from the end of the tube for the purpose of collecting food particles and for respiration. According to Ivanov (1955) the food particles collected are then digested in temporary "stomachs" formed by adjoining tentacles, or a coiled single tentacle, and then absorbed through the thin cuticle of the tentacles. This plausible explanation of feeding has some serious flaws, however. First, many species do not have cilia or an abundance of mucous glands on their tentacles, two essentials of normal tentacular feeding methods. Second, the epidermis of the tentacles is composed almost entirely of unspecialized cells and there appears to be very little enzyme activity in the region of the tentacles in the species so far examined (Southward & Southward, 1966). This does not preclude the uptake of small particulate matter by a process of micropinocytosis (Nørrevang, 1965) since the cuticle is penetrated by numerous retractable microvilli, and Gupta et al. (1966) and Gupta & Little (1969) have observed many pinocytotic vesicles in the cells beneath the cuticle. This process, however, may equally well take place along the whole length of the body. Little & Gupta (1969) have suggested that because of the restricted permeability of the tube to organic molecules the space between the tube and the body wall may be acting as a digestive chamber. In this connection it may be significant that the long post-annular gonadal region appears to be well supplied with zymogen-secreting cells as well as with cells displaying pinocytotic activity (Gupta & Little, 1970).

Although there is still some discussion as to whether uptake of small organic particles by pinocytosis takes place on a sufficiently large scale to be of use to the animal, there is no doubt that some of the smaller pogonophores are capable of taking up dissolved organic matter through the epidermis in considerable amounts. This ability is not uncommon amongst free-living benthic soft-bodied Eumetazoa, but only as a supplement to normal feeding with a digestive tract (see A. J. Southward, 1975, for a recent review of the subject). It would appear that the ability to take up amino acids and glucose is several orders of magnitude higher at normal ambient concentrations in pogonophores than in other marine invertebrates that have been investigated (A. J. Southward, 1975). Small molecules such as amino acids and glucose (but not protein) diffuse through the tubes of pogonophores very rapidly. Thus it is feasible that the decayed organic matter present in the sediments in which the tubes are buried contributes many of the nutrients required by the animals.

It would appear that the pogonophore integument and its derivatives have a number of unique features and functions. Even so, many of the epidermal cell types are found throughout the animal kingdom. The presence of chitin as a structural component in the setae and tube, however, strongly suggests protostome rather than deuterostome affinities (Florkin, 1966; Hunt, 1970). Within the protostomes the annelids have a cuticle very similar to that of pogonophores.

ACKNOWLEDGEMENTS

I am grateful to Mr C. Ogden and Mr D. Claugher for assistance with transmission electron microscopy and for discussions relating to fine structure. Mr R. Harris skilfully dried some material for scanning electron microscopy.

REFERENCES

Bailey, A. J. (1968). The nature of collagen. In *Comprehensive biochemistry.* **26**B: 297–423. Florkin, M. & Stotz, E. H. (eds). Amsterdam: Elsevier Publishing Co.

Bairati, A. (1972). Collagen: an analysis of phylogenetic aspects. *Boll. Zool.* **39**: 205–248.

Blackwell, J., Parker, K. D. & Rudall, K. M. (1965). Chitin in pogonophore tubes. *J. mar. biol. Ass. U.K.* **45**: 659–661.

Boilly, B. (1967). Contribution à l'étude ultrastructurale de la cuticle épidermique et pharyngienne chez une annelide polychète (*Syllis amica* Quatrefages). *J. Microsc.* **6**: 469–484.

Bouligand, Y. (1967). Les soies et les cellules associées chez deux Annélides Polychètes. Étude en microscopie photonique à contraste de phase et en microscopie électronique. *Z. Zellforsch. mikrosk. Anat.* **79**: 332–363.

Bouligand, Y. (1972). Twisted fibrous arrangements in biological materials and cholesteric mesophases. *Tissue & Cell* **4**: 189–217.

Brocco, S. L., O'Clair, R. M. & Cloney, R. A. (1974). Cephalopod integument: the ultrastructure of Kölliker's organs and their relationship to setae. *Cell Tiss. Res.* **151**: 293–308.

220 J. DAVID GEORGE

Brown, S. C. & McGee-Russell, S. (1971). *Chaetopterus* tubes: ultrastructural architecture. *Tissue & Cell* **3**: 65–70.

Bubel, A. (1973). An electron-microscope investigation into the cuticle and associated tissues of the operculum of some marine serpulids. *Mar. Biol. Berl.* **23**: 147–164.

Caullery, M. (1914). Sur les Siboglinidae, type nouveau d'Invertébrés recueilli par l'expédition du Siboga. *C. r. hebd. Séanc. Acad. Sci., Paris* **158**: 2014–2017.

Coggeshall, R. E. (1966). A fine structural analysis of the epidermis of the earthworm, *Lumbricus terrestris* L. *J. Cell Biol.* **28**: 95–108.

Croll, N. A. (1970). *The behaviour of nematodes, their activity, senses and responses.* London: Edward Arnold.

Defretin, R. (1971). The tubes of polychaete annelids. In *Comprehensive biochemistry* **26C**: 713–747. Florkin, M. & Stotz, E. H. (eds). Amsterdam: Elsevier Publishing Co.

Dilly, P. N. (1971). Keratin-like fibres in the hemichordate *Rhabdopleura compacta*. *Z. Zellforsch. mikrosk. Anat.* **117**: 502–515.

Dorsett, D. A. & Hyde, R. (1969). The fine structure of the compound sense organs on the cirri of *Nereis diversicolor*. *Z. Zellforsch. mikrosk. Anat.* **97**: 512–527.

Fawcett, D. W. (1966). *An atlas of fine structure. The cell, its organelles and inclusions.* London: W. B. Saunders Co.

Florkin, M. (1966). *A molecular approach to phylogeny.* Amsterdam: Elsevier Publishing Co.

Foucart, M. F., Bricteux-Gregoire, S. & Jeuniaux, C. (1965). Composition chimique du tube d'un pogonophore (*Siboglinum* sp). et des formations squelettiques de deux pterobranchs. *Sarsia* **20**: 35–41.

George, J. D. (1973). The Pogonophora and their affinities. *Microscopy.* **32**: 242–252.

George, J. D. (1975). Observations on the pogonophore, *Siboglinum fiordicum* Webb from Fanafjorden, Norway. *Rep. Underwat. Ass.* (N.S.) **1**: 17–26.

George, J. D. & Southward, E. C. (1973). A comparative study of the setae of Pogonophora and polychaetous Annelida. *J. mar. biol. Ass. U.K.* **53**: 403–424.

Gubb, D. (1975). A direct visualisation of helicoidal architecture in *Carcinus maenas* and *Halocynthia papillosa* by scanning electron microscopy. *Tissue & Cell* **7**: 19–32.

Gupta, B. L. & Little, C. (1969). Studies on Pogonophora II. Ultrastructure of the tentacular crown of *Siphonobrachia*. *J. mar. biol. Ass. U.K.* **49**: 717–741.

Gupta, B. L. & Little, C. (1970). Studies on Pogonophora. 4. Fine structure of the cuticle and epidermis. *Tissue & Cell* **2**: 637–696.

Gupta, B. L. & Little, C. (1975). Ultrastructure phylogeny and Pogonophora. *Z. Zool. Syst. Evolforsch.* Sonderheft (1975): 45–63.

Gupta, B. L., Little, C. & Philip, A. M. (1966). Studies on Pogonophora. Fine structure of the tentacles. *J. mar. biol. Ass. U.K.* **46**: 351–372.

Gustus, R. M. & Cloney, R. A. (1972). Ultrastructure similarities between setae of brachiopods and polychaetes. *Acta zool., Stockh.* **53**: 229–233.

Hama, K. (1960). The fine structure of some blood vessels of the earthworm *Eisenia foetida*. *J. biophys. biochem. Cytol.* **7**: 717–724.

Hunt, D. (1970). *Polysaccharide-protein complexes in invertebrates.* London and New York: Academic Press.

Ivanov, A. V. (1952). [New Pogonophora from Far Eastern seas]. *Zool. Zh.* **31**: 372–391. [In Russian.]

Ivanov, A. V. (1955). On external digestion in Pogonophora. *Syst. Zool.* **3**: 174–176.

Ivanov, A. V. (1963). *Pogonophora*. London and New York: Academic Press.

Jägersten, G. (1952). Studies on the morphology, larval development and biology of *Protodrilus*. *Zool. Bidr. Upps.* **29**: 426–511.

Jägersten, G. (1956). Investigations on *Siboglinum ekmani*, n. sp. encountered in Skagerak. With some general remarks on the group Pogonophora. *Zool. Bidr. Upps.* **31**: 211–252.

Jeuniaux, C. (1963). *Chitine et chitinolyse*. Paris: Masson.

Knapp, M. F. & Mill, P. J. (1971). The fine structure of ciliated sensory cells in the epidermis of the earthworm, *Lumbricus terrestris*. *Tissue & Cell* **3**: 623–626.

Lee, D. (1972). The structure of the helminth cuticle. *Adv. Parasit.* **10**: 347–379.

Little, C. & Gupta, B. L. (1969). Studies on Pogonophora III. Uptake of nutrients. *J. exp. Biol.* **51**: 759–773.

Lumsden, R. D. (1975). Surface ultrastructure and cytochemistry of parasitic helminths. *Expl Parasit.* **37**: 367–339.

Lyons, K. M. (1966). The chemical nature and evolutionary significance of monogenean attachment sclerites. *Parasitology* **56**: 63–100.

Moritz, K. & Storch, V. (1970). Über den Aufbau des Integumentes der Priapuliden und der Sipunculiden (*Priapulus caudatus* Lamark, *Phascolion strombi* Montagu). *Z. Zellforsch. mikrosk. Anat.* **105**: 55–64.

Nørrevang, A. (1965). Structure and function of the tentacle and pinnules of *Siboglinum ekmani* Jägersten (Pogonophora), with special reference to the feeding problem. *Sarsia* **21**: 37–47.

Nørrevang, A. (1974). Photoreceptors of the phaosome (hirudinean) type in a pogonophore. *Zool. Anz.* **193**: 297–304.

Orrhage, L. (1971). Light and electron microscope studies of annelid setae. *Acta zool., Stockh.* **52**: 157–169.

Orrhage, L. (1973). Light and electron microscope studies of some brachiopod and pogonophoran setae. *Z. Morph. Tiere* **74**: 253–270.

Potswald, H. E. (1971). A fine structural analysis of the epidermis and cuticle of the oligochaete *Aelosoma bengalense* Stephenson. *J. Morph.* **135**: 185–212.

Richards, K. S. (1974a). The ultrastructure of the cuticle of some British lumbricids (Annelida). *J. Zool., Lond.* **172**: 303–316.

Richards, K. S. (1974b). The histochemistry of the small granular, proteinaceous cells (albumen cells) of the epidermis of some lumbricids. (Annelida: Oligochaeta). *Ann. Histochim.* **19**: 239–251.

Sleigh, M. A. (1962). *The biology of cilia and flagella*. Oxford: Pergamon Press.

Southward, A. J. (1975). On the evolutionary significance of the mode of feeding of Pogonophora. *Z. Zool. Syst. Evolforsch.* Sonderheft (1975): 77–85.

Southward, E. C. (1963). Pogonophora. *Oceanogr. mar. Biol.* **1**: 405–428.

Southward, E. C. (1971). Recent researches on the Pogonophora. *Oceanogr. mar. Biol.* **9**: 193–220.

Southward, E. C. (1972). On some Pogonophora from the Caribbean and the Gulf of Mexico. *Bull. mar. Sci.* **22**: 739–776.

Southward, E. C. (1973). The distribution of glycogen in the tissues of *Siboglinum atlanticum* (Pogonophora). *J. mar. biol. Ass. U.K.* **53**: 665–671.

Southward, E. C. (1975a). Fine structure and phylogeny of the Pogonophora. *Symp. zool. Soc. Lond.* No. 36: 235–251.

Southward, E. C. (1975b). A study of the structure of the opisthosoma of *Siboglinum fiordicum*. *Z. Zool. Syst. Evolforsch.* Sonderheft (1975): 64–76.

Southward, E. C. & Southward, A. J. (1966). A preliminary account of the general and enzyme histochemistry of *Siboglinum atlanticum* and other Pogonophora. *J. mar. biol. Ass. U.K.* **46**: 579–616.

Storch, V. & Welsch, U. (1970). Über die Feinstruktur der Polychaeten-Epidermis (Annelida). *Z. Morph. Tiere* **66**: 310–322.

Storch, V. & Welsch, U. (1972). Über Bau und Entstehung der Mantelstacheln von *Lingula unguis* L. (Brachiopoda). *Z. wiss. Zool.* **183**: 181–189.

Towe, K. M. & Lowenstam, H. A. (1967). Ultrastructure and development of iron mineralization in the radular teeth of *Cryptochiton stelleri* (Mollusca). *J. Ultrastruct. Res.* **25**: 84–92.

Webb, M. (1964a). The posterior extremity of *Siboglinum fiordicum*. (Pogonophora). *Sarsia* **15**: 33–36.

Webb, M. (1964b). A new bitentaculate pogonophoran from Hardangerfjorden, Norway. *Sarsia* **15**: 49–55.

Webb, M. (1965). Additional notes on the adult and larva of *Siboglinum fiordicum* and on the possible mode of tube formation. *Sarsia* **20**: 21–34.

Webb, M. (1971). The morphology and formation of the pogonophoran tube and its value in systematics. *Z. Zool. Syst. Evolforsch.* **9**: 169–181.

Symp. zool. Soc. Lond. (1977) No. 39, 223.

CHAIRMAN'S SUMMING UP ON LOWER ANIMALS

T. E. HUGHES

Cox Green Cottage, Rudgwick, Sussex, England

This collection of excellent papers emphasizes the range of structures constituting the integument. This diversity ranges from ciliated epithelium, through the syncytial covering of parasitic platyhelminths to the secreted coverings of nematodes and pogonophores. What emerges from these diverse findings may perhaps rashly be summarized as follows. In arthropods and molluscs a thin non-soluble membranous layer is first formed under which the epidermis can get on with the elaboration of a complex exoskeleton or shell. In some instances this boundary layer is secreted as a sheet and in some others as smaller units which then join up. This basic system is retained in the Oligochaeta and Pogonophora, both groups in which the epidermis is active but perhaps in need of physical insulation from the environment. In parasitic platyhelminths the plasma membrane of the covering syncytium is a sufficient boundary to the skin and develops complex properties in gut parasites. The nematodes illustrate their isolationist position, not only by possessing a cuticle secreted by cells remote from the surface, but also by having no limiting membranous layer under which the tropocollagen particles could be secreted without the hazard of dispersal before they are aggregated into collagen. Nevertheless, evidently this is not a problem as collagen formation occurs in the cuticle.

One observation from this collection of papers is that microvilli on epidermal cells, which are often present, require further attention. Their presence in pogonophoran epidermis may be associated with feeding but in other instances their function requires explanation.

Symp. zool. Soc. Lond. (1977) No. 39, 225–268.

EPIDERMAL BREEDING TUBERCLES AND BONY CONTACT ORGANS IN FISHES

BRUCE B. COLLETTE

Systematics Laboratory,
National Marine Fisheries Service,
National Museum of Natural History,
Washington DC, USA

SYNOPSIS

Breeding tubercles are epidermal structures which function primarily in facilitating contact between individual fishes during spawning. Tubercles are present on some species in at least 17 families of bony fishes in five orders: Salmoniformes (Salmonidae, Plecoglossidae, Osmeridae and Retropinnidae); Gonorhynchiformes (Kneriidae and Phractolaemidae); Cypriniformes (Characidae, Lebiasinidae, Parodontidae, Cyprinidae, Gyrinocheilidae, Psilorhynchidae, Catostomidae, Homalopteridae and Cobitidae); Scorpaeniformes (Cottocomephoridae); and Perciformes (Percidae). Analogous dermal structures, contact organs, are present on the scales or fin rays of eight families in three orders: Atheriniformes (Belonidae, Oryziatidae, Cyprinodontidae, Anablepidae and Poeciliidae); Cypriniformes (Characidae and Gasteropelecidae); and Scorpaeniformes (Cottidae).

There are three types of roughening structures: tubercles consisting of aggregations of non-keratinized epidermal cells; tubercles containing substantial numbers of fully keratinized cells that are organized to form a discrete, usually conical cap; and contact organs which are bony outgrowths from fin rays or scales. In most species, breeding tubercles and contact organs are present only on the male or are much better developed on the male than on the female. Development of these roughening structures is apparently controlled by pituitary and gonadal hormones. They begin to develop before the spawning season, reach their maximum extent just before or during the spawning season, and then regress.

Breeding tubercles or contact organs develop only on freshwater or inshore marine spawning species. These structures probably originally evolved to enable breeding individuals to maintain close contact during spawning to ensure fertilization of the eggs, which is particularly important in fishes that spawn in fast-moving water. Of the 24 families with roughening structures, 21 belong to groups of fishes with cycloid scales. Only three families belong to the Acanthopterygii, which usually have ctenoid scales. The structure of contact organs and ctenii is remarkably similar leading to the hypothesis that ctenoid scales may have evolved in higher fishes to permanently replace the contact organs and breeding tubercles found during the breeding season in lower fishes.

INTRODUCTION

Fishes that employ external fertilization when they spawn in moving waters must maintain close enough proximity so that sperm can reach the eggs. If body friction is low owing to a mucous coating and if the water is moving rapidly relative to the fish, proximity may be difficult to maintain because one fish will slide against the other. To prevent this and enable the male and female to stay in close contact long enough to ensure successful fertilization, two types of temporary roughening structures have evolved in primitive euteleostean fishes—epidermal breeding tubercles and dermal contact organs. Many advanced euteleostean fishes have ctenoid scales which are remarkably similar in structure to contact organs. This paper has two purposes. First, to summarize information on the structure, occurrence and function of breeding tubercles and contact organs and to add new data since the review by Wiley & Collette (1970). Second, to consider if the structural similarity between contact organs and ctenoid scales indicates reasons for the evolution of ctenoid scales.

Morphology

Most studies have been made on various species of Cyprinidae but there are papers on tubercles of Cobitidae (Jakubowski & Oliva, 1967), *Plecoglossus altivelis* (Ebina, 1929), and *Osmerus* (Richardson, 1942) and on contact organs of Oryziatidae (Oka, 1931). In addition to their summary of the literature, Wiley & Collette (1970) described and illustrated the structure of tubercles and contact organs in 45 species belonging to 20 families. An additional 15 species were briefly described.

Comparisons of nuptial tubercle morphology and histology have revealed significant differences among and within taxonomic categories. Because of the extent and nature of these differences, it is obvious that "nuptial tubercles" and their functional analogs, contact organs, have evolved independently in a variety of fish groups. Nuptial tubercles may be divided into three groups on the basis of their structure. (1) Tubercles consisting of aggregations of non-keratinized epidermal cells (if keratinization is present, it is confined to the most superficial layers of cells and may form a light covering). (2) Tubercles containing substantial numbers of fully keratinized cells organized to form a discrete, usually conical, cap; a major component of the tubercle. (3) Contact organs composed of dermal bony outgrowths or spicules projecting from a fin ray or scale margin and surrounded by the epidermis, through which the bony outgrowths may protrude.

These studies deal with the histological structure of breeding tubercles, yet what may be functionally significant is the surface structure. Recent studies include scanning electron micrographs (SEM) of sexually dimorphic roughening structures: Skelton (1974) on tubercles of *Oreodaimon quathlambae* (Cyprinidae) and Yamamoto & Egami (1974) on the contact organs of *Oryzias latipes*

(Oryziatidae). Several recent papers have also used SEM on scale structure, such as DeLamater & Courtenay (1973, 1974) and Lanzing & Higginbotham (1974). A preliminary survey by Ralph Yerger (pers. comm.) of the surface characteristics of breeding tubercles and contact organs by scanning electron microscopy indicates that this technique might produce useful results. SEM pictures from his survey are included in the present work under the Cyprinidae (pectoral fin breeding tubercles in *Notropis*) and the Cyprinodontidae (contact organs from the fin rays of *Fundulus* and the snout scales of *Lucania*).

The ability to produce keratinized epidermal structures is important to tetrapods adapting to a terrestrial existence. A great variety of keratinized structures has evolved: desiccation resistant scales in reptiles; avian feathers for flight and insulation; mammalian hair; and warts, tubercles, claws, nails and horns that serve many functions. Comparatively few fishes, however, have developed keratinized structures. Some authors (e.g. Burgess, 1956) have stated that it is unlikely that a keratinized layer is ever found in fish epidermis. Breeding tubercles are frequently composed of substantial amounts of keratin. (Similar epidermal tubercles occur on the scales of many colubrid snakes.) Other examples of keratinized structures are the horny teeth of cyclostomes, the sharp jaws in many species of herbivorous minnows, and horny teeth on the lips of the young in others, the frictional surface of the adhesive apparatus in various homalopterids, cyprinids and silurids, and the occipital organ in the gonorhynchiform genus *Kneria*.

The process of keratinization in breeding tubercles appears essentially the same in most fishes. Epidermal cells are produced by mitoses in a columnar to cuboidal stratum germinativum next to the basement membrane. Cells in more superficial layers hypertrophy and become polygonal. They are characterized by large vesicular nuclei with one or more prominent nucleoli and abundant, often granular, acidophilic cytoplasm. Well developed intercellular spaces and many intercellular bridges usually lie between the hypertrophied cells. The transition between hypertrophied cells and the keratinized layer is so abrupt that the transitional stage is rarely observed. During keratinization nuclei disappear or persist as pyknotic remnants in the flattened, irregular cells of the keratinized layer. The keratin becomes pale orange to red, in Mallory's triple stain. Undifferentiated epidermal cells of the germinal layer have pale blue cytoplasm that becomes darker blue as cells hypertrophy and accumulate prekeratin granules, and violet in the largest cells before keratinization. The nuclei of hypertrophied cells contain prominent, darkly stained nucleoli. Spearman (1973: 69) has mentioned finding bound phospholipids in *Leuciscus* (Cyprinidae) tubercles, which is characteristic of many keratinized cells. The histochemistry of epidermal keratinization of a catfish (*Bagarius*, Sisoridae) has recently been studied (Mittal & Banerjee, 1974).

FUNCTION

Breeding tubercles are present in regions of the male that come in contact with the female or other males. They have three inferred primary functions: maintenance of body contact between the sexes during spawning; defence of nests and territories; and stimulation of the females in breeding (see Reighard, 1903, 1904, 1910a,b, 1943). They may also function in sex and species recognition in some species. Males of species with well developed tubercles are more likely to fight and hold territories (Hubbs & Cooper, 1936; Raney, 1947). There is little evidence to support suggestions that tubercles protect body and fin surfaces in nest building, hold to the substrate during oviposition, tend the nest and eggs, or that anterior head tubercles are used for scooping out the redd.

Contact organs are also present on those parts of the body and fins of the male which are directly in contact with the female during prespawning or during the spawning act. The correlation between contact organ location and behaviour suggests that they may be tactile, enabling the male to determine his exact position relative to the female (Foster, 1967). There is some morphological evidence that contact organs are tactile receptors. Vital staining with methylene blue of the anal fin rays of *Oryzias latipes* showed better innervation of the contact organ-bearing fin rays of the male than of the female which lacks contact organs (Egami & Nambu, 1961). The anal fin contact organs of males of the African cyprinodont *Nothobranchius guentheri* each receive a lateral branch from a nerve fibre which runs the length of the fin ray (see Foster, 1967: 556).

CONTROL OF DEVELOPMENT

In most fishes, breeding tubercles and contact organs originate before the spawning season and reach their maximum extent just before or during it, to then break off, slough, become eroded, or gradually regress. The gonads and the pituitary seem to be the main organs that affect development of these nuptial structures. Many authors have studied the effects of hormones on breeding colours, gonads, and ovipositor lengths in fishes (see summaries in Breder & Rosen, 1966) but most have ignored the effects on breeding tubercles or contact organs. Nuptial structure development and control is known mainly from Japanese research on breeding tubercles in the Cyprinidae and contact organs in the Japanese medakà, *Oryzias latipes*. Information is also available for the Cobitidae and Plecoglossidae.

Gonadectomy prevents the development of nuptial structures or causes those already present to regress more quickly than usual in two species of minnows, *Oryzias*, and a loach (see Wiley & Collette, 1970). Female *Oryzias* develop contact organs after testis transplantation (Okada & Yamashita, 1944). Tubercles appeared on males of the bluntnose minnow (*Pimephales notatus*) after intraperitoneal injection of pituitary extract from unsexed carp and from frogs, sheep and humans (Ramaswami & Hasler, 1955); testosterone propionate stimulated tubercles to develop in both sexes. Wiley & Collette (1970: 150) summarized reports of several hormones that cause the development of nuptial structures in females (whether or not they normally develop them) in the Cobitidae, *Oryzias* and Cyprinidae. Smith (1974) added α-methyltestosterone in *Pimephales promelas* to this list. Esterone and thiourea slightly inhibit the development of contact organs of the female *Oryzias* maintained in solutions of testosterone propionate (Egami, 1954a, 1957). The relative androgenic potency of various steroids in causing the development of contact organs on the anal fins of femal *Oryzias* is in the following order: 19-norethylnyltestosterone > methyltestosterone > 11-ketotestosterone > androstenedione > androsterone > testosterone propionate > testosterone (Arai, 1964, 1967; Hishida & Kawamoto, 1970; Kawamoto, 1969, 1973).

Temperature and light play a role in the development of nuptial structures. Contact organs develop faster at higher temperatures in androgen-treated females of *Oryzias* (Egami, 1954b). Breeding tubercles appeared on male goldfish (*Carassius auratus*) within two weeks after increase in light from eight to 12 hours a day and disappeared three to four weeks after a decrease from 12 to eight hours (Pickford & Atz, 1957: 469). Tubercles developed most quickly at a certain optimum of light duration in *Plecoglossus altivelis* (Shiraishi & Takeda, 1961).

VALUE IN SYSTEMATICS

Patterns of distribution of breeding tubercles and contact organs aid our understanding of phyletic relationships. Similar distributions of contact organs or tubercles suggest similar reproductive behaviour patterns, and behavioural similarities in turn may suggest phylogenetic relationships. Behavioural patterns themselves are valuable but are difficult to use because live material is required. Studies that utilized tuberculation as a systematic character are numerous in the Cyprinidae (see Wiley & Collette, 1970: 169). Other groups where tubercles have proved useful in classification include Salmonidae (Koelz, 1929; Vladykov, 1970), Cobitidae (Vladykov, 1935), and Percidae (Collette, 1965).

In the Cyprinodontidae, Newman (1907, 1909) related contact organ function and structure to breeding biology, and Stenholt Clausen (1967) considered the phylogenetic implications of contact organ distribution in several African genera. Foster (1963, 1967) found contact organs valuable characters in his long-term studies on the evolution of reproductive behaviour in cyprinodontoids. The structure and distributional pattern of contact organs are useful characters in characin taxonomy (see Fink, 1976; Fink & Weitzman, 1974).

OCCURRENCE

Breeding tubercles and contact organs are restricted to bony fishes belonging to the cohort Euteleostei of Greenwood, Rosen, Weitzman & Myers (1966), and they are not known to occur in any of the more primitive elopomorph, clupeomorph or osteoglossomorph fishes. Thus, the potential for the development of these structures was apparently present in ancestral euteleosteans and has manifested itself in diverse groups of living Euteleostei. Tubercles are present on some species in at least 17 families of fishes in five orders: Salmoniformes (Salmonidae, Plecoglossidae, Osmeridae and Retropinnidae): Gonorhynchiformes (Kneriidae and Phractolaemidae); Cypriniformes (Characidae, Lebiasinidae, Parodontidae, Cyprinidae, Gyrinocheilidae, Psilorhynchidae, Catostomidae, Homalopteridae and Cobitidae); Scorpaeniformes (Cottocomephoridae); and Percifomes (Percidae). Analogous dermal structures, contact organs, are present on the scales or fin rays of eight families in three orders: Atheriniformes (Belonidae,

Oryziatidae, Cyprinodontidae, Anablepidae and Poeciliidae); Cypriniformes (Characidae and Gasteropelecidae); and Scorpaeniformes (Cottidae). In most species, breeding tubercles or contact organs are only present or are much better developed on males.

SALMONIFORMES

Salmonoidei–Salmonoidea

Salmonidae

The Salmonidae includes three subfamilies (Norden, 1961): Salmoninae (trouts and salmons), Thymallinae (graylings) and Coregoninae (whitefishes). Tubercles have been reported for two species of Salmoninae, in numerous species of Coregoninae but in no Thymallinae.

Salmoninae

Five genera are recognized for the approximately 33 species of Salmoninae (Norden, 1961): *Brachymystax, Hucho, Salvelinus, Salmo* and *Oncorhynchus*. Some authors separate the monotypic *Cristivomer* from *Salvelinus*. Pappenheim (1909) reported tubercles on males of *Hucho hucho* (Linnaeus) at spawning time. Vladykov (1954, 1970) found both sexes of *Cristivomer namaycush* (Walbaum) are tuberculate and he (1954) illustrated tubercles on the scales anterior to the anal fin of a breeding male. Males of the Atlantic salmon, *Salmo salar* Linnaeus, and the sea trout, *Salmo trutta trutta* Linnaeus, develop rough and thickened skin during the breeding season (Menzies, 1931; Stokłosowa, 1966). As Stokłosowa indicated, the thickened skin may be an adaptation functionally analogous to tuberculation in other fishes. Yamazaki (1972) studied the histology of the thickened skin produced in Pacific salmon (*Oncorhynchus*) by oral administration of methyltestosterone. In the experimental groups the total thickness of the epidermis became four times thicker than in controls owing to hypertrophy of epithelial cells and cell division in the stratum germinativum.

Thymallinae

There are no reports of tubercles for this subfamily of four species in the genus *Thymallus*.

Coregoninae

Three genera are presently recognized (Norden, 1961): *Prosopium* (six species), *Coregonus* (about 20, including *Leucichthys*) and *Stenodus* (one). Tubercles have been reported on males of species in each genus and on females of some species. They are present in at least three of the six species of round whitefishes, *Prosopium* (see Wiley & Collette, 1970). Both sexes may be tuberculate with tubercles concentrated on several scale rows above and below the lateral line and extending out onto the fins in highly tuberculate males. Many publications recorded tubercles in European species of *Coregonus* (see Wiley & Collette, 1970). The first and the most complete descriptions in North American *Coregonus* were by Koelz (1929) who described their distribution for each population of each species of Great Lakes *Coregonus* (including *Leucichthys*) where breeding material was available. Tubercles are concentrated on the lateral scales for several rows above and below the lateral line. In some species, tubercles extend onto virtually all the scales. Both sexes are usually tuberculate with better development in the males. Hart (1930) and Fabricius & Lindroth (1954) described tubercles and spawning behaviour in species of *Coregonus* (see also Wiley & Collette, 1970). Berg (1948) noted the presence of tubercles on the head and sides of *Stenodus leucichthys* (Güldenstädt) males during the spawning season. Alaskan *Stenodus* are not known to develop tubercles but Alt (1971) described and figured tubercles in hybrid *Stenodus leucichthys* × *Coregonus pidschian*.

Koelz (1929) and Vladykov (1970) have used breeding tubercles as a systematic character at the generic and subgeneric level in the Coregoninae.

Wiley & Collette (1970) described tubercles in *Prosopium williamsoni* (Girard) and *Coregonus clupeaformis* (Mitchill). They are formed by hyperplasia, a local thickening of the epidermis over the scale due to increase in cell number. All cells above a plane parallel to the scale surface are keratinized and form a hemispheroid layer 184 μm thick and 556 μm wide. It is significant that cell hypertrophy plays little or no part in development of the tubercle in contrast with other keratinized tubercles.

Osmeroidea

Tubercles of *Plecoglossus*, the various smelts, and the retropinnids all have very similar morphology, the chief difference being in shape and size. All are characterized by slight to moderate amounts of cellular hypertrophy and none to slight amounts of keratinization in the surface layers. *Mallotus catervarius* is unusual in that the largest hypertrophied cells are those nearest the stratum germinativum, the reverse of the usual situation.

Rosen (1974) used this similarity in breeding tubercles as one of a series of characters that related the Retropinnidae to the Osmeridae and Plecoglossidae. He also added the neotenic non-tuberculate Salangidae to these three families to form the super-family Osmeroidea, the sister group of the Salmonoidea in the Salmonoidei.

Plecoglossidae

The ayu, *Plecoglossus altivelis* (Temminck and Schlegel), of rivers in Japan, China and Korea, is the only species in this family. Jordan & McGregor (1925) first reported the breeding male *Plecoglossus* to have tubercles on the anal fin rays. The "nuptial organs" in adult males cover almost the entire body surface—head, gill covers, scales, adipose fin and rays of all the other fins. These tubercles differ from those of cyprinids because they lack an outer cornified layer. Ebina (1929) also found large unicellular glands in *Plecoglossus* tubercles. Females also develop tubercles (Ebina, 1930; Matsui, 1950) but they are not as widely distributed on the body nor as well developed. Shiraishi & Takeda (1961) reported on the effect of photoperiodicity on the development of tubercles in this species.

Wiley & Collette (1970) described and illustrated scale and fin tubercles of *Plecoglossus*. Tubercles are wider than high (360× 213 μm in an anal fin tubercle). They form by hypertrophy of epidermal cells above the cuboidal germinal layer. Most hypertrophied cells are somewhat flattened and in section they are spindle-shaped with the longitudinal axes oriented parallel to the basement membrane. Surface cells are squamous but much thicker than in ordinary epithelium (8–13 μm v. 2 μm). Keratinization is slight.

Osmeridae

The smelt family includes six genera and ten species (McAllister, 1963). They are found in boreal and subarctic waters of the northern hemisphere and are marine, anadromous or freshwater dwellers. They spawn over sandy areas in fresh or salt water. Males are smaller than females, frequently have longer paired fins than females, and may develop enlarged scales along the lateral line. There are reports of breeding tubercles developing during the spawning season on the head, scales and fins of males of all ten species (McAllister, 1963; Wiley & Collette, 1970). Histological descriptions of tubercles have been published for four genera— *Osmerus* (Richardson, 1942), and *Spirinchus, Thaleichthys* and *Mallotus* (Wiley & Collette, 1970).

Smelt tubercles are formed largely by cellular hypertrophy, and hyperplasia in *Thaleichthys* tubercles. One or two surface cell layers of squamous epithelial cells keratinize in some smelts (seen with Mallory's triple stain). Lepidotrichia underlying fin tubercles are modified by the deposition of additional bone on the outer surface.

Retropinnidae

This family contains the monotypic New Zealand genus *Stokellia* and five species of *Retropinna* in New Zealand, Australia, Tasmania and the Chatham Islands (McDowall, 1969). Some species are confined to fresh water, others are estuarine, or marine, but all spawn in fresh water (McDowall, 1969). Wiley & Collette (1970) summarized reports of tubercles for *Stokellia anisodon* (Stokell) and *Retropinna retropinna* (Richardson). As in the Osmeridae, males have larger dorsal, anal, pectoral and pelvic fins than females. Tubercles develop on the scales and fins of breeding males and females but are better developed in males (McDowall, 1972).

Tubercles of *R. retropinna* are hemispherical and are formed by an aggregation of slightly hypertrophied cells that are about 5 μm in diameter. There is no evidence of keratinization. Tubercles of *R. chathamensis* Stokell (= *R. retropinna*) and *Stokellia anisodon* are similar to those of *R. retropinna* (see Wiley & Collette, 1970).

GONORHYNCHIFORMES

Chanoidei

Several species in two families (Kneriidae and Phractolaemidae) of the suborder Chanoidei, develop keratinized nuptial structures. In *Kneria*, males of several species develop small breeding tubercles and an "occipital organ" that functions during breeding and is keratinized on the surface. In *Phractolaemus*, tubercles consist of a heavy conical cap of keratinized epithelium supported by a core of hypertrophied epithelial cells.

Kneriidae

The Kneriidae comprise small African freshwater fishes of two genera (*Kneria* and *Parakneria*) and about a dozen species that live in fast-moving streams (Poll, 1965; Peters, 1967). *Kneria* is characterized by possessing a sexually dimorphic occipital organ in the opercular region and many fine breeding tubercles on the dorsum of the head and body. The female also develops small tubercles.

Peters (1967) described the structure of the occipital organ and breeding tubercles in *Kneria*. In section, a small tubercle resembles a transverse section of the ridges in the occipital organ, which is formed by fusion of small tubercles. Peters concluded that the occipital organ acts as a clasper to hold the sexes in close contact during breeding in swiftly flowing waters. *Parakneria*, which live on the bottoms of streams, lack the occipital organ.

Phractolaemidae

This African freshwater family contains one species with two subspecies, *Phractolaemus ansorgei ansorgei* Boulenger and *P. a. spinosus* Pellegrin, (Thys van den Audenaerde, 1961a). Several literature reports of tubercles date back to the original description. However, it was not until later that the tubercles were identified as sexually dimorphic structures. Males have four tusk-like circumorbital tubercles and prominent spine-like tubercles on three rows of nine scales each above the lateral line. Smaller, less conspicuous tubercles are on the anal and caudal fin rays and posteriorly on several rows of scales above and below the lateral line. The female also has small tubercles on many lateral body scales, the caudal fin rays and head, but none are as well developed as on the male. Thys van den Audenaerde (1961a: figs 2–5, 1961b) summarized information on *Phractolaemus* tubercles. The circumorbital tubercles of the male are probably used in fighting, whereas the lateral tubercles of both sexes probably aid in maintaining contact during spawning.

Wiley & Collette (1970) described postorbital, opercular and caudal peduncle tubercles in *Phractolaemus*. Each type has a well-developed keratinized cap ranging in thickness from 5 μm in a microscopic opercular tubercle in the female to 337 μm in a large postorbital tubercle from the male (Fig. 1). The orbital and caudal peduncle tubercles have a well developed vascular system of capillary loops that extend into the hypertrophied layer.

CYPRINIFORMES

There are three main groups of Ostariophysi. Some authors place the catfishes in a separate order (Siluriformes) from the minnows

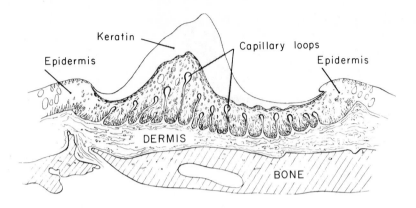

FIG. 1. Diagrammatic drawing of a section through a postorbital tubercle of *Phrac-tolaemus ansorgei*. The hypertrophied epithelium supporting the keratinized cap is vascularized by blood vessels from the dermis. (From Wiley & Collette, 1970: fig. 1.)

and characins; others (e.g. Roberts, 1973a) consider all three groups as suborders of the Cypriniformes. Representatives of several families of Characoidei have tubercles and/or contact organs, all six families of Cyprinoidei develop breeding tubercles, and non-sexually dimorphic structures, similar in structure to tubercles, are present in a few families of Siluroidei (see Wiley & Collette, 1970). In many species of the catfish family Loricariidae, breeding males develop long spines on the sides of the head, the predorsal region, and the upper surface of the pectoral and pelvic fins (see, for example, Isbrücker 1973a,b). It is not yet clear if these spines are analogous to contact organs but the situation merits further study.

Characoidei

Of the 16 families of characins, contact organs are present in many species of Characidae and in at least five species of Gasteropelecidae and breeding tubercles are probably present in all species of Parodontidae, at least five species of Lebiasinidae, and some species of Characidae, sometimes occurring simultaneously on fish with contact organs. Tubercles and contact organs occur only on males in the Characoidei as far as is known. Although they are widely reported in the taxonomic literature on characins, there appear to be no histological studies (other than Wiley & Collette, 1970) and no experimental work on them, which seems odd in view of the great popularity of the group with aquarists.

Characidae

Males of many species of characids develop specialized bony fin-ray contact organs that serve to hold the sexes in close contact during the active and sometimes violent movements of the spawning act. Some glandulocaudine characids, in which fertilization is internal (Nelson, 1964), have these structures well developed on the anal, caudal and pelvic fins. Structurally, characid contact organs are similar to those in the Cyprinodontidae and Cottidae. The earliest reference to contact organs in the Characidae according to Roberts (1973b) is that of Jenyns (1842) who reported "asperities" on the anal fin of species of *Astyanax* and *Cheirodon* and rightly concluded they were sexually dimorphic characters of the male. Characin hooks have also been reported by Eigenmann, Fowler, Schultz, Böhlke and Géry although their biological significance was not often mentioned (see Wiley & Collette, 1970). Fink & Weitzman (1974) were apparently the first to report seasonal variation in characin hooks. They found that *Cheirodon affinis* (Meek and Hildebrand) had retrose hooks on the anal and pelvic fin rays of males collected between March and July but that hooks were absent in specimens collected in October and January. Weitzman & Thomerson (1970) recognized two types of contact organs in the glandulocaudine *Hysteronotus*: strong hooks, one per ray segment on the anal fin, and small, slender, easily broken spinelets, one or more per segment on the anal and pelvic fin rays. Fink & Weitzman (1974) also recognized these two types of contact organs but as hooks and spinules. They found hooks on the anal and pelvic fin rays of males of four species of *Cheirodon* (also on the caudal rays of a fifth species), hooks on the caudal fin rays of at least three species of *Saccoderma*, but spinules on the anal and pelvic fin rays of *Carlana eigenmanni* (Meek). *Phenagoniates macrolepis* (Meek & Hildebrand), which they felt was unrelated to the other cheirodontines in the paper, lacks hooks and spinules. Fink (1976) described the spinules in his new *Eretmobrycon bayano* and contrasted them with the hooks and spinules on other characids. Géry (1973) found all four new species in his new genus *Tyttobrycon* had hooks on the anal fins in males. *T. hamatus* is particularly unusual in being among the smallest of the characoids (maximum length of females 17 mm S.L.), yet having a very strong hook on each side of the last simple ray and the first branched ray in the anal fins of males. Representative hooks and spinules from anal fins of males of three species of characids and one gasteropelecid are shown in Fig. 2. The maximum distribution of contact organs in the Characidae appears to be in *Bryconamericus peruanus* (Müller and Troschel) which has hooks on all fins supported by rays (Böhlke, 1958: 112).

Epidermal breeding tubercles occur in some species of Characidae and may occur simultaneously with dermal contact organs, [reported by Meek & Hildebrand (1916: 284) in the original description of *Bryconamericus cascajalensis* in a reference overlooked by Collette & Wiley (1970): "Breeding males with small bluish tubercles on head and margins of scales. . . . Fins in breeding males with barbs, making them rough to the touch"]. Fink (1976) recently found breeding tubercles present in males of some species of *Bryconamericus* and absent in others suggesting that the character may be useful in systematics. Breeding tubercles are distributed all over the head and body of an apparently undescribed species of *Bryconamericus* from the Pacific drainage of Ecuador, and two undescribed species related to *Ceratobranchia* from the Amazon basin of Ecuador (Roberts, 1973a: 379). I have examined material of one of the latter two species that Weitzman and Böhlke refer to the genus *Monotocheirodon*. This species is superficially very similar to some members of the cyprinid genus *Notropis* in body shape, pigment, pattern and distribution of breeding tubercles. Tubercles are concentrated on the head-snout, lower jaw, upper jaw, interorbital region, branchiostegal rays, opercle and preopercle and are also present on scales above the lateral line extending posteriorly to the dorsal fin. All appear to be simple without a well developed keratinized cap.

Hooks on the anal fin rays of *Astyanax fasciatus* were described by Wiley & Collette (1970). The contact organs are formed by proximally directed, sharp bony processes growing from the fin rays. They are arranged in rows along the fin rays and have an epidermal investment through which the points may penetrate under pressure.

Gasteropelecidae

There are three genera and about ten species of South American freshwater hatchet fishes (Weitzman, 1954). Contact organs are present on the posterior surface of some anal fin rays in at least five species—*Gasteropelecus maculatus* Steindachner, *G. sternicla* (Linnaeus), *Carnegiella marthae* Myers, *C. strigata* (Günther) and *C. vesca* Fraser-Brunner—in two of the three genera. I was unable to find any contact organs in the limited available material of the two species of *Thoracocharax*. The only literature reference to contact organs in the Gasteropelecidae is that of Weitzman (1954: 225)

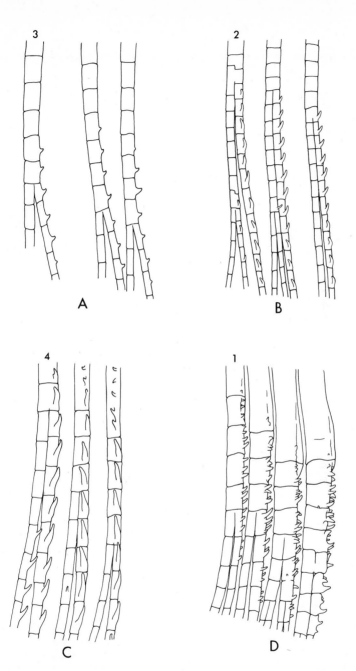

FIG. 2. Anal fin contact organs ("hooks") in four genera of characoid fishes (A, Gasteropelecidae; B–D, Characidae). A. *Carnegiella strigata*, branched rays 3–5. B. *Astyanax mexicanus* (Filippi), branched rays 2–4. C. *Eretmobrycon bayano* Fink, branched rays 4–6. D. *Cheirodon* sp., branched rays 1–4.

who reported them on anal rays 6–16 in males of *Carnegiella vesca* and illustrated them on the sixth anal ray. Contact organs are absent from the first few rays in the fin, present on rays 3–7 to continue posteriorly as far as rays 11–26, and then are absent from the last 6–20 rays depending on species and relative maturity. The contact organs appear as small spines, usually one per segment per side, but sometimes two or three, or even as many as six, may develop on the posterior surface of the rays. The spines start on segment 2–7 of a fin ray and continue to segment 2–5 from the distal end of the fin. When a ray is branched, contact organs are present only on the postero-lateral surface of the posterior branch. The simple contact organs on branched rays 3–5 of the anal fin of a male *Carnegiella strigata* are shown in Fig. 2A.

Parodontidae

Myers (1930) first reported tubercles from the snout and internasal regions in his new *Parodon apolinari*. Tubercles occur on ten species of Parodontidae—*Apareiodon affinis* (Steindachner), seven species of *Parodon* and two species of *Saccodon* (Wiley & Collette, 1970).

In *Parodon hilarii* Reinhardt, small tubercles on the snout and head form by keratinization of several layers of cells into a simple cap supported by hypertrophied cells beneath (Wiley & Collette, 1970); they resemble the simple tubercles of other cypriniform fishes, especially some in the family Cyprinidae.

Lebiasinidae

This small family of small to moderate-sized predacious South American characins has two subfamilies: Lebiasininae and Pyrrhulininae. Tubercles occur on five species in the two tribes of the Pyrrhulininae, Pyrrhulinini and Nannostomini (Wiley & Collette, 1970).

Pyrrhulinini

Small tubercles are arranged in a row along the posterior margins of some lateral scales of males in this tribe. They resemble retropinnid tubercles, being formed by hyperplasia and lacking a keratinized layer. They are hemispheroid in shape and in section are 79 μm high and 182 μm wide with ten–12 cell layers. A section of a *Copeina* tubercle is almost identical to the *Pyrrhulina* tubercle but smaller (52 μm high, 91 μm wide, with about ten cell layers). The breeding habits of these species are not known but they probably spawn with their bodies pressed together laterally.

Nannostomini

The tribe Nannostomini contains 11 small species which are not known to exceed 44·5 mm S.L. (Weitzman & Cobb, 1975). Their tubercle pattern is strikingly different from that in the Pyrrhulinini. Tubercles appear to be restricted to the ventral parts of the head of males in this tribe. Wiley & Collette (1970) reported tubercles on males of *Nannostomus bifasciatus* Hoedeman, 27–43 mm S.L. At maximum development, they covered the ventral surface of the head with the largest ones on the lower jaw. Weitzman & Cobb (1975) counted about 150 tubercles on one male in this series. They also figured tiny tubercles on the ventral surface of the head of a male *N. minimus* Eigenmann. Rows of tubercles occur on the ventral margins of the infraorbital bones and the ventral margins of the hyoid arch of a large male *N. unifasciatus* (Steindachner) (Wiley & Collette, 1970). Detailed information on the breeding habits of these species is lacking but tubercles of male *N. bifasciatus* contact the head and dorsum of the female during courtship (Nieuwenhuizen, 1964).

Tubercles from *Nannostomus bifasciatus* are formed by hypertrophy of epithelial cells into low mounds that are about 160–180 μm in diameter and 65–80 μm high from basement membrane to tip. The hypertrophied cells reach about 13 μm diameter and have large, vesicular nuclei. A few cells at the tip of some tubercles stained red with Mallory's triple stain, indicating some keratinization. No distinct keratinized cap is formed, however, as in tubercles of the Parodontidae (Wiley & Collette, 1970).

Cyprinoidei

Members of all six families in the suborder Cyprinoidei develop breeding tubercles: Cyprinidae, Gyrinocheilidae, Psilorhynchidae, Catostomidae, Homalopteridae (including Gastromyzonidae) and Cobitidae.

Cyprinidae

The large family Cyprinidae (about 2000 species), containing about ten subfamilies (Bănărescu, 1968) with many different and divergent adaptations, is widely distributed over the North American, Eurasian and African continents. Breeding tubercles have been more widely studied in minnows than in any other family. Wiley & Collette (1970) summarized the most important references by geographic area. More than 100 genera contain tuberculate species.

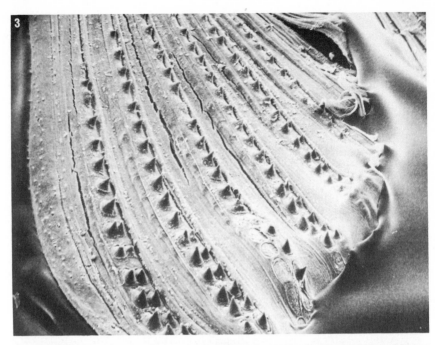

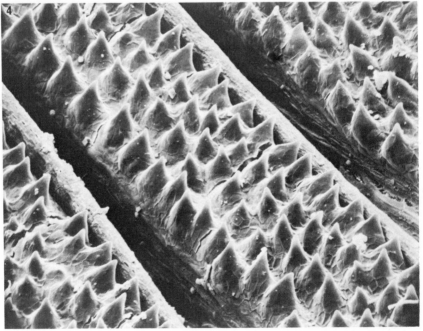

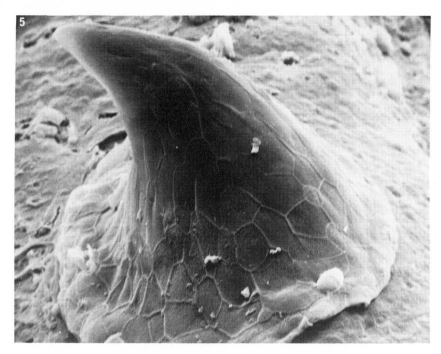

FIGS 3–5. Scanning electron micrographs of pectoral fin breeding tubercles in *Notropis* (Cyprinidae). (3) *N. lutipinnis* (Jordan and Brayton), × 12. (4) *N. petersoni* Fowler, × 122. (5) *N. chrosomus* (Jordan), × 375.

Most morphological and histological work on nuptial tubercles has been done on species of Cyprinidae. Such studies include those on breeding tubercles of the goldfish, *Carassius auratus* (Linnaeus), which consist of two types of cells (Tozawa, 1923). In the formation of breeding tubercles, the number of cell layers increases from the normal 15–20 to 25–30. Layers of hypertrophied cells bulge exteriorly to form the tubercle and internally form a pocket in the dermis. The hypertrophied cells are covered with a cornified cap, 90–150 μm thick, composed of scaly cornified cells with pycnotic nuclei or without nuclei. Similar structure has been reported for the breeding tubercles of other cyprinids (Tozawa, 1929; Sato, 1935; Kimura & Tao, 1937; Aisa, 1958, 1959). Scanning electron micrographs of the tubercles of a minnow, *Oreodaimon quathlambae* (Barnard), were presented by Skelton (1974). SEM pictures of pectoral fin breeding tubercles are included here as Figs 3–5.

Wiley & Collette (1970) described tubercles from 14 genera of Cyprinidae: *Acrossocheilus, Barbus, Campostoma, Clinostomus, Garra,*

Labeo, Leuciscus, Nocomis, Notropis, Onychostoma, Phenacobius, Pseudorasbora, Semotilus and *Varichorhinus*. Nuptial tubercle structure in cyprinids is extremely variable between species. Those with the simplest structure are minute ones (*Phenacobius mirabilis*), and the small ones which are found on the pectoral fin surfaces of many other species. These tubercles show epithelial hypertrophy and hyperplasia, those on the surface keratinizing to form a cap of compact cells supported internally by a core of hypertrophied epithelial cells. The largest tubercles with a similar degree of simplicity are found in *Leuciscus, Barbus* and *Pseudorasbora*; here tubercles do not exceed one mm in height and consist simply of a conical keratinized cap supported by an internal core of hypertrophied epithelium. Larger tubercles in the North American genera *Pimephales, Nocomis, Campostoma* and *Semotilus* are more complex because of vascularized dermal papillae which extend into the epithelial core and the presence (as in *Campostoma*) of a keratinized cap of several distinct layers. In these tubercles, dermal papillae are accompanied by a layer of the stratum germinativum and probably serve to provide nutrition to the rapidly growing epidermal cells of the tubercle as well as increasing the number of germinative cells required for rapid growth characteristic of developing tubercles.

In some Eurasian and African cyprinids (*Labeo* and *Garra*), tubercles form as keratinized caps supported by hypertrophied and hyperplastic epithelium of underlying pit or sac-like epithelial invaginations. Penetrating throughout the hypertrophied cells of the tubercle pit are numerous vascularized dermal papillae which, in this type, are devoid of any accompanying germinal epithelium. The significance of the vascularized sac-like structure cannot be determined with certainty; however, it appears to function in the maintenance of a relatively large epithelial structure over an extended reproductive period.

The epithelial-pit tubercles appear to be distinct from those in cyprinids which do not develop a pit. Intermediate forms exist, however, and the series represented successively by *Pseudorasbora parva, Nocomis leptocephalus, Onychostoma leptura, Garra taeniata, Garra gotyla* and *Labeo annectens* may illustrate an evolutionary sequence of epithelial-pit tubercles. In *Pseudorasbora*, the keratinized cap is supported by a simple core of hypertrophied epithelium. In *Nocomis*, the core is supplied by vascularized dermal papillae accompanied by a stratum germinativum, in *Onychostoma* and succeeding examples, the dermal papillae lack accompanying germinativum. In *Garra taeniata*, a rather open epithelial pit is developed, becoming deeper and more flask-shaped in *G. gotyla* and comparatively deep and narrow in *Labeo*.

Studies of distribution patterns of breeding tubercles as systematic characters in the Cyprinidae are summarized by Wiley & Collette (1970). Other similar recent papers include those by Lachner & Jenkins (1971) in *Nocomis*, Hubbs & Miller (1974) in *Dionda*, and Snelson & Pflieger (1975) in subspecies of *Notropis umbratilis* (Girard).

Additional information on Cyprinidae is available (see Wiley & Collette, 1970) on tubercles in females of 35 species of minnows and male hybrids of 16 different combinations. Others have dealt with the increase in tuberculation as the spawning season progresses: Kimura & Tao (1937) in three species of Chinese minnows, Koehn (1965) in the American *Notropis lutrensis* (Baird and Girard), Lachner & Jenkins (1971) in *Nocomis*, and Wallace (1973) and Ross (1974) in *Ericymba buccata* (Cope). In all cases maximum tubercle development occurs at the height of the spawning season. More is known about the breeding behaviour of minnows than about any other family with tuberculate species (see Reighard, Raney, and others, summarized by Wiley & Collette, 1970). Tubercles are concentrated on the head and snout of many species and in several species are employed in protecting the nest from other fishes.

Gyrinocheilidae

The Gyrinocheilidae is one of the most peculiar cyprinoid families in its mouth structure, absence of pharyngeal teeth, and presence of both exhalent and inhalent gill openings (Hora, 1923; Smith, 1945). This South-East Asian family consists of the genus *Gyrinocheilus* with two species—*G. aymonieri* (Tirant) and *G. pennocki* (Fowler). In raising the group to family level, Hora (1923) noted the tubercles that stud the proboscis of *G. aymonieri* (as *G. kaznakovi* Berg). Other reports of tubercles were made by Fowler (1937), Smith (1945) and Wiley & Collette (1970). In *G. aymonieri*, tubercles begin in juveniles. Prominent rostral tubercles are present in both sexes and become largest in females.

Sections of a large rostral tubercle of *G. aymonieri* reveal a number of unique structural features. The tubercle consists of an invagination of epithelium into a thickened pad of collagenous connective tissue, forming a sac or pit-like structure similar to that in some of the cyprinid fishes. There the similarity ends. At the surface the functional tubercle comprises a solid cone of keratinized epithelial cells. It is not a hollow keratinized cone filled with and supported by a core of hypertrophied epithelium. Below the functional tubercle a second, fully formed replacement apparently will move to the surface to replace the functional one when it is lost (Fig. 6). Below the replacement may be one or two aggregations of hypertrophied epithelial cells in the process of keratinizing to form additional replacements. The *Gyrinocheilus* tubercle pit is highly vascularized by a series of parallel, vertically oriented blood vessels that give off numerous capillaries which anastomose into a complex network that completely encloses and penetrates the peripheral layers of the tubercle epidermis. An additional unique feature is that all the epithelial cells in the pit contributing to tubercle formation are binucleate. The very fine, minute tubercles common in the male do not develop from a pit and are not vascularized but have a morphology similar to that of cobitid and homalopterid tubercles. Binucleate cells are not as apparent in these small tubercles as they are in the large ones but are seen in some sections (see Wiley & Collette, 1970).

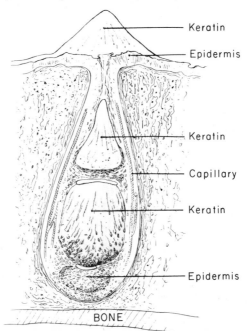

Fig. 6. Diagrammatic drawing of a section through a *Gyrinocheilus aymonieri* snout tubercle showing developing replacement tubercles. (From Wiley & Collette, 1970: fig. 7.)

Psilorhynchidae

This is a small family of peculiar fishes from the Himalayas and the Assam hills of India, Burma and Nepal, assigned by various authors to the Cyprinidae, Cobitidae and Homalopteridae but now considered a distinct family (Hora & Mukerji, 1935; Hora, 1952). Four species, all in the genus *Psilorhynchus*, are recognized (Menon & Datta, 1964). There are reports of small tubercles on the snout and head of *P. homaloptera* (Hora & Mukerji, 1935) and *P. pseudecheneis* (Menon & Datta, 1964). The latter included photographs which clearly show tubercles all over the top of the head and on the dorsal surface of the pectoral fin rays.

Tubercles from the operculum, pectoral fin and scales of male *Psilorhynchus homaloptera* Hora and Mukerji are very similar to tubercles in the Cobitidae and Homalopteridae in shape, size and structure (Wiley & Collette, 1970).

Catostomidae

The suckers are a predominantly North American family of 12 genera and about 80 species of medium to large size freshwater fishes. There are reports (see Wiley & Collette, 1970) of breeding tubercles on males of species in all genera except the now extinct *Lagochila lacera* Jordan and Brayton and the Chinese *Myxocyprinus asiatius* (Bleeker). Tubercles are usually present on most of the lateral surface of the fish—scales, anal, dorsal and caudal fins, and sides of the head. They also occur in females of several genera but they are smaller and not as widespread. Several workers used tubercle distribution as a systematic character (Hubbs, 1930; Branson, 1962; Branson & McCoy, 1966; Huntsman, 1967). Madsen (1971) described tubercles in female *Carpiodes*, McSwain & Gennings (1972) spawning in *Minytrema*, and Koch (1973) tubercles in *Chasmistes*.

Moxostoma erythrurum (Rafinesque) and *Erimyzon sucetta* (Lacépède) differ from each other in tubercle morphology (Wiley & Collette, 1970). Those of *M. erythrurum* are simply mounds of cells formed by epithelial hypertrophy and hyperplasia with keratinization of the tissue above a plane parallel to the surface. In contrast, snout tubercles of *E. sucetta* have a solid keratinized cone supported by vascularized hypertrophied epithelium and closely resemble some of the larger cyprinid tubercles.

Homalopteridae

This family of small loach-like fishes inhabits torrential streams of

248 BRUCE B. COLLETTE

South-East Asia. Silas (1953) recognized two families: the Homalopteridae with 12 genera and 53 species, and the Gastromyzonidae with 16 genera and 31 species. Greenwood *et al.* (1966) considered them one family.

Homalopterids of both sexes often have breeding tubercles scattered over the entire body. Although superficially like those of cyprinids, homalopterid tubercles differ in that the keratinized cap is composed of a single layer of cells but the hypertrophied cells beneath are enlarged to about the same size, are in the same stage of keratinization, and form a well defined, uniform layer destined to become another keratin cap. Tubercles apparently persist and this type of growth enables replacement.

Homalopterinae

Several earlier workers noted or figured tubercles without clearly pointing out they were breeding tubercles. Wiley & Collette (1970) summarized the literature and added additional tuberculate species. Tubercles are now known for species in six genera: *Balitoria, Balitoropsis, Bhavania, Hemimyzon, Homaloptera* and *Sinogastromyzon*. They are present on females in some species. Most species have tubercles on the snout or dorsal surface of the head; some frequently extend farther posteriorly, especially in males.

Tubercles on *Balitoropsis barschi* Smith and *Hemimyzon formosanum* (Boulenger) described by Wiley & Collette (1970) are similar to those on *Balitoria brucei* Gray, *Sinogastromyzon wui* Fang, *S. sanhoensis* Fang and *Bhavania australis* (Jerdon).

Gastromyzoninae

Tuberculation in the Gastromyzoninae is very similar to that in the Homalopterinae. Tubercles for six genera: *Beaufortia, Gastromyzon, Glaniopsis, Liniparhomaloptera, Prograstromyzon* and *Pseudogastromyzon*, have been reported by Wiley & Collette (1970), who also described and illustrated the histology of tubercles of *Gastromyzon borneensis* Günther and *Progastromyzon griswoldi* (Hora and Jayaram).

Cobitidae

The loaches are Eurasian freshwater fishes placed in three subfamilies (Bănărescu, 1968): Botiinae (two genera, about ten species), Cobitinae (15 genera, about 25 species), and Noemacheilinae (several genera, more than 100 species). Sexual dimorphism has long been known in the Cobitinae and

Noemacheilinae but the earliest reports mention only the "lamina circularis," a fleshy pad on the upper surface of the pectoral fin in males. Tubercles have been reported for more than 25 species, mostly in *Noemacheilus*, in seven genera (see Wiley & Collette, 1970): *Acanthophthalmus, Barbatula, Cobitis, Diplophysa, Lefua, Misgurnus* and *Noemacheilus*. Loaches develop tubercles on the head and the upper surface of the pectoral fin. The testes and the hormone methyldihydrotestosterone are involved in the development of tubercles in *Misgurnus* (Kobayashi, 1951).

Breeding tubercles in three species of *Noemacheilus* have been described by Jakubowski & Oliva (1967) and Wiley & Collette (1970). Cobitid tubercles are most similar to homalopterid tubercles as hypertrophied cells beneath the keratinized cap all enlarge to about the same size, are at the same stage of keratinization, and form a well defined, uniform layer destined to become another keratin cap. Homalopterid tubercles persist for a long time and the pectoral fin tubercles of loaches such as *Noemacheilus* seem permanent (P. Bănărescu, pers. comm.).

ATHERINIFORMES

Exocoetoidei

Belonidae

The 30 species of epipelagic fishes comprising the needlefish family Belonidae are found in freshwaters, estuaries and marine habitats; but most are marine. Needlefishes range in size from 42 to 950 mm body length (end of opercle to caudal base). Four genera (*Belonion, Potamorrhaphis, Pseudotylosurus* and *Xenentodon*) are restricted to freshwater as are a few species of *Strongylura*. *Pseudotylosurus angusticeps* (Günther) has spine-bearing scales (see Wiley & Collette, 1970; Collette, 1974). Posteriorly, the scales have more and larger spines. They are present in both sexes from 93 mm body length. It is not known whether these spines are seasonal. Probably the spines are contact organs that develop in breeding individuals of both sexes. Their presence in *Pseudotylosurus* further links the Belonidae with other atheriniform fishes.

A scale of *P. angusticeps* had three contact organs projecting from its posterior border. The shortest contact organ in the centre was 101 μm long and the longest 202 μm long (see Wiley & Collette, 1970).

Cyprinodontoidei

Contact organs, as bony dermal outgrowths of the scale margin or fin ray, are found in at least four of the eight families recognized in the suborder Cyprinodontoidei: Oryziatidae, Cyprinodontidae, Anablepidae and Poeciliidae. The term contact organ was first employed by Newman (1907, 1909) in his studies of North American Cyprinodontidae. Numerous subsequent papers refer to them in this family. Their development has been well studied experimentally in the Japanese medaka *Oryzias latipes* (Temminck and Schlegel) (see Wiley & Collette, 1970).

Oryziatidae

This family of seven species of rice fishes or medakas of the genus *Oryzias* (Rosen, 1964) is found in fresh and brackish water from India to Japan. Contact organs, "papillary processes" are known to occur only in the Japanese medaka, *Oryzias latipes*, but have apparently not been recorded from any of the other six species.

In *Oryzias latipes*, contact organs develop as males reach maturity to remain throughout the year (Oka, 1931; Okada & Yamashita, 1944), and become slightly reduced in winter (Egami, 1954c: 7). Oka (1931) discussed their histological structure and development and found that their size continues to increase as the male grows. The contact organs develop as bony processes of the fin ray and have a mesenchyme-filled axial space continuous with that in the centre of the fin ray. Yamamoto & Egami (1974) described them using scanning electron micrographs. Histology of contact organs induced on the anal fin rays of female *Oryzias* by oral ethisterone was described by Uwa (1975). Yamamoto (1975) summarized the secondary sex characters and aspects of biology of *O. latipes*.

Cyprinodontidae

The killifishes are a large family (about 45 genera and 300–400 species) of oviparous top-minnows found in shallow fresh, estuarine and marine waters of North and South America, Europe, Africa and Asia (Foster, 1967). Myers (1955) recognized seven subfamilies, one of which (Oryziatinae) was subsequently raised to family level. Sexually mature males of most cyprinodontids have contact organs on the fin rays and scales (Foster, 1963, 1967; Stenholt Clausen, 1967); chapter 1 of Stenholt Clausen's paper is entitled "Ctenoidy, a nearly universal character in the cyprinodonts". There are records of contact organs for the Fundulinae,

Cyprinodontinae, Orestiatinae, Rivulinae and Procatopodinae (including Lamprichthyinae) but not for the African Pantanodontinae.

Newman (1907, 1909) first studied contact organs in detail in three species of Fundulinae and one species of Cyprinodontinae. Apparently overlooking Newman's papers, Fowler (1916) described scale and fin ray contact organs (as "spinules") in six species of *Fundulus* plus *Lucania* and *Cyprinodon*, as did Ermin (1946) in the Anatolian cyprinodontine *Kosswigichthys asquamatus* Sözer, a species with body scales reduced to only 15 or 20 and yet with contact organs on them in males. Miller (1956) compared the distribution of contact organs on the scales and fins of five American genera of Cyprinodontinae: *Cyprinodon, Floridichthys, Garmanella, Jordanella* and *Cualac*. Literature records for the Fundulinae and Cyprinodontinae were summarized by Wiley & Collette (1970). Since then, Hastings & Yerger (1971) reported contact organs in males of *Adinia xenica* (Jordan and Gilbert) and described their function in clasping the female during spawning. Contact organs occur on the scales and anal fin rays of *Cyprinodon bovinus* Baird and Girard (Echelle & Miller, 1974).

The Orestiatinae is a subfamily of 20 species, all in the genus *Orestias*, of Lake Titicaca and other high Andean lakes and rivers. Tchernavin (1944) reported sharp, curved spines on the dorsal, anal and pectoral fins of males of eight species, and spines were also present on the scales of one species. Where females also have spines, they are less well developed though present in larger specimens.

Contact organs are well known in the annual killifishes of the subfamilies Rivulinae and Procatopodinae. Stenholt Clausen (1967) found contact organs in all procatopodine genera (except *Procatopus*): *Aplocheichthys, Hypsopanchax, Plataplochilus, Poropanchax* and *Lamprichthys tanganicus* which he transferred to the Procatopodinae. Contact organs are present in *Aphyosemion, Roloffia* and *Nothobranchius* of the Old World Rivulinae but absent in *Aplocheilus* and *Epiplatys*. He included photographs of "ctenoid" scales of seven species and pelvic fin contact organs of *Poropanchax normani* (Ahl). The distribution and shape of contact organs in these two subfamilies proved useful systematic characters. Miller & Hubbs (1974) used minute slender contact organs on the scales of males of *Rivulus robustus* as a diagnostic character of their new species.

Contact organs seem to be permanent in a number of species of

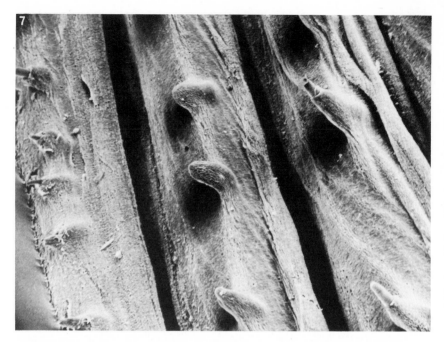

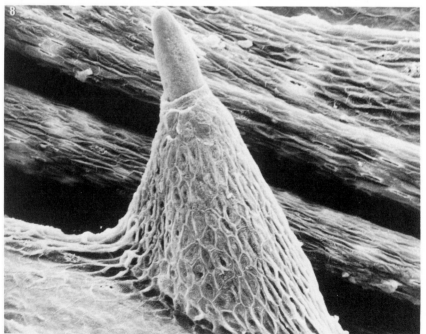

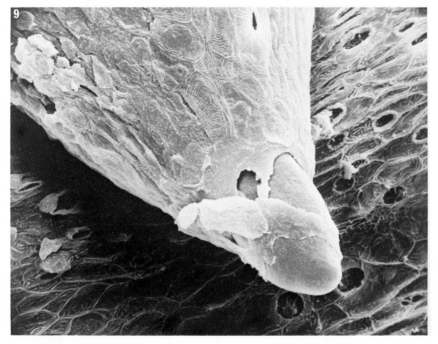

FIGS 7–9. Scanning electron micrographs of fin contact organs in *Fundulus seminolis* Girard (Cyprinodontidae). (7) Proximal section of anal fin, ×64. (8) Distal portion of anal fin, ×310. (9) Distal surface of right pelvic fin, ×645.

African cyprinodonts (Stenholt Clausen, 1967). They occur in all full-grown males of those species possessing them, and in *Lamprichthys*, *Plataplochilus* and two species of *Hypsopanchax*, even in full-grown females too, irrespective of season.

Contact organs in *Fundulus heteroclitus* (Linnaeus) and *Cynolebias whitei* Myers were described and illustrated by Wiley & Collette (1970). Those of *Fundulus* are very similar to the descriptions by Newman (1907, 1909). Sections of contact organs in *F. stellifer* (Jordan) and *F. catenatus* (Storer) are essentially identical except for size. Scanning electron micrographs of contact organs of the fin in *Fundulus* (Figs 7–9) and snout contact organs in *Luciana parva* (Baird) (Figs 10–12) are very similar to those for *Oryzias* (Yamamoto & Egami, 1974).

Anablepidae

Three species of viviparous four-eyed fishes (*Anableps*) occur in fresh and brackish waters of Central America and northern South

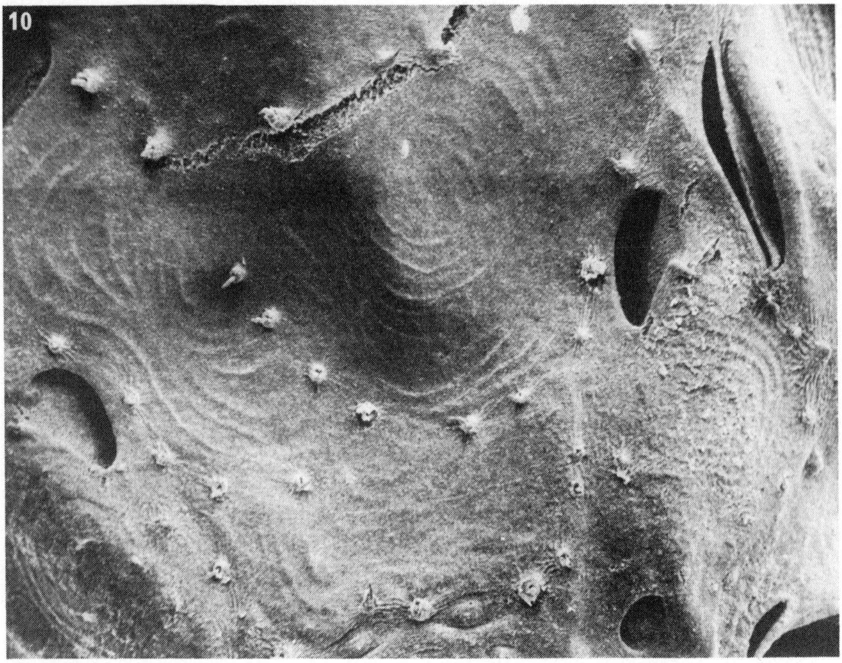

FIGS 10–12. Scanning electron micrographs of snout contact organs in *Lucania parva* (Baird) (Cyprinodontidae). (10) ×34. (11) ×136. (12) ×750.

America. Contact organs occur on the posterior margins of the scales of all three species (see Wiley & Collette, 1970). When present in both sexes, they extend further dorsally and ventrally in males. Fowler (1916) figured contact organs in both sexes of *Anableps anableps* (Linnaeus).

Poeciliidae

The Poeciliidae, which are small viviparous top-minnows in fresh and brackish waters of the New World from north and central United States south to northern Argentina, include guppies, platies, swordtails and mollies. Rosen & Bailey (1963) recognized three subfamilies (two monotypic), five tribes, 21 genera and 138 species; about 20 additional species have been described or resurrected since then. In spite of extensive behavioural and genetic work on the family, contact organs were mentioned only in *Poeciliopsis* (Wiley & Collette, 1970) although *Xenodexia ctenolepis* Hubbs of the Xenodexiinae was known to have "ctenoid" scales all over the body of males, females and juveniles (Hubbs, 1950).

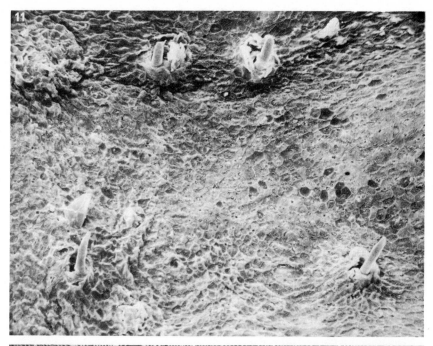

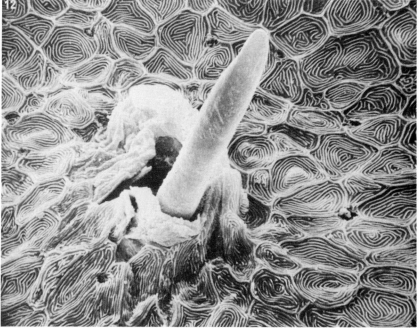

Contact organs occur on the heads of males in three genera of two tribes: *Poecilia* in the Poeciliini, *Poeciliopsis* and *Phallichthys* in the Heterandriini. Males of all species in the subgenus *Poecilia* except the gynogenetic Amazon molly *P.* (*P.*) *formosa* (Girard) have snout contact organs (Wiley & Collette, 1970). Two additional species in the subgenus—*P. mexicanus* (Steindachner) and *P. butleri* Jordan—also have contact organs across the rostrums of breeding males (Schultz & Miller, 1971). Contact organs are not mentioned by Miller (1975) in the original descriptions of *P. chica* and *P. catemaconis* but examination of some paratypes of the former species (USNM 214088) confirms their presence. They have not been found in other subgenera, *Lebistes*, *Pamphorichthys* and *Limia*.

Contact organs from the snout of a male *Poecilia sphenops* Valenciennes appeared identical in structure to those of species of *Fundulus* (Wiley & Collette, 1970: fig. 11A).

SCORPAENIFORMES

Cottoidei

Cottidae

Several species of marine sculpins develop contact organs. They occur on the inside surfaces of the pectoral and pelvic fin rays of species in three genera: *Gymnocanthus*, *Myoxocephalus* and *Triglops* (Wiley & Collette, 1970).

Contact organs on the posterior surface of the pectoral fin rays of males of *Myoxocephalus scorpius* (Linnaeus) are bifurcate structures supported internally by bony processes from the fin ray. They incline proximally and are very heavily constructed, suggesting that they are used during mating to clasp the female (Wiley & Collette, 1970). Cowan (1970) compared contact organs on the pectoral and pelvic fins of two additional species of *Myoxocephalus*—*M. polyacanthocephalus* (Pallas) and *M. jaok* (Cuvier and Valenciennes). They are also described and figured on the ventral surface of the pelvic fin rays in males of *Melletes papilio* Bean. Here the structures are long, slender and weak (Wiley & Collette, 1970).

Cottocomephoridae

This freshwater family of eight genera and 17 species, mostly confined to Lake Baikal in Siberia, is an offshoot of the Cottidae and considered only a subfamily of the Cottidae by some authors.

Large round pearl-like tubercles of "epithelialen Ursprunges" develop on the inner side of the pectoral fin rays of male *Cottocomephorus grewingki* (Dybowski) during the spawning period (Berg, 1907). Later, Berg (1949: 1174) reported epithelial tubercles on the pectoral fin rays of male *C. comephoroides* Berg.

On the basis of the close relationships of the Cottocomephoridae to the Cottidae, Wiley & Collette (1970) erroneously concluded that these sexually dimorphic structures were similar to those in the Cottidae. However, examination of *C. grewingki* (from Dr A. N. Svetovidov) subsequent to that paper shows that Berg was correct. Well developed tubercles on the distal three-quarters of pectoral fin rays 2 or 3 to 17 or 19 (of 19–21 rays) of three mature males (152–180 mm S.L.) are best developed on rays 7–18, on the distal half of the fin. The tubercles are in a single row of ten–14 tubercles per ray, a little more elongate than Berg portrayed (1907: pl. 3, fig. 1b). They are absent from the pelvic fins. The tubercles do not take up alizarin, are loosely attached over the fin ray, are not continuous with the segment of the fin ray and thus are clearly epidermal breeding tubercles and not dermal contact organs.

Maiboroda, Chernyaev & Fedorova (1975) have shown that epidermal breeding tubercles develop on the pectoral fins of male *C. grewingki* and *C. inermis* (Jakowlew).

PERCIFORMES

Percoidei

Percidae

Among approximately 163 species of perches and darters of this freshwater family, breeding tubercles are present in about 50 species in five genera in two tribes—the North American Etheostomatini and the similarly adapted European Romanichthyini. The relatively few (14) early reports of tubercles in this family were summarized by Collette (1965). Since then, they have been reported in *Etheostoma boschungi* (Wall & Williams, 1974). Breeding tubercle distribution proved to be a useful systematic character at tribal, generic and specific levels in the Percidae (Collette, 1963, 1965; Wiley & Collette, 1970). Williams (1975) reported tubercles on the pelvic fins of males of all six species of the subgenus *Ammocrypta*, including his two new ones. They occur on the anal fins of four species and *A. clara* Jordan and Meek also has tubercles on the lowermost three or four rays in the caudal fin.

Breeding tubercles in two genera of each tribe were described by Wiley & Collette (1970): *Romanichthys valsanicola* Dumitrescu, Bănărescu and Stoica, and *Zingel streber* (Siebold) in the Romanichthyinae; and *Percina evides* (Jordan and Copeland) and *Etheostoma swannanoa* Jordan and Evermann in the Etheostomatini. Percid tubercles form by hyperplasia and moderate hypertrophy of epidermal cells to form conical mounds of tissue. In mature structures, the surface cells are somewhat keratinized to form a thin, rugose covering. Instead of tubercles, breeding males of some darters develop thickened ridges of epidermis along the rays of some of the fins. These ridges of *Etheostoma swannanoa*, a darter with tubercles on the body, appear identical to a fin-ray tubercle of *Percina evides*. A rugose covering on the surface of both tubercles and ridges suggests good frictional properties to make them effective in maintaining contact between spawning individuals.

DISCUSSION

Chondrichthyan fishes (sharks, skates and chimaeras) may be able to avoid the problem of needing to maintain contact because they all practice internal fertilization. The pelvic fins of males are modified into intromittent organs—claspers or myxopterygia—for this purpose. Furthermore, both sexes of sharks are covered with rough placoid scales. The placoid scale cover is essentially absent in the Holocephali (chimaeras) but males of a number of species have a club-shaped organ (tentaculum) on the forehead, whose suggested function is to assist holding the female during copulation. Skates and rays have the scale covering greatly reduced or absent. Adult males of many species of Rajidae develop one to five rows of alar spines on the dorsal side of the outer part of each pectoral (Bigelow & Schroeder, 1953), which may assist in holding the female during copulation (Libby & Gilbert, 1960). Some species also develop spines in the pelvic region. Pelvic fin denticles present in both sexes of *Raja ocellata* Mitchill occur only in females of the smaller *R. erinacea* Mitchill (Templeman, 1965; McEachran & Musick, 1973). Both alar and pelvic spines develop at the same time as other sexually dimorphic structures involved in reproduction, such as calcification of clasper cartilages (McEachran & Musick, 1973).

Most chondrostean fishes have large rhomboid bony plates which should not be slippery. Even *Polyodon*, the paddlefish, generally considered to be naked, is not slippery but has tiny denticles in the skin (Weisel, 1975).

Roughening structures like breeding tubercles or contact organs are not known in primitive malacopterygian fishes (elopomorphs, clupeomorphs and osteoglossomorphs). In several families of three more-advanced orders of malacopterygian fishes (Salmoniformes, Gonorhynchiformes and Cypriniformes), breeding tubercles are frequently present, especially in species that live or spawn in freshwater or intertidal areas. Contact organs are present in several families of the Atheriniformes and Cypriniformes.

In addition to having contact organs on the fin rays of males of some species of five families of Atheriniformes, three genera have "ctenoid" scales: *Xenodexia* (Poeciliidae), *Lamprichthys* (Cyprinodontidae) and *Pseudotylosurus* (Belonidae). These structures are not sexually dimorphic and do not appear to vary seasonally in these species. The presence of "typical" ctenoid scales in members of these three lines of atherinomorph fishes is evidence that contact organs have evolved independently and become genetically fixed in several lines of fishes as permanent non-dimorphic contact organs. Additional evidence of their independent origin (and of breeding tubercles) comes from the presence of both types of structures in the Characoidei and Cottoidei.

Data on a cyprinodontid are of interest. The monotypic Anatolian cyprinodontine *Kosswigichthys asquamatus* Sözer has body scales greatly reduced in number and size—15–20 scales, 85–190 μm in diameter—yet contact organs are present on most scales in males (Ermin, 1946: 250–258). Perhaps *Kosswigichthys* has not become completely naked because the few remaining scales are needed to bear contact organs which are important in reproductive behaviour.

An advanced characteristic of many groups of Acanthopterygii (and Paracanthopterygii) is the possession of ctenoid scales. Within the Acanthopterygii, species in the suborders Perciformes and Scorpaeniformes develop breeding tubercles or contact organs. There are three major freshwater families within the suborder Percoidei—Percidae, Centrarchidae and Cichlidae. Why are many species of only the Percidae tuberculate? Neither tubercles nor contact organs are present in the Centrarchidae and Cichlidae which are moderate-sized fishes living in predominantly lentic habitats. The larger lentic species of Percinae (*Perca* and *Gymnocephalus*) and Luciopercinae (*Stizostedion*) also lack tubercles. It is the small species which compose the Romanichthyini and Etheostomatini that develop tubercles and most of these spawn in stream riffles. Tubercles apparently evolved independently in each tribe in addition to ctenoid scales in response to the strong selective pressure to keep the spawning pairs together in fast-moving water.

Two families of Scorpaeniformes, suborder Cottoidei, develop roughening structures. Some estuarine species of Cottidae develop contact organs and at least three species of the freshwater Lake Baikal Cottocomephoridae develop breeding tubercles.

Coral reef fish communities are dominated by spiny-rayed, ctenoid-scaled acanthopterygian fishes. Smith & Tyler (1972) considered that the increased strength and durability of fin rays and scales in this habitat is to protect the fishes against this rough calcareous environment. John D. McEachran (pers. comm.) has suggested an alternative explanation. Perhaps the widespread occurrence of ctenoid scales in coral reef fishes, which have extended breeding seasons, provides these fishes with permanent roughening structures. The selective value would be high in regions with extended breeding seasons whereas temporary roughening structures would be more advantageous in regions with a short breeding season.

It has been postulated that the primary function of spines on ctenoid scales is to modify the boundary layer and make it turbulent, thereby to lower resistance to movement through the water (Aleev, 1963; Burdak, 1968). While this may now be a function of ctenoid scales, it seems unlikely that they originally evolved for this reason. The fastest swimming fishes (Scombridae, Istiophoridae, Xiphiidae) have reduced scales or have lost the scale cover entirely. Hora (1922) suggested that ridges and tubercles of some Indian hill stream fishes (Homalopteridae, Sisoridae) might have a hydrodynamic function.

There appear to be no fundamental structural differences between cycloid scales with contact organs and ctenoid scales. Three tropical genera in three different families of atherinomorph fishes have what appear to be genetically fixed, permanent contact organs. The widespread occurrence of ctenoid scales in acanthopterygian fishes testifies to the selective value of the character. I believe that ctenoid scales are genetically fixed contact organs whose original function was to keep members of spawning groups in close contact with each other.

ACKNOWLEDGEMENTS

Dr Ralph M. Yerger kindly permitted me to use the SEM photographs in this study. His work was done with a grant from the Florida State University Committee on Faculty Research Support.

Robert W. Hastings performed the technical work and Ron Parker was the SEM operator. Dr A. N. Svetovidov made three tuberculate specimens of *Cottocomephorus grewingki* available for study. William L. Fink read the section on Characoidei and called my attention to several important references and specimens. Dr Stanley H. Weitzman permitted me to examine his cleared and stained specimens of Gasteropelecidae for contact organs. Figure 2 was drawn by Keiko Hiratsuka Moore. James E. Böhlke, Daniel M. Cohen, Walter R. Courtenay, Jr., John D. McEachran, Stanley H. Weitzman and Martin L. Wiley read drafts of the paper and suggested improvements, most of which have been incorporated into the paper. This does not imply that they agree with all I have presented.

REFERENCES

Aisa, E. (1958). Contributo allo studio dei cosiddetti "tubercoli nuziali" in *Rutilus rubilius*. Ricerche macroscopiche ed istologiche. *Veterinaria Ital.* **9**: 736–741.

Aisa, E. (1959). I tubercoli nuziali in *Rutilus rubilio* Bp. var. *rubella* (*trasimenicus*) Bp. del Lago Trasimeno. Osservazioni macroscopiche ed istologiche. *Boll. Zool.* **26**: 601–606.

Aleev, Yu. G. (1963). *Function and gross morphology in fish.* Akad. Nauk SSSR Sevastopol. Biol. Sta. [In Russian, U.S. Department of Commerce translation TT 67-51391.]

Alt, K. T. (1971). Occurrence of hybrids between inconnu, *Stenodus leucichthys nelma* (Pallas), and humpback whitefish, *Coregonus pidschian* (Linnaeus) in Chatanika River, Alaska. *Trans. Am. Fish. Soc.* **100**: 362–365.

Arai, R. (1964). Comparison of the effects of androgenic steroids on production of pearl organs in the female Japanese bitterling and of papillary processes on anal-fin rays in the female medaka. *Bull. natn. Sci. Mus. Tokyo* **7**: 91–94.

Arai, R. (1967). Androgenic effects of 11-ketotestosterone on some sexual characteristics in the teleost, *Oryzias latipes*. *Annotnes zool. jap.* **40**: 1–5.

Bănărescu, P. (1968). Recent advances in teleost taxonomy and their implications on freshwater zoogeography. *Rev. roumaine Biol.* (*Zool.*) **13**: 153–160.

Berg, L. S. (1907). Die Cataphracti des Baikal-Sees (Fam. Cottidae, Cottocomephoridae und Comephoridae). *Wiss. Ergeb. Zool. Exped. Baikal-See 1900–1902.* No. 3, 1–75.

Berg, L. S. (1948, 1949). The freshwater fishes of the U.S.S.R. and adjacent countries. *Fauna USSR* No. 27, 3 vol., 4th ed. (Office Tech. Serv. Trans. No. 61-31218, 63-11056, 63-11057).

Bigelow, H. S. & Schroeder, W. C. (1953). Fishes of the western North Atlantic Part 2. Sawfishes, guitarfishes, skates and rays. Chimaeroids. Sears Found. Mar. Res. Mem. **1**. New Haven, Conn.: Sears Foundation.

Böhlke, J. E. (1958). Studies on fishes of the family Characidae—No. 14. A report on several extensive recent collections from Ecuador. *Proc. Acad. nat. Sci. Philad.* **110**: 1–121.

Branson, B. A. (1962). Observations on the distribution of nuptial tubercles in some catostomid fishes. *Trans. Kans. Acad. Sci.* **64**: 360–372.

Branson, B. A. & McCoy, C. J., Jr. (1966). Observations on breeding tubercles in *Xyrauchen texanus* (Abbott). *SWest. Nat.* **11**: 301.

Breder, C. M. & Rosen, D. E. (1966). *Modes of reproduction in fishes.* Garden City, N.Y.: Natural History Press.

Burdak, V. D. (1968). [The functional significance of ctenoid scales in fish.] *Zool. Zh.* **47**: 732–738. [In Russian, translated by British Library, RTS 7919.]

Burgess, G. H. O. (1956). Absence of keratin in teleost epidermis. *Nature, Lond.* **178**: 93–94.

Collette, B. B. (1963). The subfamilies, tribes, and genera of the Percidae (Teleostei). *Copeia* **1963**: 615–623.

Collette, B. B. (1965). Systematic significance of breeding tubercles in fishes of the family Percidae. *Proc. U.S. natn. Mus.* **117**: 567–614.

Collette, B. B. (1974). South American freshwater needlefishes (Belonidae) of the genus *Pseudotylosurus. Zool. Meded.* **48**: 169–186.

Cowan, G. I. M. (1970). A morphological comparison of two closely related species of the genus *Myoxocephalus* (Pisces: Cottidae) with notes on their life histories and ecology. *Can. J. Zool.* **48**: 1269–1281.

DeLamater, E. D. & Courtenay, W. R., Jr. (1973). Studies on scale structure of flatfishes. I. The genus *Trinectes*, with notes on related forms. *Proc. A. Conf. SEast. Assoc. Game Fish Comm.* **27**: 591–608.

DeLamater, E. D. & Courtenay, W. R., Jr. (1974). Fish scales as seen by scanning electron microscopy. *Fla Sci.* **37**: 141–149.

Ebina, K.-I. (1929). Nuptial organ of the salmonoid fish, *Plecoglossus altivelis* T. & S. *J. Imp. Fish. Inst., Tokyo* **25**: 23–25.

Ebina, K.-I. (1930). Occurrence of the nuptial organ in the female of the salmonoid fish, *Plecoglossus altivelis* T. & S. *J. Imp. Fish. Inst., Tokyo* **26**: 21–23.

Echelle, A. A. & Miller, R. R. (1974). Rediscovery and redescription of the Leon Springs pupfish, *Cyprinodon bovinus*, from Pecos County, Texas. *SWest. Nat.* **19**: 170–190.

Egami, N. (1954a). Effects of hormonic steroids on the formation of male characteristics in females of the fish, *Oryzias latipes*, kept in water containing testosterone propionate. *Annotnes zool. jap.* **27**: 122–127.

Egami, N. (1954b). Influence of temperature on the appearance of male characters in females of the fish, *Oryzias latipes*, following treatment with methyldihydrotestosterone. *J. Fac. Sci. Univ. Tokyo* (Sect. 4 Zool.) **7**: 280–298.

Egami, N. (1954c). Geographic variations in the male characters of the fish, *Oryzias latipes. Annotnes zool. jap.* **27**: 7–12.

Egami, N. (1957). Inhibitory effect of thiourea on the development of male characteristics in females of the fish, *Oryzias latipes*, kept in water containing testosterone propionate. *Annotnes zool. jap.* **30**: 26–30.

Egami, N. & Nambu, M. (1961). Factors initiating mating behavior and oviposition in the fish, *Oryzias latipes. J. Fac. Sci. Univ. Tokyo* (Sect. 4 Zool.) **9**: 263–278.

Ermin, R. (1946). Schuppenreduktion bei Zahnkarpfen (Cyprinodontidae). *Istanb. Univ. Fen Fak. Mecm.* (B) **11**: 217–272.

Fabricius, E. & Lindroth, A. (1954). Experimental observations on the spawning of whitefish, *Coregonus lavaretus* L., in the stream aquarium of the Holle Laboratory at River Indalsälven. *Rept Inst. Freshw. Res. Drottningholm* **35**: 105–112.

Fink, W. L. (1976). A new genus and species of characid fish from the Bayano River basin of Panama (Pisces: Cypriniformes). *Proc. biol. Soc. Wash.* **88**: 331–344.

Fink, W. L. & Weitzman, S. H. (1974). The so-called cheirodontin fishes of Central America with descriptions of two new species (Pisces: Characidae). *Smithson. Contrib. Zool.* No. 172: 1–46.

Foster, N. R. (1963). Reproductive behavior patterns and functional anatomy of some American oviparous cyprinodont fishes. *Int. congr. Zool.* **16**(1): 158 [Abstract].

Foster, N. R. (1967). Trends in the evolution of reproductive behavior in killifishes. *Studies Trop. Oceanogr.* **5**: 549–566.

Fowler, H. W. (1916). Some features of ornamentation in the killifishes or toothed minnows. *Am. Nat.* **50**: 743–750.

Fowler, H. W. (1937). Zoological results of the third de Schauensee Siamese Expedition. Part VIII, Fishes obtained in 1936. *Proc. Acad. nat. Sci. Philad.* **89**: 125–264.

Géry, J. (1973). New and little-known Aphyoditeina (Pisces, Characoidei) from the Amazon Basin. *Stud. Neotrop. Fauna* **8**: 81–137.

Greenwood, P. H., Rosen, D. E., Weitzman, S. H. & Myers, G. S. (1966). Phyletic studies of teleostean fishes, with a provisional classification of living forms. *Bull. Am. Mus. nat. Hist.* **131**: 341–455.

Hart, J. L. (1930). The spawning and early life history of the whitefish, *Coregonus clupeaformis* (Mitchill), in the Bay of Quinte, Canada. *Contr. Can. Biol. Fish.* (N.S.) **6**(7): 165–214.

Hastings, R. W. & Yerger, R. W. (1971). Ecology and life history of the diamond killifish *Adinia xenica* (Jordan and Gilbert). *Am. Midl. Nat.* **86**: 276–291.

Hishida, T. & Kawamoto, N. (1970). Androgenic and male-inducing effects of 11-ketotestosterone on a teleost, the medaka (*Oryzias latipes*). *J. exp. Zool.* **173**: 279–283.

Hora, S. L. (1922). Structural modification in the fish of mountain torrents. *Rec. Indian Mus.* **24**: 31–61.

Hora, S. L. (1923). On a collection of fish from Siam. *J. nat. Hist. Soc. Siam* **6**: 143–184.

Hora, S. L. (1952). Functional divergence, structural convergence and preadaptation exhibited by the fishes of the cyprinoid family Psilorhynchidae Hora. *J. Bombay nat. Hist. Soc.* **50**: 880–884.

Hora, S. L. & Mukerji, D. D. (1935). Fish of the Naga Hills, Assam. *Rec. Indian Mus.* **37**: 381–404.

Hubbs, C. L. (1930). Materials for a revision of the catostomid fishes of eastern North America. *Misc. Publs Univ. Mich. Mus. Zool.* No. 20: 1–47.

Hubbs, C. L. (1950). Studies of cyprinodont fishes. XX. A new subfamily from Guatemala, with ctenoid scales and a unilateral pectoral clasper. *Misc. Publs Mus. Zool. Univ. Mich.* **78**: 1–28.

Hubbs, C. L. & Cooper, G. P. (1936). Minnows of Michigan. *Bull. Cranbrook Inst. Sci.* No. 8: 1–84.

Hubbs, C. L. & Miller, R. R. (1974). *Dionda erimyzonops*, a new, dwarf cyprinid fish inhabiting the Gulf coastal plain of Mexico. *Occ. Pap. Mus. Zool. Univ. Mich.* No. 671: 1–17.

Huntsman, G. R. (1967). Nuptial tubercles in carpsuckers (*Carpiodes*). *Copeia* **1967**: 457–458.

Isbrücker, I. J. H. (1973a). Status of the primary homonymous South American catfish, *Loricaria cirrhosa* Perugia, 1897, with remarks on some other loricariids (Pisces, Siluriformes, Loricariidae). *Annali Mus. civ. Stor. nat. Giacomo Doria* **79**: 172–191.

Isbrücker, I. J. H. (1973b). Redescription and figures of the South American mailed catfish, *Rineloricara lanceolata* (Günther, 1860) (Pisces, Siluriformes, Loricariidae). *Beaufortia* **21**: 75–89.

Jakubowski, M. & Oliva, O. (1967). Note on pearl organs on the stone loach, *Noemacheilus barbatulus* (Linnaeus, 1758) (Osteichthyes, Cobitidae). *Věst. čsl. Spol. zool.* **31**: 25–27.

Jenyns, L. (1842). Fish. In *The zoology of the voyage of H.M.S. Beagle.* Part IV, 1–72. Darwin, C. (ed.). London.

Jordan, D. S. & McGregor, E. A. (1925). Family Plecoglossidae. In Record of fishes obtained by David Starr Jordan in Japan, 1922, by D. S. Jordan and C. L. Hubbs, *Mem. Carneg. Mus.* **10**(2): 147–149.

Kawamoto, N. (1969). Effects of androstenedione, 19-norethynyltestosterone, progesterone, and 17α-hydroxyprogesterone, upon the manifestation of secondary sex characters on the medaka, *Oryzias latipes. Development Growth Diff.* **11**: 89–103.

Kawamoto, N. (1973). Androgenic potencies of androsterone, methyltestosterone, testosterone propionate, and testosterone upon the manifestation of papillary processes in the female medaka, *Oryzias latipes. Zool. Mag. Tokyo* **82**: 36–41. [In Japanese with English abstract.]

Kimura, S. & Tao, Y. (1937). Notes on the nuptial coloration and pearl organs in Chinese fresh-water fishes. *Shanghai Sizenkagaku Kentkyusyo Iho* **6**: 277–318. [In Chinese, translated by Tchaw-ren Chen, NMFS Syst. Lab. Translation no. 66.]

Kobayashi, H. (1951). Experimental studies on the sexual characters of the loach, *Misgurnus anguillicaudatus* (Cantor). *Annotnes zool. jap.* **24**: 212–221.

Koch, D. L. (1973). Reproductive characteristics of the cui-ui lakesucker (*Chasmistes cujus* Cope) and its spawning behavior in Pyramid Lake, Nevada. *Trans. Am. Fish. Soc.* **102**: 145–149.

Koelz, W. (1929). Coregonid fishes of the Great Lakes. *Bull. U.S. Bur. Fish.* **43**: 297–643.

Koehn, R. K. (1965). Development and ecological significance of nuptial tubercles on the red shiner, *Notropis lutrensis. Copeia* **1965**: 462–467.

Lachner, E. A. & Jenkins, R. E. (1971). Systematics, distribution, and evolution of the chub genus *Nocomis* Girard (Pisces, Cyprinidae) of eastern United States, with descriptions of new species. *Smithson. Contr. Zool.* No. 85: 1–97.

Lanzing, W. J. R. & Higginbotham, D. R. (1974). Scanning microscopy of surface structures of *Tilapia mossambica* (Peters) scales. *J. Fish Biol.* **6**: 307–310.

Libby, E. L. & Gilbert, P. W. (1960). Reproduction in the clear-nosed skate, *Raja eglanteria. Anat. Rec.* **138**: 365.

Madsen, M. L. (1971). The presence of nuptial tubercles on female quillback (*Carpiodes cyprinus*). *Trans. Am. Fish. Soc.* **100**: 132–134.

Maiboroda, A. A., Chernyaev, G. A. & Fedorova, S. V. (1975). Morphohistological features of the changes in the skin and pectoral fins at the formation of the spawning livery of Baikal sculpins of the genus *Cottocomephorus* (Cottidae). *Zool. Zh.* **54**(a): 1340–1346. [In Russian with English abstract.]

Matsui, I. (1950). On the morphological dissimilarity of ayu (*Plecoglossus altivelis* T. & S.) in the circumstantial difference, sex and scales circuli and the discrimination of "pond-cultured ayu" and "natural ayu". *Jap. J. Ichthyol.* **1**: 17–24.

McAllister, D. E. (1963). A revision of the smelt family, Osmeridae. *Bull. natn. Mus. Can.* No. 191: 1–53.

McDowall, R. M. (1969). Relationships of galaxioid fishes with a further discussion of salmoniform classification. *Copeia* **1969**: 796–824.

McDowall, R. M. (1972). The taxonomy of estuarine and brackish-lake *Retropinna* from New Zealand (Galaxioidei: Retropinnidae). *Jl R. Soc. New Zealand* **2**: 501–531.

McEachran, J. D. & Musick, J. A. (1973). Characters for distinguishing between immature specimens of the sibling species *Raja erinacea* and *Raja ocellata* (Pisces: Rajidae). *Copeia* **1973**: 238–250.

McSwain, L. & Gennings, R. M. (1972). Spawning behavior of the spotted sucker *Minytrema melanops* (Rafinesque). *Trans. Am. Fish. Soc.* **101**: 738–740.

Meek, S. E. & Hildebrand, S. F. (1916). The fishes of the fresh waters of Panama. *Publs Field Mus. nat. Hist.* (Zool. Ser.) **10**(15): 1–374.

Menon, A. G. K. & Datta, A. K. (1964). Zoological results of the Indian Cho-Oyu expedition (1958) in Nepal. Part 7.—Pisces (concluded). *Psilorhynchus pseudecheneis*, a new cyprinid fish from Nepal. *Rec. Indian Mus.* **59**: 253–255.

Menzies, W. J. M. (1931). *The salmon. Its life story.* Edinburgh and London: Wm. Blackwood and Sons Ltd.

Miller, R. R. (1956). A new genus and species of cyprinodontid fish from San Luis Potosi, Mexico, with remarks on the subfamily Cyprinodontinae. *Occ. Pap. Mus. zool. Univ. Mich.* No. 581: 1–17.

Miller, R. R. (1975). Five new species of Mexican poeciliid fishes of the genera *Poecilia*, *Gambusia*, and *Poeciliopsis*. *Occ. Pap. Mus. zool. Univ. Mich.* No. 672: 1–44.

Miller, R. R. & Hubbs, C. L. (1974). *Rivulus robustus*, a new cyprinodontid fish from southeastern Mexico. *Copeia* **1974**: 865–869.

Mittal, A. K. & Banerjee, T. K. (1974). A histochemical study of the epidermal keratinization in the skin of a fresh-water teleost *Bagarius bagarius* (Ham.) (Sisoridae, Pisces). *Mikroskopie* **30**: 337–348.

Myers, G. S. (1930). Fishes from the upper Rio Meta Basin, Colombia. *Proc. biol. Soc. Wash.* **43**: 65–71.

Myers, G. S. (1955). Notes on the classification and names of cyprinodont fishes. *Trop. Fish Mag.* **1955** (March): 7.

Nelson, K. (1964). Behavior and morphology in the glandulocaudine fishes (Ostariophysi, Characidae). *Univ. Calif. Publs Zool.* **75**: 59–152.

Newman, H. H. (1907). Spawning behavior and sexual dimorphism in *Fundulus heteroclitus* and allied fish. *Biol. Bull. mar. biol. Labs Woods Hole* **12**: 314–348.

Newman, H. H. (1909). Contact organs in the killifishes of Woods Hole. *Biol. Bull. mar. biol. Labs Woods Hole* **17**: 170–180.

Nieuwenhuizen, A. V. D. (1964). *Tropical aquarium fish: their habits and breeding behavior.* Translated by Alfred Leutscher. New York: D. Van Nostrand Co., Inc.

Norden, C. R. (1961). Comparative osteology of representative salmonid fishes, with particular reference to the grayling (*Thymallus arcticus*) and its phylogeny. *J. Fish. Res. Bd Can.* **18**: 679–791.

Oka, T. B. (1931). On the processes on the fin-rays of the male of *Oryzias latipes* and other sex characters of this fish. *J. Fac. Sci. Imp. Univ. Tokyo* (Sect. 4 Zool.) **2**: 209–218.

Okada, Y. K. & Yamashita, H. (1944). Experimental investigation of the manifestation of secondary sexual characters in fish, using the medaka, *Oryzias latipes* (Temminck & Schlegel) as material. *J. Fac. Sci. Imp. Univ. Tokyo* (Sect. 4 Zool.) **6**: 383–437.

Pappenheim, P. (1909). Pisces (inkl. Cyclostomata), Fische. *Süsswasserfauna Dtl.* 1: 90–201.

Peters, N., Jr. (1967). Opercular- und Postopercularorgan (Occipitalorgan) der Gattung *Kneria* (Kneriidae, Pisces) und ein Vergleich mit verwandten Strukturen. *Z. Morph. Ökol. Tiere* 59: 381–435.

Pickford, G. E. & Atz, J. W. (1957). *The physiology of the pituitary gland of fishes.* New York: N.Y. Zool. Soc.

Poll, M. (1965). Contribution à l'étude des Kneriidae et description d'un nouveau genre, le genre *Parakneria* (Pisces, Kneriidae). *Mém. Acad. R. belg.* 36(4): 1–28.

Ramaswami, L. S. & Hasler, A. D. (1955). Hormones and secondary sex characters in the minnow, *Hyborhynchus. Physiol. Zool.* 28: 62–68.

Raney, E. C. (1947). Subspecies and breeding behavior of the cyprinid fish *Notropis procne* (Cope). *Copeia* 1947: 103–109.

Reighard, J. (1903). The function of the pearl organs of the Cyprinidae. *Science, N.Y.* 17: 531.

Reighard, J. (1904). Further observations on the breeding habits and on the function of the pearl organs in several species of Eventognathi. *Science, N.Y.* 19: 211–212.

Reighard, J. (1910a). The pearl organs of American minnows in their relation to the factors of descent. *Science, N.Y.* 31: 472.

Reighard, J. (1910b). Methods of studying the habits of fishes with an account of the breeding habits of the horned dace. *Bull. U.S. Bur. Fish.* 28: 1111–1136.

Reighard, J. (1943). The breeding habits of the river chub, *Nocomis micropogon* (Cope). *Pap. Mich. Acad. Sci. Arts Lett.* 28: 397–423.

Richardson, L. L. (1942). The occurrence of nuptial tubercles on the female of *Osmerus mordax* (Mitchill). *Copeia* 1942: 27–29.

Roberts, T. R. (1973a). Interrelationships of ostariophysans. *Zool. J. Linn. Soc.* 53 (Suppl. 1): 373–395.

Roberts, T. R. (1973b). The glandulocaudine characid fishes of the Guayas Basin in western Ecuador. *Bull. Mus. comp. Zool.* 144: 489–514.

Rosen, D. E. (1964). The relationships and taxonomic position of the halfbeaks, killifishes, silversides, and their relatives. *Bull. Am. Mus. nat. Hist.* 127: 219–267.

Rosen, D. E. (1974). Phylogeny and zoogeography of salmoniform fishes and relationships of *Lepidogalaxias salamandroides. Bull. Am. Mus. nat. Hist.* 153: 265–326.

Rosen, D. E. & Bailey, R. M. (1963). The poeciliid fishes (Cyprinodontiformes), their structure, zoogeography, and systematics. *Bull. Am. Mus. nat. Hist.* 126: 1–76.

Ross, D. F. (1974). Tuberculation of the silverjaw minnow, *Ericymba buccata. Copeia* 1974: 271–272.

Sato, M. (1935). Note on the nuptial coloration and pearl organs of *Tribolodon hakonensis* (Günther). *Sci. Rep. Tohoku Univ.* (Ser. 4 Biol.) 10: 499–514.

Schultz, R. J. & Miller, R. R. (1971). Species of the *Poecilia sphenops* complex (Pisces: Poeciliidae) in Mexico. *Copeia* 1971: 282–290.

Shiraishi, Y. & Takeda, T. (1961). The influence of photoperiodicity on the maturation of ayu-fish, *Plecoglossus altivelis. Bull. Freshw. Fish. Res. Lab., Tokyo* 11: 69–84. [In Japanese with English summary.]

Silas, E. G. (1953). Classification, zoogeography and evolution of the fishes of the cyprinoid families Homalopteridae and Gastromyzonidae. *Rec. Indian Mus.* **50**: 173–263.

Skelton, P. H. (1974). On the life colours and nuptial tubercles of *Oreodaimon quathlambae* (Barnard, 1938) (Pisces, Cyprinidae). *Ann. Cape Prov. Mus. (Nat. Hist.)* **9**: 215–222.

Smith, C. L. & Tyler, J. C. (1972). Space resource sharing in a coral reef fish community. *Sci. Bull. Los Angeles Co. Nat. Hist. Mus.* **14**: 125–170.

Smith, H. M. (1945). The fresh-water fishes of Siam, or Thailand. *Bull. U.S. natn. Mus.* No. 188: 1–622.

Smith, R. J. F. (1974). Effects of 17α-methyltestosterone on the dorsal pad and tubercles of fathead minnows (*Pimephales promelas*). *Can. J. Zool.* **52**: 1031–1038.

Snelson, F. F., Jr. & Pflieger, W. L. (1975). Redescription of the redfin shiner, *Notropis umbratilis*, and its subspecies in the central Mississippi River basin. *Copeia* **1975**: 231–249.

Spearman, R. I. C. (1973). *The integument. A textbook of skin biology.* London: Cambridge Univ. Press.

Stenholt Clausen, H. (1967). *Tropical old world cyprinodonts.* Kobenhaven: Akad. Forlag.

Stokłosowa, S. (1966). Sexual dimorphism in the skin of sea-trout, *Salmo trutta*. *Copeia* **1966**: 613–614.

Tchernavin, V. V. (1944). A revision of the subfamily Orestiinae. *Proc. zool. Soc. Lond.* **114**: 140–233.

Templeman, W. (1965). Some resemblances and differences between *Raja erinacea* and *Raja ocellata*, including a method of separating mature and large-immature individuals of these two species. *J. Fish. Res. Bd Can.* **22**: 899–912.

Thys van den Audenaerde, D. F. E. (1961a). Existence de deux races geo-graphiques distinctes chez *Phractolaemus ansorgei* Blgr. 1901 (Pisces, Clupei-formes). *Bull. Acad. R. Sci. Outre-Mer* **7**: 222–251.

Thys van den Audenaerde, D. F. E. (1961b). L'anatomie de *Phractolaemus ansorgei* Blgr. et la position systématique des Phractolaemidae. *Ann. Mus. R. Afr. centr.*, (8° Zool.), No. 103: 101–167.

Tozawa, T. (1923). Studies on the pearl organs of the goldfish. *Annotnes zool. jap.* **10**: 253–263.

Tozawa, T. (1929). Experiments on the development of the nuptial coloration and pearl organs of the Japanese bitterling. *Folia anat. jap.* **7**: 407–417.

Uwa, H. (1975). Formation of anal-fin processes at the anterior margin of joint plates induced by treatment with androgen in adult females of the medaka, *Oryzias latipes. Zool. Mag., Tokyo* **84**: 161–165. [In Japanese with English abstract.]

Vladykov, V. D. (1935). Secondary sexual dimorphism in some Chinese cobitid fishes. *J. Morph.* **57**: 275–302.

Vladykov, V. D. (1954). Taxonomic characters of the eastern North American chars (*Salvelinus* and *Cristivomer*). *J. Fish. Res. Bd Can.* **11**: 904–932.

Vladykov, V. D. (1970). Pearl tubercles and certain cranial peculiarities useful in the taxonomy of coregonid genera. In *Biology of coregonid fishes*: 167-193. Lindsey, C. C. and Woods, C. S. (eds). Winnipeg: Univ. Manitoba Press.

268   BRUCE B. COLLETTE

Wall, B. R., Jr. & Williams, J. D. (1974). *Etheostoma boschungi*, a new percid fish from the Tennessee River drainage in northern Alabama and western Tennessee. *Tulane Stud. Zool. Bot.* **18**: 143–182.
Wallace, D. C. (1973). Reproduction of the silverjaw minnow, *Ericymba buccata* Cope. *Trans. Am. Fish. Soc.* **102**: 786–793.
Weisel, G. F. (1975). The integument of the paddlefish, *Polyodon spathula. J. Morph.* **145**: 143–150.
Weitzman, S. H. (1954). The osteology and the relationships of the South American characid fishes of the subfamily Gasteropelecinae. *Stanford Ichthy. Bull.* **4**: 213–263.
Weitzman, S. H. & Cobb, J. S. (1975). A revision of the South American fishes of the genus *Nannostomus* Günther (family Lebiasinidae). *Smithson. Contrib. Zool.* No. 186: 1–36.
Weitzman, S. H. & Thomerson, J. E. (1970). A new species of glandulocaudine characid fish, *Hysteronotus myersi*, from Peru. *Proc. Calif. Acad. Sci.* (4) **38**(8): 139–156.
Wiley, M. L. & Collette, B. B. (1970). Breeding tubercles and contact organs in fishes: Their occurrence, structure, and significance. *Bull. Am. Mus. nat. Hist.* **143**: 143–216.
Williams, J. D. (1975). Systematics of the percid fishes of the subgenus *Ammocrypta*, genus *Ammocrypta*, with descriptions of two new species. *Bull. Alabama Mus. nat. Hist.* No. 1: 1–56.
Yamamoto, M. & Egami, N. (1974). Fine structure of the surface of the anal fin and the processes on its fin rays of male *Oryzias latipes. Copeia* **1974**: 262–265.
Yamamoto, T. (1975). *Medaka (killifish) biology and strains.* Stock Culture Biol. Field Series. Tokyo: Keigaku Publ. Co.
Yamazaki, F. (1972). Effects of methyltestosterone on the skin and the gonad of salmonids. *Gen. comp. Endocrinol.* Suppl. 3: 741–750.

Symp. zool. Soc. Lond. (1977) No. 39, 269–289.

THE ANURAN TADPOLE SKIN: CHANGES OCCURRING IN IT DURING METAMORPHOSIS AND SOME COMPARISONS WITH THAT OF THE ADULT

H. FOX

Department of Zoology, University College London, London, England

SYNOPSIS

The fine structure and the degeneration of the skin of larvae and adults of *Rana temporaria* and *Xenopus laevis* have been described. Throughout ontogeny there is a high degree of similarity in their skin structure and fate, and the epidermis and dermis are considered to be a unified dynamic system. New cell types and functional properties (physiological and biochemical) arise at specific intervals in ontogeny (especially at climax), as the larval skin structure grades almost imperceptibly into that of the froglet and thence adult. Differences recognized in the skin of the larval tail, of its body and of the adult, are considered to be of less importance than the overriding and fundamental similarities, which they share and which persist throughout life.

INTRODUCTION

Since the earlier descriptions by light microscopy of amphibian larval and adult skin (Howes, 1947; Noble, 1954; Andrews, 1959), use of the electron microscope has revealed a wealth of ultrastructural detail (see among others Leeson & Threadgold, 1961; Voûte, 1963; Parakkal & Matoltsy, 1964; Farquhar & Palade, 1965, 1966; Fox, 1972a, 1974a; Spearman, 1973; Lavker, 1974; Whitear, 1974, 1975). The present account is concerned with the ultrastructure of anuran skin from different regions of the larva and the adult. Examples are drawn mainly from *Rana temporaria* and *Xenopus laevis*, and an attempt is made to show that larval epidermis and dermis represent stages in the development of skin which grade into those of the adult. There is thus no need to postulate any fundamental changes in skin structure and function throughout ontogeny.

It is true nevertheless, that there are differences between larval and adult skin of amphibians; these will be described in the succeeding pages. Furthermore, specializations occur in epidermal tissue; for example the heavily cornified digital pads of *Hyla cinerea* (Ernst, 1973a,b), the horny jaws of the larval *Rana pipiens* (Luckenbill, 1965) and the evanescent larval cement glands (Eakin, 1963;

Perry & Waddington, 1966; Lyerla & Pelizzari, 1973). Again new types of cells appear in the body (and limb) epidermis and dermis before and during metamorphic climax; though in contrast, epidermal Leydig cells of newts are lost at this time (Kelly, 1966). Yet the overall similarities of anuran skin throughout life are striking, and would appear to outweigh in importance such differences that occur. Throughout life the relatively uniform, albeit dynamic, tissues of the anuran skin can thus be claimed to have a basic structure and function.

The purpose of this account is to examine whether this hypothesis has some validity.

GENERAL DESCRIPTION OF FIGURES

All the illustrations were from skin fixed in a combined mixture of osmic acid and glutaraldehyde, except for those fixed in osmic acid alone (Palade fixative; Fig. 3), or in glutaraldehyde and post-osmicated (Fig. 12) and those specially prepared to show the localization of acid phosphatase (Figs 13–15). For further details of the electron microscopical methods used see Fox (1974a). The scale on the illustrations is 1 μm.

ABBREVIATIONS FOR FIGURES 1–15

au, autolysis; bl, basement lamellar collagen; cf, collagen fibrils; co, cornified epidermal cell; cy, cytolysome; d, desmosome; db, dense body; dl, dense cellular surface layer; ds, dense substance below presloughing cell; ic, ingested collagen in macrophage; ie, inner epidermal cell; ij, intercellular junction; ma, macrophage; oe, outermost epidermal cell; rp, reaction product registering the localization of acid phosphatase and hence lysosomal enzyme activity; tf, tonofilaments; vrp, vestigial reaction product; xa, xanthophore.

FIG. 1. *Xenopus laevis*, stage 57; tail region somewhat proximal to the tip. Non-degenerate epidermal cells above the dermal basement lamella.

FIG. 2. *X. laevis*, stages 63–64; tail stub in the distal region. Surface epidermal cellular autolysis. There is also heavy cytolysis of the inner epidermal cell, which could represent phagocytosis by an adjacent phagocytic cell or more probably a large cytolysome within an autolysing epidermal cell.

FIG. 3. *Rana temporaria*, stages 51–52; tail stub region near the tip. Outer epidermal cellular cornification preparatory to sloughing (see Fig. 7).

FIG. 4. *X. laevis*, stage 49. Epidermal cells of back skin during prometamorphosis when there is no degeneration.

FIG. 5. *R. temporaria*, stage 53. Back epidermis near the end of metamorphic climax. Note the large number of cytolysomes within cells of different layers.

FIG. 6. *X. laevis*, stages 63–64. Back epidermis at metamorphic climax. The outermost cells are cornified and ready to slough; the inner cells are somewhat electron translucent. Note the reduced dermal basement lamellar collagen and fibroblast and xanthophore.

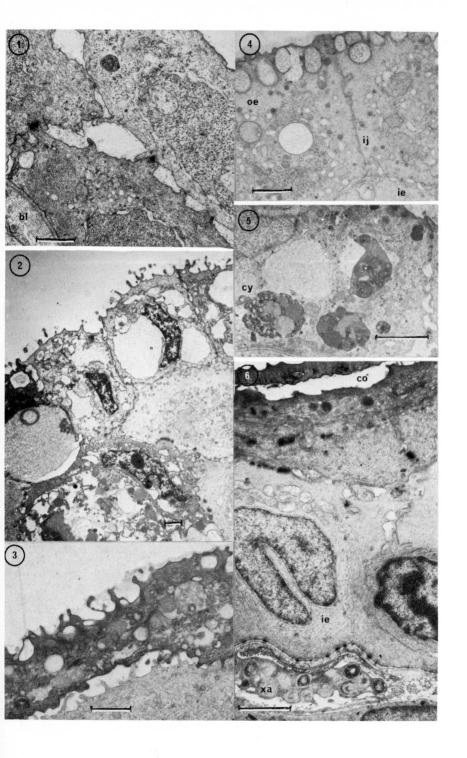

The tail

Aspects of the fine structure of the epidermis of the anuran tail, before and during metamorphic climax, have been described (see Chapman & Dawson, 1961; Leeson & Threadgold, 1961; Fox, 1972a, 1974a). In prometamorphic larvae (Etkin, 1964) of *Rana temporaria* and *Xenopus laevis*, the non-degenerate tail epidermis comprises two to three layers of cells (Weiss & Ferris, 1954; Fox, 1970, 1972a; Fox & Hamilton, 1971; see Fig. 1). In proximal tail regions there frequently appears to be a greater number of layers. This is probably due to section orientation, for examination by light and phase contrast microscopy of transverse sections (embedded in paraffin and Araldite respectively) of different regions of the anuran tail did not reveal any extra layers.

Underlying the epidermis are the adepidermal space (including lamellated bodies, Nakao, 1974) and membrane (Salpeter & Singer, 1959), and thence the orthogonally arranged collagen fibrils (each about 40–50 nm thick) of the basement lamella (see Fox, 1972a: fig. 2). The latter is about 3–4 μm wide in older larvae before climax. The number of plies (regular layers of alternating orientation) in anuran larvae is about 20 ± 2 (Weiss & Ferris, 1954, 1956), a number which may vary in different genera, for in *X. laevis* back skin (stage 55) and tail skin (stage 53) (Nieuwkoop & Faber, 1956) the basement lamellae were found to have 23 plies and there are 29 plies in back skin of a 44-mm long larva of *Rana pipiens* at stage 7 (Taylor & Kollros, 1946; see Kemp, 1963). There are anchoring filaments from the epidermal cells to the adepidermal membrane and anchoring fibrils and larger anchoring fibres, which extend from the adepidermal membrane into the basement lamellar collagen (Nakao, 1974). Their presence in tails of *Rana rugosa* is confirmed in tails of *R. temporaria*.

Outermost somewhat flattened cells of the young amphibian epidermis include ciliary and mucous cells (Edds & Sweeny, 1961; Steinman, 1968; Billet & Gould, 1971). Later in development cilia are lost (Kessel, Beams & Shih, 1974), probably soon after stage 44 in *X. laevis*; they are certainly absent at stage 47 (Fox & Hamilton, 1971). Occasionally vestiges occur even at late stages of larval ontogeny. A basal body and ciliary rootlets were recognized at the external epidermal surface of a late prometamorphic larval stage 47 (Cambar & Marrot, 1954) of *R. temporaria*. Short processes, and probably surface ridges also, develop early on from the epidermal outer surface, which is covered by a thin layer of mucus. These components remain until cell death at climax (Figs 2 and 3).

Adjacent outermost cells join laterally by tight junctions, and numerous desmosomes occur between all the epithelial cells. Typically, a well developed prometamorphic tail epidermis of *Rana* and *Xenopus* includes cells whose nuclei are variable in shape but usually flatter at the surface. Inner epidermal cells may be more spherical, cuboidal and often irregular in shape and there is some interdigitation between adjacent cells. The cytoplasm includes a granular endoplasmic reticulum, which may be quite extensive in some cells, abundant ribosomes often grouped in polysomes, mitochondria and a Golgi complex, which frequently is well developed and associated with numerous smooth-surfaced rounded vesicles–some at least are probably lysosomes (Fox, 1974a). Mucous granules, of variable electron density, line the external epidermal surface, and others occur within the cell away from the surface. All the epithelial cells contain tonofilaments, each about 7–8 nm thick, which especially in older larvae are often extremely profuse and have a felt-like appearance. Membrane-bound pigment bodies, lipid and larger lysosomes occur, the latter becoming more numerous in surface cells at late prometamorphosis (Fig. 2). The inner margins of the basal epidermal cells are lined by half-desmosomes (so-called "bobbins" of Weiss & Ferris, 1954), from which masses of tonofilaments lead almost perpendicularly into the cell. These are the Figures of Eberth (Chapman & Dawson, 1961; Fox, 1974b: fig. 2).

In addition tail epidermis includes melanophores (Bagnara, 1960), which are also present in the dermis (Gartz, 1970), Leydig cells (Pflugfelder & Schubert, 1965; Kelly, 1966), Merkel cells (*vide infra*), other granular cells which are probably immigrant polymorphonuclear neutrophils or granulocytes and distributed nerve fibres.

In general tail epidermal cells of *Rana* and *Xenopus* are similar in appearance at comparable stages of development, though even within the same genus there is some variability, especially near climax, as cellular necrosis commences at the tip. At this region there are features of incipient chromatopycnosis, cytoplasmic vacuolation and autolysis. Indeed at surprisingly relatively early stages of prometamorphosis (in *Xenopus* at stages 51–52 when there is merely a tiny hind limb bud), occasionally some outermost epidermal cells, at various levels of the tail, may be quite well advanced in the process of cornification in preparation for the major climactic necrosis.

The back skin

There are two to three layers of cells in back epidermis of *Xenopus* at stage 55 (Farquhar & Palade, 1965), an arrangement confirmed by the author in back and tail skin of *Xenopus* at stage 49 (Fig. 4) and likewise found in hind-limb skin of *Bufo* (Balinsky, 1972) and *Xenopus* (Kelley & Bluemink, 1974; Fox, unpublished). There are three epidermal cell layers at late prometamorphosis in *Rana catesbeiana* (Chapman & Dawson, 1961), two to three layers at a similar stage and up to five layers at climax in *Xenopus* and *R. temporaria*, when surface cells are sloughing (Fig. 6), although the possibility of section obliquity (*vide supra*) cannot be discounted. There are five to six layers of epidermal cells in *Ambystoma* larvae (Farquhar & Palade, 1965). Larval back and tail epidermal cells of prometamorphic *Xenopus* and *Rana* are generally similar in fine structure. Numerous back epidermal cells, especially inner ones of *Xenopus*, may, however, be somewhat electron translucent and though mitochondria are frequently seen, such profiles are mainly filamentous or fibrous and show little complexity (Fig. 6).

At climax back epidermis includes well developed melanophores and granular cells (probably immigrant blood cells, both types of cell having no desmosomes) and Leydig cells, some of which reveal an extensive granular endoplasmic reticulum alongside the large mucous vesicle. These cells are particularly well developed in *Xenopus* (Pflugfelder & Schubert, 1965). Merkel cells (Nafstad & Baker, 1973) are present; they also occur in the cloacal–tail region epidermis of climactic *Xenopus* (Fox, 1974a), in the proximal tail region of climactic *Rana temporaria* and in prometamorphic and climactic back and hind limb epidermis of *Rana* and *Xenopus* (Fox & Whitear, unpublished). Flask cells, which differentiate from epidermal cells, are present in back epidermis of a climactic stage 52 (Cambar & Marrot, 1954) *R. temporaria* (Whitear, 1975, pers. comm.). All amphibian larvae and adult perennibranchiate urodeles have epidermal neuromasts. They disappear, however, at metamorphic climax in anurans, though they are retained in the aquatic *Xenopus* (Dijkgraaf, 1963; Shelton, 1970).

The dermis of back skin of anurans at climax includes melanophores, xanthophores (Berns & Narayan, 1970; see Fig. 6), iridophores (seen in a stage 48–49 *R. temporaria*, a stage just preceding climax, Whitear, pers. comm.), granulocytes, large multicellular mucous and granular glands—which lead via ducts to the skin surface—capillaries, muscle and nerve components. Only melanophores of the chromatophore–type cells are present in both epidermis and dermis.

Tail and body dermis also include mesenchymal macrophages, which are involved in the destruction of the basement lamellar collagen (*vide infra*) and fibroblasts. The latter cells seem to play a role in the manufacture of tropocollagen whose polymerized components make up the basement lamella (Hay & Revel, 1963; Jackson, 1968; Fox, 1972a). Whether synthesis of collagen and macrophagic activity are the work of the same cells is not known.

THE SKIN OF THE ADULT

Aspects of the fine structure of adult anuran skin have been described (Voûte, 1963; Parakkal & Matoltsy, 1964; Farquhar & Palade, 1965; Lavker, 1974; Fox, 1974a; Whitear, 1974, 1975; see also Figs 10–12).

In brief there are about five to six layers of epidermal cells, joined by desmosomes. The outermost layers become keratinized at regular intervals as the stratum corneum; in *Rana temporaria* kept in a vivarium at room temperature, moulting occurs every two or three days (Whitear, 1975). Below, a second layer of cells, the granular region, includes mucous granules although these may also be recognized in the outermost epidermal cells. Middle and deeper layers have been called the stratum mucosum and stratum spinosum respectively. The basal layer or stratum germinativum, is separated from the dermis by the adepidermal space and membrane (Fig. 9). During the moulting cycle outermost epidermal cells become horny (or scaly), flattened and electron dense. The cornified cell is enveloped by a straight dense thickened membrane (see Lavker, 1974; Fox, 1974a). At first outermost cells retain various cellular components though incipient autolysis occurs (Fig. 10). Thence follows further autolysis; the tonofilaments remain, however, but fuse to a homogeneous mass. Lysosomes and lipid are recognizable and the nucleus is flattened and becomes chromatopycnotic. The morphological events of the moult have been described in *Bufo bufo* by Budtz & Larsen (1973, 1975); phases of preparation, separation, sloughing and differentiation in *Rana temporaria* were detailed by Whitear (1975).

Underlying epidermal cells, of varied shape and sometimes cuboidal with a convoluted surface, include large quantities of tonofilaments, mucous granules, which are smaller at the

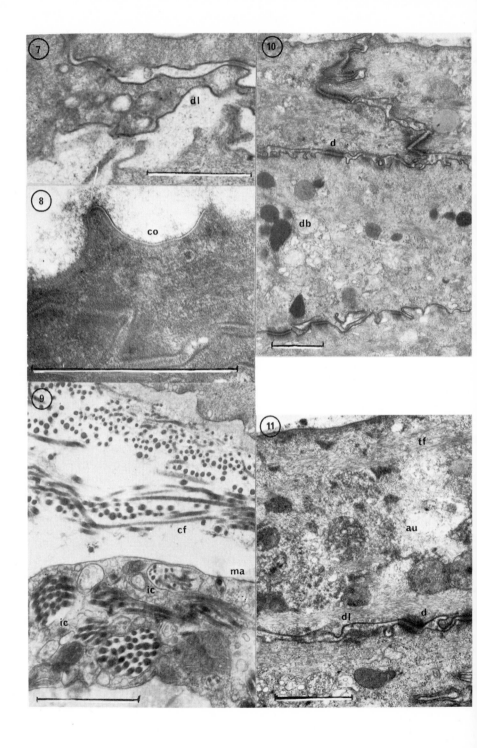

periphery, membrane-bound pigment granules, lipid, a rough and smooth endoplasmic reticulum, ribosomes, a Golgi complex and mitochondria.

The adult epidermis includes flask cells (about 10% of the cell population, Whitear, 1975), Merkel cells (about 0·3%, Nafstad & Baker, 1973), both of which have desmosomes, and other extra-epidermally derived cells which do not have them. The latter cells include melanophores, histiocytes and granular blood cells; nerve fibres are present. The dermis includes large amounts of collagen arranged in alternate bundles, fibroblasts, melanophores, xantho-phores, iridophores, dermal glands, capillaries, muscles and nerve elements.

AMPHIBIAN SKIN DEGENERATION

Throughout metamorphic climax anuran tail tissues progressively degenerate and typically in *Rana temporaria*, proceeding from the distal region proximally, more of the tail is affected. Necrosis thus becomes more widespread simultaneously with the overall reduc-tion in tail size, until the small necrotic tail stub finally disappears (see Fox, 1972a,b,c, 1973a,b,c, 1974a,b). The isolated tail of *Xenopus* degenerates *in vitro* in a manner similar to that which occurs *in vivo* (Fox & Turner, 1967) under the influence of a relatively high ambient concentration of thyroxine, triiodothyronine or thyroxine analogs (Weber, 1962; Shaffer, 1963; Frieden & Just, 1970). In *Rana*, for example, the outermost degenerate epidermal cells of the distal region of the reduced tail stub include fibrous or other dense rounded bodies, which are

FIGS 7–11. For key to abbreviations see p. 270. Scale on all figures 1 μm.
FIG. 7. *X. laevis*, stage 63. Back epidermis at the height of metamorphic climax. Outermost epidermal cells are cornified and have a dense enveloping membrane. Compare the arrangement with Figs 3, 8 and 12.
FIG. 8. *R. temporaria*, stage 54 at the end of climax. Back epidermis of newly formed young froglet. The outermost cells are cornified with the loss of various cytoplasmic organelles but tonofilaments are retained. There is an outer thickened and dense membrane enveloping the cells, a structure which also occurs in the larval tail and adult body when cells are cornified.
FIG. 9. *R. temporaria*, adult female back skin. Phagocytosis by a macrophage of dermal collagen fibrils. Presumably during life the epidermis and dermis are regularly remodelled; the surface cells of the epidermis periodically slough and new collagen fibrils are continu-ously synthesized and phagocytosed in the dermis.
FIG. 10. *R. temporaria*, adult female belly epidermis probably at the intermoult stage (Whitear, 1975). The outermost epidermal cells, however, show incipient autolysis before the more severe degeneration and cornification at moulting.
FIG. 11. *R. temporaria*, adult female belly epidermis. Severe autolysis of the outermost epidermal cells; heavier thickening of the enveloping surface membrane. The cells are probably at the preparation phase during the sloughing cycle (Whitear, 1975).

probably lysosomes, and lipid. These electron dense, flattened cells
are dehydrated and cornified, more frequently described as
keratinized. Ultimately the cell components are unrecognizable
and only the tightly packed tonofilaments, fused as a homogeneous
mass, remain.

An outer thickened dense membrane envelops the fully cornified epidermal cell (Fig. 3), a feature first recognized in adults
(Farquhar & Palade, 1965; Fox,1974a; Lavker, 1974; Whitear,
1975); here the membrane is about 20–25 nm thick, slightly thicker
than in the larva.

It is probable that the desmosomes are ultimately degraded
by lysosomal enzymes (Douglas, Ripley & Ellis, 1970), and
finally they release the cornified cells which are shed. Side by
side with the surface cellular autolysis and cornification many
inner tail epidermal cells develop large cytolysomes, which
frequently fill much of the cell. Occasionally (as in *Xenopus*)
heavy autolysis of outer and inner epidermal cells is recognized, without as yet any obvious features of cornification
(Fig. 2).

Histochemical investigation by electron microscopy reveals that
tail epidermal cells of young prometamorphic larvae of *Xenopus* at
stages 46–47 (the smallest distinguishable hind-limb buds do not
appear until stage 49, Nieuwkoop & Faber, 1956) possess discrete
lysosomal bodies positive for reaction product (a register for acid
phosphatase; see Gomori, 1952; Barka & Anderson, 1962; Fox,
1974a).

Degenerating tail epidermal cells, in different layers of *Rana*
and *Xenopus* at late prometamorphosis and climax, show reaction
product in small lysosomes, autophagic vacuoles and larger cytolysomes and also at the cell surface (Fig. 13; see also Fox, 1974a).
Reaction product is never deposited on desmosomes, tight junctions, the external epidermal surface, tonofilaments and collagen.
The primary lysosomes probably originate from the Golgi cisternae (Novikoff, Essner & Quintana, 1964; Michaels, Albright & Patt,
1971; Fox, 1974a). Heavier though similar deposition of reaction
product is found in cytolysomes of epidermal cells at climax. As in
adults little reaction product occurs in the outermost highly cornified cells, which have now practically completed their autolysis
and are mainly composed of fused tonofilamentous substance
(Figs 14 and 15).

Simultaneously with epidermal cellular degeneration the dermal collagenous basement lamella is destroyed, a process elicited

mainly by invasive mesenchymal macrophages which engulf the collagen and ingest it within heterophagic vacuoles utilizing lysosomal enzymes (Usuku & Gross, 1965; Gona, 1969; Fox, 1972a).

In addition to the qualified similarity of fine structure of the larval anuran tail and back epidermis, features of their degeneration at climax are similar (Figs 3, 6–8). A dense thickened surface membrane likewise envelopes the outermost back epidermal cells. Nevertheless though larval back epidermal cells frequently include numerous cytolysomes at climax (Fig. 5), on the whole there appears to be less major cytolysis within inner cells, compared with the tail, (Fig. 6). The mechanism is more akin to that which proceeds in the adult during the periodic and regular sloughing cycle.

Comparison of profiles of back epidermal cellular degeneration in *Rana* and *Xenopus* at climax, with those profiles demonstrating acid phosphatase activity in the epidermal cells of the larval tail, external gill filaments and the adult body of such anurans (Farquhar & Palade, 1965; Michaels *et al.* 1971; Fox, 1972a, 1974a; Lavker, 1974), strongly suggests that in all these different regions in the larva and adult lysosomal enzymes similarly initiate autolysis of cell components, for autophagic vacuoles and cytolysomes are commonplace in anuran climactic and adult back epidermal cells (Figs 5, 14 and 15).

Epidermal cells of the tail and gill filaments disappear during larval life, an important distinction from that which occurs in the climactic and adult body epidermis. The latter retain their basal germinative epidermal cells, which maintain the overall epidermal population by replenishing from below those that are shed at the surface. Nevertheless it is likely that all post-climactic epidermal cells, of whatever type above the basal layer, eventually degenerate and are shed at some occasion during the sloughing cycle. Yet little is known about the life cycles of different specialized cells of the amphibian epidermis. Whether flask cells, for example, keratinize and slough is not known; they may well be cut off from below by replacement cells thence to be shed with the slough (Whitear, 1975).

At climax all the basement lamellar collagen of the anuran tail is phagocytosed by mesenchymal macrophages (see Fox, 1972a). If the larval *Rana pipiens* is exposed to a relatively high ambient concentration of exogenous thyroxine (1 mg/litre of tap water), mesenchymal cells likewise invade the basement lamella of the back

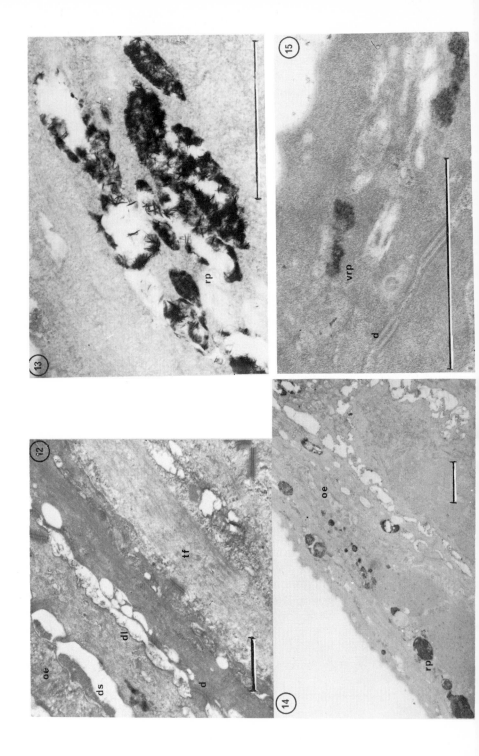

skin, detach it from the adepidermal membrane and thus separate the collagen from the epidermis. Beneath the adepidermal membrane the stratum spongiosum develops from the mesenchymal cells and the stratum compactum, or adult dermal lamella, is derived from the basement lamellar collagen plus some mesenchymal cells. Polymerization of fresh collagen fibrils and ground substance results in a new basement membrane between the adepidermal membrane and the stratum spongiosum (Kemp, 1963). It is not clear from Kemp's account whether mesenchymal cells at some stage actually phagocytose some at least of the basement lamellar collagen of the back skin, though it would appear that collagen fibrils are retained within the stratum compactum. At metamorphic climax the fibrillar collagenous zone of *Xenopus* disintegrates and the stratum spongiosum replaces it (Pflugfelder & Schubert, 1965).

In view of the striking similarity of the process in climatic larval back and tail dermis, some phagocytosis of collagen in larval back skin may be predicted, especially as new collagen is subsequently formed. Examination of climatic *Rana* and *Xenopus* back skin reveals a highly disorganized collagenous basement lamella invaded, among others, by mesenchymal macrophagic cells, in a manner similar to that which takes place in the tail. Their cytoplasmic profiles seem replete with heterophagic vacuoles of ingested degraded collagen. Phagocytosis of collagen fibrils by macrophages was also recognized in adult back skin of *Rana temporaria* (Fig. 9).

Therefore, it is reasonable to assume that at climax the basement lamellar collagen of the back skin is at least partially, perhaps even wholly, replaced by newly synthesized collagen which increases in amount in the froglet and adult.

FIGS 12–15. For key to abbreviations see p. 270. Scale on all figures 1 μm.

FIG. 12. *X. laevis*, adult male back epidermis during the sloughing period. The outermost cornified cells are in the process of being shed, probably at a stage just before separation.

FIG. 13. *R. temporaria*, stage 49 at the onset of the metamorphic climax. Heavy deposition of reaction product in the tail outer epidermal cells, near the tip. Autolysis and cornification are proceeding as the epidermal cells degenerate before sloughing.

FIG. 14. *R. temporaria*, adult female belly skin epidermis. Outermost cornified cells at the height of the sloughing cycle showing lysosomal bodies positive for reaction product. Most of the cytoplasmic components are degraded and the cornified cells would soon have been shed.

FIG. 15. *R. temporaria*, adult female back epidermis. Outermost highly cornified epidermal cell with vestigial deposition of reaction product. Most of the cellular tissue, except for the tonofilaments, has autolysed. The desmosomes, however, are still present and cells are shed only when they degrade and hence release the cells.

DISCUSSION

The,skins of the anuran larval tail and body and of the adult show many similarities, though indeed some differences occur. In terms of biochemistry, for example, they differ in their content of glycosaminoglycans, and hyaluronidase, present in prometamorphic and climactic skin of *Rana catesbeiana*, seems to be absent in skin of adults (Lipson, Cerskus & Silbert, 1971). Again in the same species the skin of the adult is less permeable to Na^+ and Cl^- ions (Alvarado & Moody, 1970) and the response of ATPase to thyroxine differs in the tadpole compared with the adult (Kawada, Taylor & Barker, 1972). In morphological terms the epidermis of the adult has more layers of cells compared with that of the tadpole, though climactic back epidermis has practically reached the adult number. The epidermis and dermis of the adult may well include a somewhat greater variety of cell types than is present in preclimactic larvae, though indeed most new cells have appeared by the time of climax. In the newt *Taricha torosa*, however, Leydig cells which are common in the epidermis of larval amphibians have disappeared at the end of metamorphosis coinciding with cornification (Kelly, 1966).

Merkel cells and melanophores are present in the larval epidermis before climax (*vide supra*); flask cells appear in the epidermis (in *Rana temporaria*, Whitear, pers. comm.) and xanthophores and iridophores in the dermis at climax. Iridophores occur in tadpoles of *R. catesbeiana* (Ide, 1973) and *R. temporaria* (Whitear, pers. comm.). Presumably in the adult a more substantial skin is necessary as an adaptation to the increase in body size and its physiological and ecological needs. Furthermore in the post-climactic and adult anurans the basal epidermal cells continue to replenish the epidermal cell population—which obviously cannot occur in the missing tail after climax—as cells are lost from the surface at intervals during the sloughing cycle.

Michaels *et al.* (1971) described epidermal cellular degeneration of the external gill filaments of the larval *Rana pipiens* to proceed by autolysis; that some epidermal cells phagocytose others and heterophils and macrophages remove necrotic debris. Likewise in the climactic tadpole tail of the dwarf tree frog *Litoria glauerti*, Kerr, Harmon & Searle (1974) described autolysis of epidermal cells which are ingested by nearby viable cells and the majority by macrophages distributed throughout the epidermis; a phenomenon they termed apoptosis.

Phagocytosis of one epidermal cell by another, or by a macrophage, is difficult to establish with any degree of certainty from static profiles of electron microscopy. Adjacent cells may indent one another and under certain conditions of section orientation a highly necrotic cell, or its remnants, may appear to be enclosed within a somewhat healthier one. "It is uncertain whether the apparently phagocytic cells were active in the process of breakdown or simply passively accommodated their dying neighbours" (Michaels et al., 1971). Again cellular autophagy and heterophagy appear extremely similar under the electron microscope and "autophagic vacuoles may indeed be difficult to distinguish from ingested apoptopic bodies that do not contain nuclear remnants" (Kerr et al., 1974).

Epidermal cells of external gill filaments of premetamorphic tadpoles appear to degenerate somewhat differently from those of the tail and body during climax and post-climax, for the superficial gill-filament epidermal cells do not cornify at this early stage of larval development (Michaels et al., 1971). Hourdry (1974) has described similar autolytic phenomena, of lysosomal nature, when the internal gill filaments of Discoglossus pictus degenerate at metamorphic climax. The extruded necrotic substance is ultimately ingested by macrophages as in the case of the external gill filament epidermal cells of Rana pipiens.

Kerr et al. (1974) are in error in assuming that secondary lysosomes are few in epidermal cells of the tail at fairly advanced stages of its regression. In Rana and Xenopus small lysomal bodies are plentiful in surface epidermal cells and indeed in inner ones too, near climax, and large autolytic cytolysomes are common, with substantial deposition of acid phosphatase, in numerous epidermal cells at climax (see Fox, 1974a).

It seems to be universally agreed, therefore, that among amphibians the epidermal cells autolyse when they degenerate. Larval epidermal cells of anurans cornify and slough from the skin surface, in a manner similar to that of the adult epidermis during the sloughing cycle (Gona, 1969; Lavker, 1974; Fox, 1974a). The complex process would hardly permit substantial phagocytosis; indeed if some macrophagic activity does occur then it is of relatively minor significance.

The extensive cytolysis in tail epidermis at climax is autophagic and lysosomal. That which occurs with inner tail cells probably provides a supplement to the autolysis and cornification of those at the skin surface, and assists in facilitating the severe and rapid epidermal destruction which occurs during tail involution.

Apart from a seemingly higher degree of cytolysis of tail epidermal cells, cellular degeneration of the larval and adult

epidermis seems to be similar. The invasion of the dermal basement lamellar collagen by mesenchymal cells, in the climactic tail
and back, is comparable, though subsequently new collagen fibrils
are synthesized and thence deposited in the body dermis of the
post-climactic froglets (Kemp, 1963). In terms of structure and
ultimate fate larval and adult amphibian skin reveal strong
similarities, such differences as there are being mainly modifications of a fundamental arrangement in adaptation to the animals'
changing size and mode of life. It is of interest that when an aquatic
environment is retained by the adult, as in the case of *Xenopus*, the
neuromasts of the aquatic larva are retained; they are lost in the
terrestrial *Rana*.

During prometamorphosis some new tail and body epidermal
cells arise to accommodate the overall increase in larval size. More
body epidermal cells are produced than are lost in the post-
climactic growing froglet. In the adult presumably epidermal cell
loss and gain are in balance in harmony with the sloughing cycle.
Only a relatively modest percentage of larval epidermal cells of
Rana and *Xenopus* appear to degenerate during prometamorphosis, judged from electron microscopical examination of various
regions of the tail and body. At late prometamorphosis the larva
ceases to grow larger and presumably epidermal numbers remain
approximately constant. It is not clear whether there is a reduction
(or cessation) in the number of newly produced tail epidermal
cells. Basal tail epidermal cells may differ from those of the body by
dying prematurely at climax, in some way due to a lower threshold
of survival to the relatively high circulatory concentration of thyroid hormones. Alternatively tail basal epidermal cells may be
basically the same as those of the body but suffer degeneration at
climax because of necrotizing influences from other tail tissues,
which lead to a failure of blood supply and innervation.

It is of interest that a particular specimen of *R. temporaria* at the
onset of climax showed massive cytolysis of the epidermis, a feature
similar to the severe necrosis of tail epidermal cells. Whether there
are regional differences in the degree of epidermal degeneration
in the climactic larval body or whether most of the body epidermis
is replaced at this time, is not known. It would seem unlikely,
however, that the basal cells are replaced; more likely they remain
and continue to provide the increased population of epidermal
cells required by the post-climactic froglet.

The fact that at climax on the whole there seems to be greater
autolysis within tail inner epidermal cells, compared with those of

the body of the larva, suggests intrinsic differences between them. Yet the necrotic milieu experienced by the tail epidermis cannot be disregarded. In *Alytes obstetricans* skin (and other tissues) of the tail homografted to the tadpole back sometimes survived metamorphosis (Delsol & Flatin, 1967). Thus tail tissues may not be specifically programmed to degenerate at climax. Perhaps tail epidermal cellular specificity and location are both involved in their climactic regression, which primarily is triggered off by those endocrinological activities occurring near and at climax (Etkin, 1970). They elicit the varied and complex cellular biochemical changes of different reacting tissues of the tail leading to its involution (Weber, 1969; Frieden & Just, 1970).

ACKNOWLEDGEMENTS

I am pleased to express my thanks to Dr Mary Whitear of the Department of Zoology, University College London, for reading the manuscript and for many discussions on the subject of this work. The technical assistance of Edwin Perry is warmly appreciated.

REFERENCES

Alvarado, R. H. & Moody, A. (1970). Sodium and chloride transport in tadpoles of the bull frog *Rana catesbeiana*. *Am. J. Physiol.* **218**: 1510–1516.
Andrews, W. (1959). *Text book of comparative histology*. New York and London: Oxford University Press.
Bagnara, J. T. (1960). Tail melanophores of *Xenopus* in normal development and regeneration. *Biol. Bull. mar. biol. Lab., Woods Hole* **118**: 1–8.
Balinsky, B. I. (1972). The fine structure of the amphibian limb bud. *Acta Embryol. exp.* **1972**, suppl.: 455–470.
Barka, T. & Anderson, P. J. (1962). Histochemical methods for acid phosphatase using hexazonium pararosanilin as complex. *J. Histochem. Cytochem.* **10**: 741-753.
Berns, M. W. & Narayan, K. S. (1970). An histochemical and ultrastructural analysis of the dermal chromatophores of the variant ranid blue frog. *J. Morph.* **132**: 169–180.
Billet, F. A. & Gould, R. P. (1971). Fine structural changes in the differentiating epidermis of *Xenopus laevis* embryos. *J. Anat.* **108**: 465–480.
Budtz, P. E. & Larsen, L. O. (1973). Structure of the toad epidermis during the moulting cycle. I. Light microscopic observations in *Bufo bufo* (L.). *Z. Zellforsch. mikrosk. Anat.* **144**: 353–368.
Budtz, P. E. & Larsen, L. O. (1975). Structure of the toad epidermis during the moulting cycle. II. Electron microscopic observations in *Bufo bufo*. *Cell Tiss. Res.* **159**: 459–483.
Cambar, R. & Marrot, B. (1954). Table chronologique du développement de la grenouille agile (*Rana dalmatina* Bon.). *Bull. biol. Fr. Belg.* **88**: 168–177.

Chapman, G. B. & Dawson, A. B. (1961). Fine structure of the larval anuran epidermis, with special reference to the figures of Eberth. *J. biophys. biochem. Cytol.* **10**: 425–435.

Delsol, M. & Flatin, J. (1967). Premieres observations d'ensemble sur des homogreffes realisées chez têtard d'*Alytes obstetricans*. *Bull. Ass. Anat. 52'nd. Réunion*, Paris–Orsay, April 1967: 398–402.

Dijkgraaf, S. (1963). The functioning and significance of the lateral-line organs. *Biol. Rev.* **38**: 51–105.

Douglas, W. H. J., Ripley, R. C. & Ellis, R. A. (1970). Enzymatic digestion of desmosome and hemidesmosome plaques performed on ultrathin sections. *J. Cell Biol.* **44**: 211–215.

Eakin, R. M. (1963). Ultrastructural differences of the oral sucker in the Pacific tree frog, *Hyla regilla*. *Devl Biol.* **7**: 169–179.

Edds, M. V. & Sweeny, P. R. (1961). Chemical and morphological differentiation of the basement lamella. In *Synthesis of molecular and cellular structures*: 111–138. Rudnick, D. (ed.). New York: Ronald Press.

Ernst, V. V. (1973a). The digital pads of the frog, *Hyla cinerea*: I. The epidermis. *Tissue & Cell* **5**: 83–96.

Ernst, V. V. (1973b). The digital pads of the frog, Hyla *cinerea*: II. The mucous glands. *Tissue & Cell* **5**: 97–104.

Etkin, W. (1964). Metamorphosis. In *Physiology of the Amphibia*: 427–468. Moore, J. A. (ed.). New York and London: Academic Press.

Etkin, W. (1970). An endocrine mechanism of amphibian metamorphosis, an evolutionary achievement. *Mem. Soc. Endocr.* No. 18: 137–155.

Farquhar, M. G. & Palade, G. E. (1965). Cell junctions in amphibian skin. *J. Cell Biol.* **26**: 263–291.

Farquhar, M. G. & Palade, G. E. (1966). Adenosine triphosphatase localization in amphibian epidermis. *J. Cell Biol.* **30**: 359–379.

Fox, H. (1970). Cilia in cloaca and hind gut of *Xenopus* Larvae seen by electron microscopy. *Archs Biol. (Liège)* **81**: 1-20.

Fox, H. (1972a). Tissue degeneration: an electron microscope study of the tail skin of *Rana temporaria* during metamorphosis. *Archs Biol. (Liège)* **83**: 373–394.

Fox, H. (1972b). Sub-dermal and notochordal collagen degeneration in the tail of *Rana temporaria*: an electron microscopic study. *Archs Biol. (Liège)* **83**: 395–405.

Fox, H. (1972c). Muscle degeneration in the tail of *Rana temporaria* larvae at metamorphic climax: an electron microscopic study. *Archs Biol. (Liège)* **83**: 407–417.

Fox, H. (1973a). Degeneration of the tail notochord of *Rana temporaria* at metamorphic climax. Examination by electron microscopy. *Z. Zellforsch. mikrosk. Anat.*138: 371–386.

Fox, H. (1973b). Degeneration of the nerve cord in the tail of *Rana temporaria* during metamorphic climax: a study by electron microscopy. *J. Embryol. exp. Morph.* **30**: 377–396.

Fox, H. (1973c). Ultrastructure of tail degeneration in *Rana temporaria*. *Folia morph. (Praha)* **21**: 109–112.

Fox, H. (1974a). The epidermis and its degeneration in the larval tail and adult body of *Rana temporaria* and *Xenopus laevis* (Amphibia: Anura). *J. Zool., Lond.* **174**: 217–235.

Fox, H. (1974b). Tail degeneration in anuran larvae. *Br. J. Herpet.* **5**: 397–404.

Fox, H. & Hamilton, L. (1971). Ultrastructure of diploid and haploid cells of *Xenopus laevis* larvae. *J. Embryol. exp. Morph.* **26**: 81–98.

Fox, H. & Turner, S. C. (1967). A study of the relationship between the thyroid and larval growth in *Rana temporaria* and *Xenopus laevis*. *Archs Biol. (Liège)* **78**: 61–90.

Frieden, E. & Just, J. J. (1970). Hormonal responses in amphibian metamorphosis. In *Biochemical actions of hormones* **1**: 1–52. Litwak, G. (ed.). New York and London: Academic Press.

Gartz, R. (1970). Adaptationsmorphologie der Melanophoren von Krallenfrosch-Larven. *Cytobiologie* **2**: 220–234.

Gomori, G. (1952). *Microscopic histochemistry; principles and practice.* Ithaca: University of Chicago Press.

Gona, A. (1969). Light and electronmicroscopic study on thyroxin-induced *in vitro* resorption of the tadpole tail fin. *Z. Zellforsch. mikrosk. Anat.* **95**: 483–494.

Hay, E. D. & Revel, J. D. (1963). Autoradiographic studies of the origin of the basement lamella. *Devl Biol.* **7**: 152–168.

Hourdry, J. (1974). Étude des branchies "internes" puis de leur régression au moment de la métamorphose, chez la larve de *Discoglossus pictus* (Otth.), amphibien anoure. *J. Miscroscopie* **20**: 165–182.

Howes, N. H. (1947). The skin of the tadpole of the common toad *Bufo bufo bufo* (L.), during metamorphosis. *Proc. zool. Soc. Lond.* **116**: 602–610.

Ide, H. (1973). Effects of ACTH on melanophores and iridophores isolated from bullfrog tadpoles. *Gen. comp. Endocr.* **21**: 390–397.

Jackson, S. F. (1968). The morphogenesis of collagen. In *Biology of collagen* **2**: 1–66. Gould, S. F. (ed.). London and New York: Academic Press.

Kawada, J., Taylor, R. E. & Barker, S. B. (1972). Changes in Na, K-ATP-ase activity of *Rana catesbeiana* tadpole epidermal tissue during thyroxine-induced metamorphosis. *Endocr. jap.* **19**: 53–57.

Kelley, R. O. & Bluemink, J. G. (1974). An ultrastructural analysis of cell and matrix differentation during early limb development in *Xenopus laevis*. *Devl Biol.* **37**: 1–17.

Kelly, D. E. (1966). The Leydig cell in larval amphibian epidermis. Fine structure and function. *Anat. Rec.* **154**: 685–700.

Kemp, N. E. (1963). Metamorphic changes of dermis in skin of frog larvae exposed to thyroxine. *Devl Biol.* **7**: 244–254.

Kerr, J. F. R., Harmon, B. & Searle, J. (1974). An electron-microscope study of cell deletion in the anuran tadpole tail during spontaneous metamorphosis with special reference to apoptosis of striated muscle fibres. *J. Cell Sci.* **14**: 571–585.

Kessel, R. G., Beams, H. W. & Shih, C. Y. (1974). The origin, distribution and disappearance of the surface cilia during embryonic development of *Rana pipiens* as revealed by scanning electron microscopy. *Am. J. Anat.* **141**: 341–359.

Lavker, R. M. (1974). Horny cell formation in the epidermis of *Rana pipiens*. *J. Morph.* **142**: 365–378.

Leeson, C. R. & Threadgold, L. T. (1961). The differentiation of the epidermis in *Rana pipiens*. *Acta anat.* **44**: 159–173.

Lipson, M. J., Cerskus, R. A. & Silbert, J. E. (1971). Glycosaminoglycans and glycosaminolglycans-degrading enzyme of *Rana catesbeiana* back skin during late stages of metamorphosis. *Devl Biol.* **25**: 198–208.

Luckenbill, L. M. (1965). Morphogenesis of the horny jaws of *Rana pipiens* larvae. *Devl Biol.* **11**: 25–49.

Lyerla, T. A. & Pelizzari, J. J. (1973). Histological development of the cement gland in *Xenopus laevis* . A light microscopic study. *J. Morph.* **141**: 491–502.

Michaels, J. E., Albright, J. T. & Patt, D. I. (1971). Fine structural observations on cell death in the epidermis of the external gills of the larval frog *Rana pipiens*. *Am. J. Anat.* **132**: 301–318.

Nafstad, P. H. & Baker, R. E. (1973). Comparative ultrastructural study of normal and grafted skin in the frog, *Rana pipiens*, with special reference to neuro-epithelial connections. *Z. Zellforsch. mikrosk. Anat.* **139**: 451–462.

Nakao, T. (1974). Some observations on the fine structure of the epidermal–dermal junction in the skin of the frog *Rana rugosa*. *Am. J. Anat.* **140**: 533–550.

Nieuwkoop, P. D. & Faber, J. (1956). *Normal table of* Xenopus laevis (*Daudin*) Amsterdam: North Holland Publ. Company.

Noble, G. K. (1954). *The biology of the Amphibia.* New York: Dover Publications.

Novikoff, A. B., Essner, E. & Quintana, N. (1964). Golgi apparatus and lysosomes. *Fedn Proc. Fedn Am. Socs exp. Biol.* **23**: 1010–1022.

Parakkal, P. F. & Matoltsy, G. (1964). A study of the fine structure of the epidermis of *Rana pipiens. J. biophys. biochem. Cytol.* **20**: 85–94.

Perry, M. M. & Waddington, C. H. (1966). The ultrastructure of the cement gland in *Xenopus laevis. J. Cell Sci.* **1**: 193–200.

Pflugfelder, O. & Schubert, G. (1965). Elektronmikroskopische Untersuchungen an der Haut von Larven-und Metamorphosestadien von *Xenopus laevis* nach Kaliumperchloratbehandlung. *Z. Zellforsch. mikrosk. Anat.* **67**: 96–112.

Salpeter, M. M. & Singer, M. (1959). The fine structure of the adepidermal reticulum in the basal membrane of the skin of the newt *Triturus. J. biophys. biochem. Cytol.* **6**: 35–40.

Shaffer, B. M. (1963). The isolated *Xenopus laevis* tail: a preparation for studying the central nervous system and metamorphosis in culture. *J. Embryol. exp. Morph.* **11**: 77–90.

Shelton, P. M. J. (1970). The lateral line system at metamorphosis in *Xenopus laevis* (Daudin). *J. Embryol. exp. Morph.* **24**: 511–524.

Spearman, R. I. C. (1973). *The integument.* Cambridge: University Press.

Steinman, R. M. (1968). An electron microscopic study of ciliogenesis in developing epidermis and trachea in the embryo of *Xenopus laevis. Am. J. Anat.* **122**: 19–52.

Taylor, A. C. & Kollros, J. J. (1946). Stages in the normal development of *Rana pipiens. Anat. Rec.* **94**: 7–24.

Usuku, G. & Gross, J. (1965). Morphologic studies of connective tissue resorption in the tail fin of metamorphosing bull frog tadpoles. *Devl Biol.* **11**: 352–370.

Voûte, C. L. (1963). An electron microscopic study of the skin of the frog (*Rana pipiens*). *J. Ultrastruct. Res.* **9**: 497–510.

Weber, R. (1962). Induced metamorphosis in isolated tails of *Xenopus* larvae. *Experientia* Basel) **18**: 84.

Weber, R. (1969). Tissue involution and lysosomal enzymes during anuran metamorphosis. In *Lysosomes in biology and pathology.* **2**: 437–467. Dingle, J. T. & Fell, H. B. (eds). Amsterdam and London: North Holland Publ. Company.

Weiss, P. & Ferris, W. (1954). Electronmicroscopic study of the texture of the basement membrane of larval amphibian skin. *Proc. natn. Acad. Sci. U.S.A.* **40**: 105–112.

Weiss, P. & Ferris, W. (1956). The basement lamella of amphibian skin. Its reconstruction after wounding. *J. biophys. biochem. Cytol.* **2** (Suppl). 275–282.
Whitear, M. (1974). The nerves in frog skin. *J. Zool., Lond.* **172**: 503–529.
Whitear, M. (1975). Flask cells and epidermal dynamics in frog skin. *J. Zool., Lond.* **175**: 107–149.

Symp. zool. Soc. Lond. (1977) No. 39, 291–313.

A FUNCTIONAL COMPARISON BETWEEN THE EPIDERMIS OF FISH AND OF AMPHIBIANS

MARY WHITEAR

Department of Zoology, University College London, London, England

SYNOPSIS

Various cell types occurring in the epidermis of fish and of amphibians are described, and their functions discussed. The majority of epidermal cells in these animals are mucigenic; the surface cells in fish and in larval amphibians secrete a mucoid cuticle. There is some evidence of contributions of lipoprotein to the cuticle. A similar mucoid layer occurs at the surface of the skin of amphibians after metamorphosis, but it is then secreted into the subcorneal space, and exposed at the surface after a moult. The second tier of cells in the epidermis of adult amphibians corresponds to the outermost layer in tadpoles or in fish. A keratinized surface layer has been reported in some teleosts. It is suggested that the primary function of keratinization is protection against abrasion.

In grown amphibians the skin glands are multicellular, but fish possess a variety of unicellular epidermal glands. A type from *Latimeria* skin is illustrated.

Differentiated epidermal cells can also be sensory; these may be grouped in end organs such as neuromasts or taste buds. In addition, fish epidermis contains scattered sensory cells which closely resemble gustatory cells; these are believed to be chemosensory. Such cells have not been observed in adult amphibians, but a type which may correspond has been found in tadpoles. A further differentiated epidermal cell, the Merkel cell, has been found in a number of species of amphibians, both larval and adult. New results suggest that Merkel cells occur also in teleost skin.

In fish and in larval amphibians the gill epithelium is an organ of importance in the regulation of salt and water balance, but in adult amphibians this function is transferred to the skin. Tadpole gills possess a cell type containing numerous mitochondria, which is also found in the skin. Chloride cells in fish have a similar distribution, but a different fine structure. In adult amphibian skin, the flask cells provide the nearest equivalent. It has been suggested that all these cell types are concerned in transport processes, but there are considerable difficulties in investigating their precise function.

INTRODUCTION

Epithelia are bounding tissues and are usually physiologically active. Consequently they are morphologically interesting because they are strictly polarized; cell differentiation and replacement take place from the inside outwards, and individual cells show directional modifications.

Many epithelia have a multiplicity of functions, and this is especially true of the skin epithelium, the epidermis, of aquatic animals. The epidermis has to be protective, and sensitive; interactions with the environment involve the transport across it of various substances, either actively or passively. These generalizations apply even to arthropods and nematodes, groups with notoriously tough integuments. Multiple functions can be reflected in morphological complexity, and the epidermis usually contains several recognizably distinct types of cell. There are two problems here: how is the epidermis programmed to produce various types of cell, and moreover to vary the complex according to the region of the body, and how can functions be ascribed to the various cell types? I shall concentrate on the second aspect, ignoring the more fundamental problem of programming. I shall also confine my remarks to epidermal cells, not considering those which are intrusive in the epidermis, such as chromatophores or blood cells, and also neglecting the dermis, interesting though it is.

PROTECTIVE FUNCTIONS, KERATINIZATION, MUCUS AND OTHER SECRETIONS

The unicellular mucous glands of fishes, and the multicellular mucous glands of amphibians, are too well known to need description here. In addition, the ordinary epithelial cells in both groups are potentially mucigenic (Parakkal & Matoltsy, 1964; Carmignani & Zaccone, 1975). One of the functions of the ordinary epithelial cells, which make up the bulk of the tissue and eventually reach the outer surface, is to produce the external mucoid layer, or mucous cuticle, which covers the skin. This layer has essentially the same nature as the "fuzz" on the surfaces of internal epithelia, and is an elaboration of the glycocalyx, which is secreted through or from the apical plasma membrane. It appears in fixed material as an array of delicate branching fibrils projecting from the outside of the apical membrane of the cell. The fibrils themselves are an artefact of fixation and do not appear in frozen material (Ito, 1974).*

The skin cuticle is quite variable in different species of fish, and on different parts of the body (Whitear, 1970). The pectoral fin rays of *Blennius pholis* bear an extracellular secretion some 10 μm thick, which is more than half the total thickness of the epidermis in the region. In life the layer is fairly soft, and whitish; in sections of fixed material (Fig. 1) it is coarsely fibrous. The reactions to different stains suggest that the coarse fibres are derived from the electron dense vesicles in the distal parts of the surface epidermal cells; the vesicles can sometimes be found passing across the apices of these cells. On the fin web, and over much of the body surface, the whitish layer is not visible in life, the fixed cuticle is thinner and does not have the coarse fibrils, and the vesicles in the surface epithelial cells are not electron dense.

*Swift & Mukherjee (1976, *J. Cell Biol.* **69**: 491–494) have since reported that fibrils can appear after freeze etching.

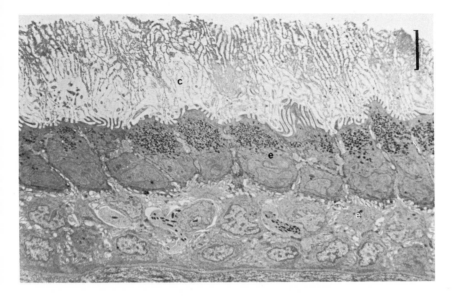

FIG. 1. Section of epidermis of a pectoral fin ray of *Blennius pholis*. Abbreviations: c, cuticle; e, epithelial cells. Scale 5 μm.

Commonly the fish skin cuticle is about 1·0 μm thick, or less, as on the body skin of *Gasterosteus aculeatus* (Fig. 2); the sheet of compacted material at the surface of the secreted layer is not always found. There are some particles of dirt stuck on the outside of the cuticle in this specimen, emphasizing its protective role even when as thin as this. In the stickleback, the surface epithelial cells do not have particularly numerous vesicles, but react to histochemical tests for acid mucopolysaccharides (Bremer, 1972).

The surface of tadpole skin has a mucoid cuticle of about the same thickness as in the stickleback; large mucous vesicles discharge into the cuticle (Fig. 3) and a compact surface layer is sometimes present.

Stereoscan or shadowed electron micrographs of the surface of the skin in amphibians and in fishes show an elegant pattern of microvillar ridges, which in fish are often arranged concentrically on each cell (Komnick & Stockem, 1969; Yamada, 1966; Collette, this symposium pp. 254–255, and other authors). It has been shown in tissue culture that the surface ridges move slowly (Bereiter-Hahn, 1971). Hawkes (1974) suggested that the microridges may aid in holding mucus on to the cell, but it is equally or perhaps more probable that the ridges are a device for providing

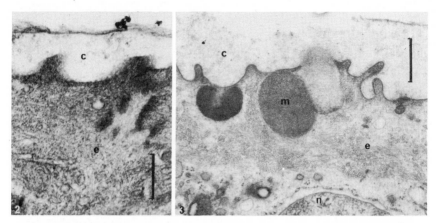

FIG. 2. Section at the surface of the epidermis of flank skin of *Gasterosteus aculeatus*. Abbreviations and scale as in Fig. 3.

FIG. 3. Section at the surface of the epidermis of back skin of a *Rana temporaria* tadpole. Abbreviations: c, cuticle; e, epithelial cell; m, mucous granule; n, nucleus. Scale 0·5 μm.

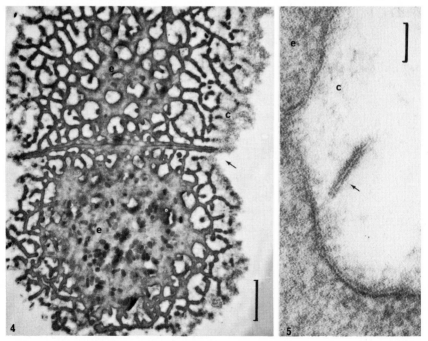

FIG. 4. Tangential section of the tip of a toe of a *Rana temporaria* tadpole. Abbreviations: c, cuticle; e, epithelial cells; the arrow indicates the zona occludens between the two cells. Scale 1 μm.

FIG. 5. Part of the surface of an outer epidermal cell from the toe of a tadpole of *Xenopus laevis*, at high magnification, showing the apical plasma membrane and a bilaminar body in the cuticle (arrowed). Abbreviations: c, cuticle; e, epithelial cell. Scale 0·05 μm.

more secretory surface. The cytoarchitecture of the ridges and terminal web region immediately below them is described in *Lebistes* by Schliwa (1975). Figure 4 is of a glancing section of the extreme tip of a tadpole's toe, showing how the microridges are embedded in the cuticle. The chemical nature of the coating layer is complex. Apart from the variations in the number and appearance of the vesicles in the apical parts of the surface cells, there is histological evidence for other contributions. If the tadpole cuticle is surveyed at high magnification, leaf-shaped bilaminar bodies can be found (Fig. 5) which are distinct from the fibrillae of the "fuzz". In the Figure the leaf-shaped structure is seen edge on; often there appears to be continuity with the outer leaflet of the plasma membrane, but the bodies may be detached and loose in the cuticle. Such bilaminar fragments have been seen also in some situations in adult amphibians and in fish. Although they are probably not precisely fragments of the plasma membrane, the artefacts of fixation are so similar that it can be supposed they represent a lipoprotein contribution to the cuticle (Whitear, in 1976a).

The section of Fig. 4 passes through the tight junction between two cells; such a *zona occludens* is normally present at the distal rim of surface epithelial cells. In adult frog skin, the surface cells are keratinized, and there are tight junctions at the distal rims of both these cells and those of the layer below (Farquhar & Palade, 1965). The section in Fig. 6 is from an individual of *Rana temporaria* which was killed when in the preparation phase of the moult cycle; the positions of the tight junctions are indicated by arrows. Although the outer cells are keratinized and dead, they still bear remnants of an external mucoid layer. By following through the events of the moult cycle, it can be deduced that this mucus was secreted early in the previous moult, between 39 and 25 hours before the frog was killed, and that it was then secreted into the subcorneal space underneath the keratinized layer. In Fig. 6 there appear to have been two phases of secretion into this space, the darker material dating from the previous moult and the paler material having come recently from the cell below, and at least partially from the dark mucous vesicles characteristic of cells of this layer.

In Fig. 6, the intercellular space below the second tier cell shows very little electron dense material, although appropriate methods such as staining with ruthenium red would show up a glycocalyx. Figure 7 shows the corresponding space between the second and third tiers from the surface, from a frog at a later stage of the moult cycle, when the second tier, or replacement layer, cells are keratinized, but the slough above is not yet shed. The intercellular

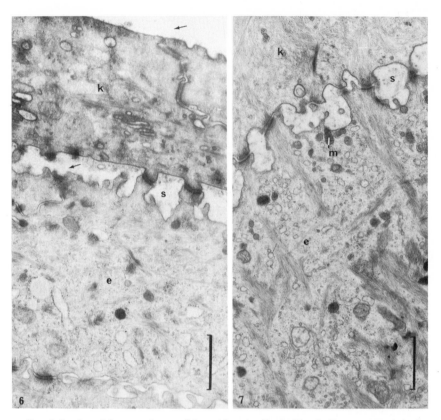

FIG. 6. Section of the outer layers of the epidermis of back skin of a *Rana temporaria* in the preparation phase of the moult cycle. The arrows indicate the positions of the tight junctions in the keratinized layer and in the replacement layer. Abbreviations: e, cell of replacement layer; k, keratinized cell; s, subcorneal space. Scale 1 μm.

FIG. 7. Section of the outer layers of the epidermis of back skin of a *Rana temporaria* in the separation phase of the moult cycle, showing a newly keratinized cell of the replacement layer and the new subcorneal space below it. Abbreviations: e, epithelial cell of third tier; k, keratinized cell of replacement layer; m, mucous granule; s, new subcorneal space. Scale 1 μm.

space below the replacement layer is the new subcorneal space and already contains secreted material; the cell above has only just keratinized, and the diagnostic shell under its plasma membrane is not yet fully thickened. Some of the material in the space may have come from the cell above before it keratinized, but mucous vesicles can be seen against the membrane of the cell below. This cell has also newly formed tight junctions with its neighbours (Whitear, 1975).

In the adult frog, then, the outer side of the second tier of epidermal cells resembles the epidermal surface of a tadpole, secreting a mucous layer and having tight junctions. In fact, this is the outer layer of living cells, so that in an amphibian after metamorphosis the physiological outer surface is not at the same place as the physical outer surface.

The keratinized layer allows water, ions and smallish molecules to pass through it, although it excludes molecules as large as ruthenium red (Nielsen, 1972; Martinez-Palomo, Erlij & Bracho, 1971). Ruthenium red will not normally stain the material in the subcorneal space, simply because it does not gain access to it; where the stain can infiltrate under the keratinized layer, as at the edge of a block, the mucus in the subcorneal space reacts to it. The external surface layer of fish epidermis also stains with ruthenium red (Lanzing & Wright, 1974), emphasizing the similarity of that secretion to the content of the subcorneal space. Amphibians have a secretion corresponding to the fish cuticle under the keratinized layer, and another, secreted previously, at the outer surface.

A subcorneal space occurs wherever the surface layers are keratinized, for instance in the toes of axolotls and of larval salamanders, although elsewhere, where their skins are not keratinized, the space between the first and second cell layers is not differentiated and the second tier cells are not united by tight junctions.

The cornification on the toes of larval urodeles is of interest because it may give a clue to the selective advantage of keratinization. It is often stated that keratinization in tetrapods is a device to prevent water loss, although associated phospholipids rather than keratin provide the actual waterproofing (Spearman, 1973). In the amphibians the thin stratum corneum is permeable to water, so that water conservation cannot be its function.

In fishes, it appears that there are three ways of guarding against potential abrasion. The thick and fibrous cuticle on some parts of *Blennius* has been mentioned; even greater development of a cuticle occurs in the gurnards, Triglidae (Whitear, 1970), and stonefish (Fishelson, 1973). Mittal and his colleagues have made interesting studies of the skins of several tropical air-breathing fishes. One of these, *Amphipnous cuchia*, is capable of leaving the water, and has numerous large mucous cells in the epidermis (Mittal & Munshi, 1971). It also has a mucus-rich layer in the dermis, so paralleling certain anurans (Elkan, 1968), but that is beyond my scope. As far as the epidermis goes, *Anguilla* provides a similar example of a fish able to leave the water and is proverbially slippery, although a tame eel does not feel particularly slimy. The catfish *Heteropneustes fossilis* also has many mucous cells in the epidermis; it does not emerge from the water voluntarily but is liable to be caught by drought (Mittal & Munshi, 1971) and is related to the well-known walking catfishes *Clarias* spp., which do wander on land. Fish are capable of making keratin even if they do not generally do so; specialized structures like breeding tubercles are keratinized (Collette, his chapter in this volume) and there have been reports of more general keratinization. In some of these cases it is doubtful if the phenomena described amount to true keratinization (Kawaguti, 1966; Fishelson, 1973; Bone & Brook, 1973) but there is histochemical evidence that the surface layer of the knifefish *Notopterus notopterus* is keratinized as a sheet, as in amphibians, although goblet mucous cells are also present (Mittal & Bannerjee, 1974a). The surface of the large catfish *Bagarius bagarius* is also partly keratinized (Mittal & Bannerjee, 1974b); these authors suggest that there may be an inverse relationship between the degree of keratinization and the number of mucous glands, one or the other mechanism providing protection.

The habitat of modern air-breathing teleosts is similar to that generally assumed for the fish ancestors of tetrapods, in stagnant, tropical fresh waters, liable to drought. The dipnoans have a mucigenic skin which is not keratinized (Kitzan & Sweeny, 1968; Pfeiffer, 1968a); they take special action to avoid desiccation, by burrowing or by making a cocoon. The amphibians, by concentrating mucus production in multicellular glands, are capable of secreting copious mucus and of having the skin keratinized in addition, so getting a double advantage in protection against abrasion.

The feet of aquatic urodele larvae which walk on the bottom, like *Salamandra salamandra*, are liable to wear and tear in a way that the general body surface, or the feet of a swimming tadpole, are not. Hence, perhaps, the premature keratinization of their toe skin. It is obvious when handling fresh skin that the epidermis of adult amphibians is much tougher than that of tadpoles or of fish, although this must depend on the strength of desmosomal attachments as well as on the nature of the surface layers. It may well be, however, that the main problems facing the early amphibians resulted from loss of the gills, and with them a major piscine mechanism for the control of salt balance, rather than from danger of direct desiccation. Ionic transport in skin and gills is discussed below (p. 303).

Both mucus secretion and keratinization of the surface layers can provide protection against attack by microorganisms. It has been suggested that an important function of the granular glands of amphibians, which in different species secrete a great variety of venomous or irritant substances, is to guard against infection (Habermehl, 1974). This does not preclude the same substances being poisonous or distasteful to larger predators.

Teleosts, and other fish, have a variety of unicellular glands other than the goblet mucous cells. There is not space to describe these fully. The ostariophysan type of club cell is thought to release an alarm substance which is detected by other individuals of the same species (see Pfeiffer, Sasse & Arnold, 1971, for references). Other types of secretory cell may, judging by their staining reactions, correspond more directly to the granular glands of amphibians, for instance, the granular glands of some catfish (Henrikson & Matoltsy, 1968). Some fish have venom glands associated with the skin (Russell, 1965). Larval urodeles have a type of unicellular secretory cell, the Leydig cell; it has been suggested that these may have a role in fluid conservation (Kelly, 1966).

In spite of an increasing number of histochemical studies, it is not always possible to classify the types of secretory cells in fish skin; even mucous cells vary in the precise nature of their secretion and in their appearance in electron micrographs. The skin of the coelacanth, *Latimeria chalumnae*, is mucigenic; Pfeiffer (1968b) described large mucous cells, and a type of serous cell confined to the pit lines of the head. Figure 8 is of a section of *Latimeria* epidermis from the base of the pectoral fin; the surface epithelial cells are bordered by an apical palisade of mucous granules. The large mucous gland cells are not shown, but there is also a smaller type of secretory cell, confined to the surface layers, and, if the interpretation of the cell with a narrow apex on the left as a juvenile stage is correct, differentiating at that level. The secretion is formed in the Golgi apparatus (Fig. 9). From its appearance this could be either a mucous cell or a serous cell; Pfeiffer's plates do not show cells of this type in the surface layers of the head epidermis.

SENSORY FUNCTIONS

In fish and in amphibians the epidermis is penetrated by nerve fibres, some of which come to free endings (Whitear, 1971a, 1974) while others are associated with differentiated epidermal cells of a sensory nature. These may be grouped, either as neuromasts or, in many species of fish, as external taste buds. These are too well

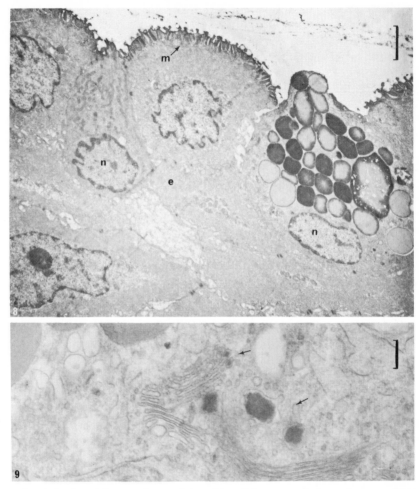

FIG. 8. Section of the outer layers of the epidermis from near the base of a pectoral fin in *Latimeria chalumnae*. The cell with the nucleus near the base, on the left, is interpreted as a juvenile stage of the cell with secretory droplets, on the right. Abbreviations: e, epithelial cell; m, mucous granules at the border of a surface epithelial cell; n, nuclei of the differentiated cells. Scale 2 µm.

FIG. 9. Part of the cytoplasm of a secretory cell as in Fig. 8, showing the formation of secretion in the Golgi apparatus (arrowed). Scale 0·02 µm.

known to pause over, except to mention that fish neuromasts may be further specialized as electroreceptors and that both types of end organ incorporate special secretory cells, which make the cupula of neuromasts and in taste buds have a more obscure role. Amphibians have neuromasts as larvae, and occasionally as adults if they remain aquatic; they do not have external taste buds. Many fish have taste buds in the skin, and in addition teleosts have modified epidermal cells, which appear to be chemoreceptors, occurring singly, scattered in the epidermis (Whitear, 1971b). Figure 10 shows such a cell from the catfish *Ictalurus melas* kindly lent by Mrs Birgitte Lane. The identification of this type of cell as a chemoreceptor is due to the close resemblance of the fine structure to that of the gustatory cells of the appropriate species, even though there is considerable variation between species. A common feature is the presence of a core of fibrillar cytoplasm penetrating into the cell below the external process; rows of vesicles lie alongside. The cells generally have a nerve fibre at the proximal end, although there is no nerve profile in Fig. 10; synaptic specializations have not been seen. When the nerve supply to the taste buds of a particular area of skin is interrupted, leading to degeneration of the taste buds, the scattered sensory cells persist (Lane, 1977).

Scattered sensory cells have not been found in adult amphibians, but a type found in *Rana temporaria* tadpoles may be chemosensory (Fig. 11). It has a process to the outside, and serial sections showed a fibrillar core beneath. The presence of nerve fibres below is not conclusive evidence of innervation because nerve fibres run everywhere between the two epidermal cell layers. This cell type is distinct from those previously described from electron microscopical studies of tadpole skin, although it could correspond to a type described by Meyer (1962), see Whitear (1976b).

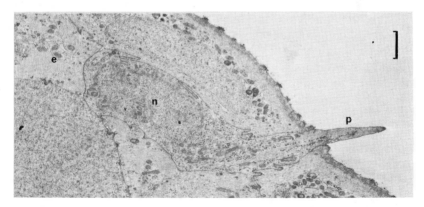

FIG. 10. Section of the outer layers of the epidermis of flank skin of *Ictalurus melas*, with a chemosensory cell. Abbreviations: e, epithelial cell; n, nucleus of sensory cell; p, distal process of sensory cell. Scale 1 μm. Micrograph lent by Birgitte Lane.

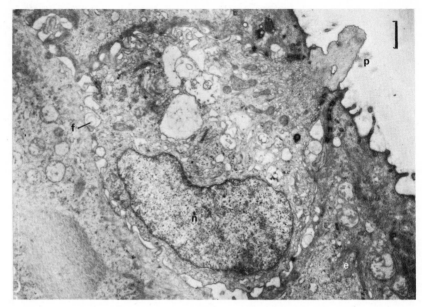

Fig. 11. Section of a differentiated cell in the epidermis of back skin of a *Rana temporaria* tadpole. Abbreviations: e, surface epithelial cell; f, nerve fibre profile; n, nucleus of differentiated cell; p, distal process. Scale 1 μm.

Merkel cells, which are assumed to be concerned in tactile reception, are found in the epidermis of amphibians, both larval and adult, and have much the same characteristics as in higher tetrapods (Hulanicka, 1910, 1913; Nafstad & Baker, 1973; Winkelmann & Breathnach, 1973). Epithelial Merkel cells can be recognized by the relatively small ratio of cytoplasm to nucleus, and by the presence of granules or dense-cored vesicles and of characteristic finger-like processes which push into adjacent cells. There is a synaptic association with nerve fibres. Figure 12 shows part of a Merkel cell from digital skin of a *Salamandra salamandra* larva, with some granules and a peripheral process. Delicate longitudinal fibrillae in the process extend into the cytoplasm of the Merkel cell. The nerve profile here is not at a synapse.

Merkel cells have not previously been reported from fish, but Fig. 13, again of *Ictalurus* epidermis and lent by Birgitte Lane, shows a rounded cell, with relatively scanty cytoplasm, two peripheral processes, and adjacent nerve fibre profiles. It also contains cored vesicles, not visible at this magnification, although the core is not so dense as in the tetrapods. These observations extend the distribution of Merkel cells to the teleosts (Lane, 1977).

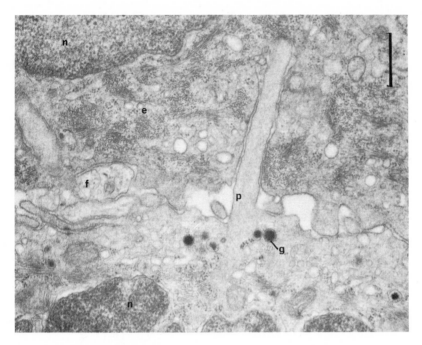

FIG. 12. Section in the basal layer of the epidermis of digital skin of a *Salamandra salamandra* larva, showing part of a Merkel cell. Abbreviations: e, basal layer epidermal cell; f, nerve fibre profile; g, dense granule of Merkel cell; n, nuclei; p, peripheral process of Merkel cell. Surface of skin towards the right. Scale 0·5 μm.

TRANSPORT IN THE EPIDERMIS

The surface epidermal cells of tadpoles, which have already been mentioned in connection with mucous secretion, have a peculiarity; they often have a central bleb (Fig. 14). At first sight this looks like secretory activity, but comparison with other epithelia suggests that alternatively this could be evidence of intake to the cell, either pinocytotic or phagocytotic (see for instance Enders & Nelson, 1973). However, this is speculative. There are also scattered ciliated cells (Billett & Courtenay, 1973); in the axolatl these persist on the external gills even in the fully grown animal.

A major difference in the skin physiology of amphibians as compared with fish is that in adult amphibians the skin takes over the ionic regulatory mechanisms which in tadpoles and in fish are performed by the gill epithelium (see Maetz, 1974, for references). This is separate from differences in the permeability of the skin which may also exist (Alvarado & Moody, 1970). In fish, specialized

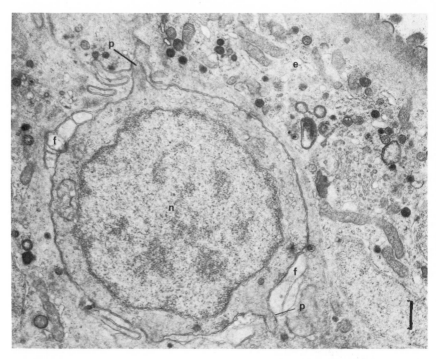

FIG. 13. Section in the outer layers of the epidermis of flank skin of *Ictalurus melas*, with a cell interpreted as a Merkel cell. Abbreviations: e, surface epithelial cell; f, nerve fibre profiles; n, nucleus of Merkel cell; p, peripheral processes. Scale 0·5 μm. Micrograph lent by Birgitte Lane.

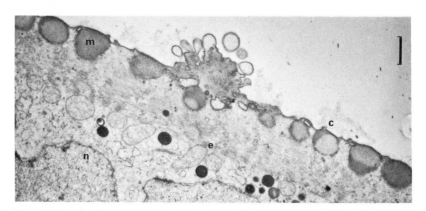

FIG. 14. Section of a surface epidermal cell of back skin of a *Rana temporaria* tadpole, with a bleb. Abbreviations: c, cuticle; e, epithelial cell; m, mucous granule; n, nucleus. Scale 1 μm.

cells of the gill epithelium, the chloride cells, have long been implicated in transport processes, although their exact role is still not determined (Motais & Garcia-Romeu, 1972). Chloride cells occur also in the oral and skin epidermis of many species of teleost (see Whitear, 1971b). They are recognized by a characteristic system of branching tubules in the cytoplasm, which are in continuity with the cell surface and not part of the endoplasmic reticulum (Nakao, 1974; Komuro & Yamamoto, 1975) and possess numerous mitochondria.

Figure 15 is from the head skin of a *Rana temporaria* tadpole; the cell on the right has a different arrangement of microridges from that on the left, also a thinner external surface layer, and small dense apical granules instead of the normal large mucous granules. This cell represents one of the epidermal cell types described by Billett & Gould (1971). Such cells have more mitochondria than the ordinary epidermal cells, and are commoner in the epithelium of the external and internal gills than in the skin. Similar cells occur in axolotl skin (Fährmann, 1971) and in the adult oral skin of a number of species (Whitear, 1975 and unpublished observations). It has been suggested that the mitochondria-rich cells of tadpole gills are concerned with osmoregulation (Hourdry, 1974).

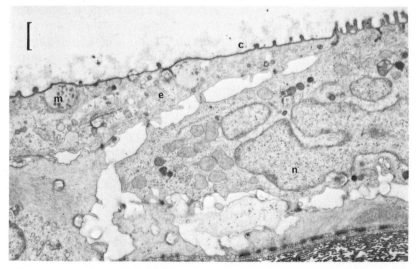

FIG. 15. Section of epidermis of head skin of a *Rana temporaria* tadpole, to contrast a mitochondria-rich cell, on the right, with an ordinary surface epithelial cell. Abbreviations: c, cuticle; e, surface epithelial cell; m, mucous granule; n, nucleus of mitochondria-rich cell. Scale 1 μm.

It should not be assumed that all "mitochondria-rich cells" are necessarily of the same type, in the sense that they perform similar functions. In Fig. 8, the cell on the left was interpreted as a juvenile stage of the secretory cell type, because, apart from the presence of the secretory droplets, the detailed structure of the cytoplasm was indistinguishable, but it has got many mitochondria. Fish chloride cells contain many mitochondria but have branching cytoplasmic tubules and may have an apical invagination, specializations which are not found in amphibian mitochondria-rich cells. These morphological differences suggest that the internal physiology of the two cell types is not the same, even if they prove to have analogous functions. Whether the well known mitochondria-rich cells of the amphibian urinary bladder are related to those of the tadpole gills is an open question. In adult amphibian external skin the nearest equivalent is the flask cell (Fig. 16). These illustrate very well the difficulty of ascribing function to a particular cell type. They have been known for over a century and are still mysterious. It is only recently that they have been implicated in osmoregulation or in transport processes (Lodi, 1971; Guardabassi, Campantico & Olivero, 1972; Voûte, Hänni & Ammann, 1972; Rosen & Friedley, 1973; Whitear, 1972, 1975; Voûte, Thummel & Brenner, 1975).

Flask cells first appear during metamorphosis as the epidermis becomes keratinized, which is also the time that the external skin takes over the ionic regulatory functions formerly carried out by the gill epithelium (Boonkoom & Alvarado, 1971; Alvarado & Moody, 1970). The most investigated transport process in amphibian skin is the active transport of sodium, but it is not necessary to assume that the flask cells are especially concerned with that. The variations in sodium transport during an induced moult *in vitro* can be explained in terms of changes in the replacement layer cells and those immediately below them, even though during the moult the apices of the flask cells degenerate and are reorganized again afterwards. Part of the difficulty over flask cells is that they are so variable: some, like that in Fig. 16, have a complex ridged apex, which at higher magnifications shows a layer of ordered material under the apical membrane. This layer is apparently of the same structure as that occurring on coated vesicles. Other flask cells, even in the same individual, can have a relatively flat apex, or the apical ridges may be fused together (Whitear, 1975).

There have been reports that the morphology of the flask cells is affected by keeping animals in a salt-rich medium when the cells are said to be less well developed (Guardabassi *et al.*, 1972; Voûte *et*

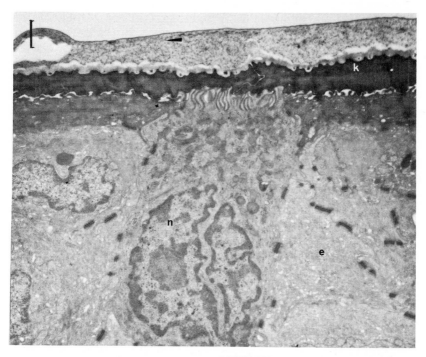

FIG. 16. Section of epidermis of *Xenopus laevis* back skin, with a flask cell. Abbreviations: e, epithelial cell; k, keratinized cell; n, nucleus of flask cell. Scale 1 μm.

al., 1972). Figure 16 is taken from a *Xenopus laevis* which had been kept for four days in 0·05% NaCl, but even after a month in 0·75% NaCl flask cells have every appearance of being active. Some flask cells have the complex apex with a layer under the membrane, whether the animal has been kept in saline or in distilled water (Whitear, unpublished observations). Some new data, however, have brought out more resemblances between the flask cells and the mitochondria-rich cells of the oral epithelium than had been noticed previously (Whitear, 1975).

The amphibian flask cells have an astonishing similarity to the insect "chloride cells" described by Komnick & Wichard (1975, and earlier references) which are also mitochondria-rich, lose the apex at moulting, and may possess a ridged apex with the same type of layer under the membrane. The insect cells have been shown to absorb salts from the external solution (Komnick, Rhees & Abel, 1972) and their reaction to osmium tetroxide–silver lactate solution, supposed to show the distribution of chloride in the tissues, resembles that of the frog flask cells to dilute silver nitrate solution (Whitear, 1972). Osmium tetroxide–silver lactate applied to frog skin gives a picture similar to the Ranvier technique in the epidermis (Van Lennep & Komnick, 1971), although these authors do not mention the flask cells. It remains to be discovered which of the several transport paths in amphibian skin goes through the flask cells, but it is becoming increasingly probable that they are in some way involved. One guess about their individual physiology is that it is incompatible with a destiny of keratinization. It has been suggested that the chloride cells of fish gills are primarily extra-renal excretory cells, even though they are concerned also with salt regulation (Motais & Garcia-Romeu, 1972) and it should be considered whether the flask cells are concerned with the movement of something larger than inorganic ions.

Here it is worth going back to the mucous cuticle. In Fig. 16 the material on the outside of the skin is mucus from the skin glands, which is clearly distinct from the external layer on the surface cells. It has been suggested that this mucus, and that in the subcorneal space, acts as an ion trap (Van Lennep & Komnick, 1971) or has some other function in the transport process (Larsen, 1972). The properties of mucus as an ion trap can vary from place to place; the secretion at the apex of fish chloride cells reacts to histochemical tests for sodium and chloride when the cuticle on the adjacent respiratory cells does not (Bierther, 1970).

It is usually assumed that the presence of mucus on the skin is connected with water conservation. There are species differences in the functioning of the skin glands; in some anurans such as *Rana catesbeiana* the mucous glands discharge spontaneously so as to keep a film of mucus over the skin, while in some other species and particularly in the aquatic *Xenopus laevis* this does not happen (Lillywhite, 1975). Skin glands are discharged when *Xenopus* is caught, which accounts for the secretion in Fig. 16. If *Rana temporaria* is killed quickly by pithing, the mucous glands do not usually discharge appreciably.

The mucous glands have functions other than the protective ones mentioned above (p. 298). Frogs produce alkaline skin secretions containing various salts, to counteract the acidification of the skin resulting from carbon dioxide excretion (Friedman, LaPrade, Aiyawar & Huf, 1967). In practice it is difficult to separate the action of mucous glands from that of granular glands; although Lindley (1969) found that granular gland secretion did not affect the electrical properties of the skin, there is a possibility that water

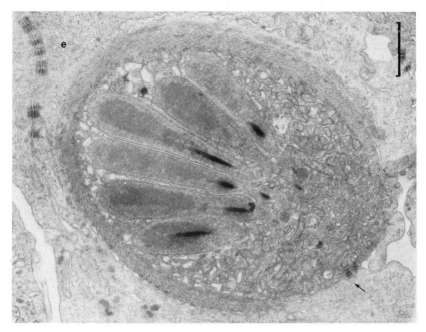

FIG. 17. Section of epidermis of *Gasterosteus aculeatus*, with a rodlet cell. The surface of the epidermis is to the right. There are desmosomes between the rodlet cell and the epithelial cell adjacent to it (arrowed). e, Epidermal cell. Scale 1 μm. Micrograph lent by P. Phromsuthirak.

and electrolytes are recycled (Watlington & Huf, 1971). Perhaps this might be significant in skin exposed to air, which has not got the possibility of absorbing salts from the external medium. Active transport of sodium continues in skin with the outer surface blotted *in vitro*, at least for a time; Andersen & Zerahn (1963) used this technique to measure the size of the sodium transport pool, and showed that marked sodium was transferred to the inside of the skin in a matter of minutes. It seems unlikely that the sodium pump shuts down when a frog is out of water; skin transport mechanisms could still draw on a salt store in secreted mucus, whether this is of the external surface layer or derived from skin glands. Is it possible that the presence of a keratinized stratum corneum, retaining the secretion in the subcorneal space, could have been a factor in the original adjustment of physiological mechanisms which took place when the ancestral amphibians emerged onto land? The endocrine control of salt and water balance in anurans in different environmental situations is discussed by Scheer, Mumbach & Thompson (1974).

CONCLUSION

This survey of the diversity of cell types found in the epidermis of
fish and amphibians is by no means exhaustive. There are few cases
where the functions of particular cells can be precisely defined.
One last example will be added, although with some reservations.
Figure 17 is of a micrograph kindly lent by Mr Pramarn Phromsuthirak, and shows a structure likely to be seen by anyone working
on fish tissues. The section is from epidermis of *Gasterosteus
aculeatus*. There has been argument for 70 years as to whether the
cell with the rod-like contents belongs to the fish or is a sporozoan
parasite (see Leino, 1974; Flood, Nigrelli & Gennaro, 1975). Here,
there are undoubted desmosomes between it and the neighbouring epidermal cells, as reported by Leino from other situations.
Nevertheless, personally I find it easier to believe in an intracellular
parasite than in a secretory cell type which occurs sporadically in
numerous species and in sites as diverse as external and internal
epithelia and also in the endothelium of the vascular system. The
existence of such structures adds another whole dimension to the
subject of cell diversity: that of potential pathological changes.

REFERENCES

Alvarado, R. H. & Moody, A. (1970). Sodium and chloride transport in tadpoles of
    the bullfrog *Rana catesbeiana. Am. J. Physiol.* **218**: 1510–1516.
Andersen, B. & Zerahn, K. (1963). Method for non-destructive determination of
    the sodium transport pool in frog skin with radiosodium. *Acta physiol. scand.*
    59: 319–329.
Bereiter-Hahn, J. (1971). Licht- und elektronenmikroskopische Untersuchungen
    zur Funktion von Tonofilamenten in den Epidermiszellen von Fischen.
    Cytobiol. **4**: 73–102.
Bierther, M. (1970). Die Chloridzellen des Stichlings. *Z. Zellforsch. mikrosk. Anat.*
    107: 421–446.
Billett, F. S. & Courtenay, T. H. (1973). A stereoscan study of the origin of ciliated
    cells in the embryonic epidermis of *Ambystoma mexicanum. J. Embryol. exp.
    Morph.* **29**: 549–558.
Billett, F. S. & Gould, R. P. (1971). Fine structural changes in the differentiating
    epidermis of *Xenopus laevis* embryos. *J. Anat.* **108**: 465–480.
Bone, Q. & Brook, C. E. R. (1973). On *Schedophilus medusophagus* (Pisces:
    Stromateoidei). *J. mar. biol. Ass. U.K.* **53**: 753–761.
Boonkoom, V. & Alvarado, R. H. (1971). Adenosine triphosphatase activity in
    gills of larval *Rana catesbeiana. Am. J. Physiol.* **220**: 1820–1824.
Bremer, V. H. (1972). Einige Untersuchungen zur Histochemie der sezernieren-
    den Elemente der Teleostier-Epidermis. *Acta histochem.* **43**: 28–40.
Carmignani, M. P. A. & Zaccone, G. (1975). Histochemical analysis of epidermal
    cells and mucous cells in the skin of *Torpedo ocellata* Rafinesque. *Acta
    histochem.* **52**: 100–110.
Elkan, E. (1968). Mucopolysaccharides in the anuran defence against dessication.
    J. Zool., Lond. **155**: 19–53.

Enders, A. C. & Nelson, D. M. (1973). Pinocytotic activity of the uterus of the rat. *Am. J. Anat.* **138**: 277–300.

Fährmann, W. (1971). Die Morphodynamik der Epidermis des Axolotls (*Siredon mexicanum* Shaw) unter dem Einfluss von exogen applizierten Thyroxin. I. Die Epidermis des neotenen Axolotls. *Z. mikrosk.-anat. Forsch.* **83**: 472–506.

Farquhar, M. G. & Palade, G. E. (1965). Cell junctions in amphibian skin. *J. Cell Biol.* **26**: 263–291.

Fishelson, L. (1973). Observations on skin structure and sloughing in the stone fish *Synanceja verrucosa* and related fish species as a functional adaptation to their mode of life. *Z. Zellforsch. mikrosk. Anat.* **140**: 497–508.

Flood, M. T., Nigrelli, R. F. & Gennaro, J. F. (1975). Some aspects of the ultrastructure of the 'Stabchendrüsenzellen', a peculiar cell associated with the bulbus arteriosus and with other fish tissues. *J. Fish Biol.* **7**: 129–138.

Friedman, R. T., LaPrade, N. S., Aiyawar, R. M. & Huf, E. G. (1967). Chemical basis for the [H⁺] gradient across frog skin. *Am. J. Physiol.* **212**: 962–972.

Guardabassi, A., Campantico, E. & Olivero, M. (1972). Effect of environmental changes on the skin and pituitary of *Xenopus laevis* Daudin specimens treated and untreated with prolactin. *Monit. zool. ital.* (*N.S.*) **6**: 129–146.

Habermehl, G. G. (1974). Venoms of Amphibia. In *Chemical zoology* **9**: 161–183. Florkin, M. & Scheer, B. T. (eds). London and New York: Academic Press.

Hawkes, J. W. (1974). The structure of fish skin. I. General organization. *Cell Tiss. Res.* **149**: 147–158.

Henrikson, R. C. & Matoltsy, A. G. (1968). The fine structure of teleost epidermis. III. Club cells and other cell types. *J. Ultrastruct. Res.* **21**: 222–232.

Hourdry, J. (1974). Étude des branchies "internes" puis de leur régression au moment de la métamorphose, chez la larve de *Discoglossus pictus* (Otth), amphibien anoure. *J. Microscopie* **20**: 165–182.

Hulanicka, R. (1910). Recherches sur les terminaisons nerveuses de la peau de *Rana esculenta. Bull. int. Acad. Sci. Lett. Cracovie* (B) **1909**: 687–703.

Hulanicka, R. (1913). Recherches sur l'innervation de la peau de *Triton cristatus. Bull. int. Acad. Sci. Lett. Cracovie* (B) **1912**: 400–404.

Ito, S. (1974). Form and function of the glycocalyx on free cell surfaces. *Phil. Trans. R. Soc.* (B) **268**: 55–66.

Kawaguti, S. (1966). Electron microscopy on the cornification of the epidermis of the fish scale with special reference to the mucous cell. *Biol. J. Okayama Univ.* **12**: 47–56.

Kelly, D. E. (1966). The Leydig cell in larval amphibian epidermis. Fine structure and function. *Anat. Rec.* **154**: 685–700.

Kitzan, S. M. & Sweeny, P. R. (1968). A light and electron microscope study of the structure of *Protopterus annectens* epidermis. I. Mucus production. *Can. J. Zool.* **46**: 767–772.

Komnick, H., Rhees, R. W. & Abel, J. H. (1972). The function of ephemerid chloride cells. Histochemical, autoradiographic and physiological studies with radioactive chloride on *Callibaetis. Cytobiol.* **5**: 65–82.

Komnick, H. & Stockem, W. (1969). Oberfläche und Verankerung des stratum corneum an mechanisch stark beanspruchten Körperstellen beim Grasfrosch. *Cytobiol.* **1**: 1–16.

Komnick, H. & Wichard, W. (1975). Histochemischer nachweis von Chloridzellen bei Wasserwanzen (Hemiptera: Hydrocorisae) und ihre Feinstruktur bei *Hesperocorixa sahlbergi* Fieb. (Hemiptera: Corixidae). *Int. J. Insect Morphol. Embryol.* **4**: 89–105.

312   MARY WHITEAR

Komuro, T. & Yamamoto, T. (1975). The renal chloride cell of the fresh-water catfish *Parasilurus asotus*, with special reference to the tubular membrane system. *Cell Tiss. Res.* **160**: 263–271.

Lane, E. B. (1977). *Structural aspects of skin sensitivity in the catfish* Ictalurus. Ph.D. Thesis: University of London.

Lanzing, W. J. R. & Wright, R. G. (1974). The ultrastructure of the skin of *Tilapia mossambica* (Peters). *Cell Tiss. Res.* **154**: 251–264.

Larsen, E. H. (1972). Characteristics of aldosterone stimulated transport in isolated skin of the toad, *Bufo bufo* (L.). *J. ster. Biochem.* **3**: 111–120.

Leino, R. L. (1974). Ultrastructure of immature, developing, and secretory rodlet cells in fish. *Cell Tiss. Res.* **155**: 367–381.

Lillywhite, H. B. (1975). Physiological correlates of basking in amphibians. *Comp. Biochem. Physiol.* **52A**: 323–330.

Lindley, B. D. (1969). Nerve stimulation and electrical properties of frog skin. *J. gen. Physiol.* **53**: 427–449.

Lodi, G. (1971). Histoenzymologic characterization of the flask cells in the skin of the crested newt under normal and experimental conditions. *Atti Accad. Sci. Torino* **105**: 561–570.

Maetz, J. (1974). Aspects of adaptation to hypo-osmotic and hyper-osmotic environments. In *Biochemical and biophysical perspectives in marine biology* **1**: 1–167. Malins, D. C. & Sargent, J. R. (eds). London and New York: Academic Press.

Martinez-Palomo, A., Erlij, D. & Bracho, H. (1971). Localization of permeability barriers in the frog skin epithelium. *J. Cell Biol.* **50**: 277–287.

Meyer, M. (1962). Kegel- und andere Sonderzellen der larvalen Epidermis von Froschlurchen. *Z. mikrosk.-anat. Forsch.* **68**: 79–131.

Mittal, A. K. & Bannerjee, T. K. (1974a). Structure and keratinization of the skin of a fresh-water teleost *Notopterus notopterus* (Notopteridae, Pisces). *J. Zool., Lond.* **174**: 341–355.

Mittal, A. K. & Bannerjee, T. K. (1974b). A histochemical study of the epidermal keratinization in the skin of a fresh-water teleost *Bagarius bagarius* (Ham.) (Sisoridae, Pisces). *Mikroskopie* **30**: 337–348.

Mittal, A. K. & Munshi, J. S. D. (1971). A comparative study of the structure of the skin of certain air-breathing fresh-water teleosts. *J. Zool., Lond.* **163**: 515–532.

Motais, R. & Garcia-Romeu, F. (1972). Transport mechanisms in the teleostean gill and amphibian skin. *Ann. Rev. Physiol.* **34**: 141–176.

Nafstad, P. H. J. & Baker, R. E. (1973). Comparative ultrastructural study of normal and grafted skin in the frog, *Rana pipiens*, with special reference to neuroepithelial connections. *Z. Zellforsch. mikrosk. Anat.* **139**: 451–462.

Nakao, T. (1974). Fine structure of the agranular cytoplasmic tubules in the lamprey chloride cells. *Anat. Rec.* **178**: 49–61.

Nielsen, R. (1972). The effect of polyene antibiotics on the aldosterone induced changes in the sodium transport across isolated frog skin. *J. ster. Biochem.* **3**: 121–128.

Parakkal, P. F. & Matoltsy, A. G. (1964). A study of the fine structure of the epidermis of *Rana pipiens*. *J. Cell Biol.* **20**: 85–94.

Pfeiffer, W. (1968a). Die Fahrenholzschen Organe der Dipnoi und Brachiopterygii. *Z. Zellforsch. mikrosk. Anat.* **90**: 127–147.

Pfeiffer, W. (1968b). Über die Epidermis von *Latimeria chalumnae* J. L. B. Smith 1939 (Crossopterygii, Pisces). *Z. Morph. Tiere* **63**: 419–427.

Pfeiffer, W., Sasse, D. & Arnold, M. (1971). Die Schreckstoffzellen von *Phoxinus phoxinus* und *Morulius chrysophakedion* (Cyprinidae, Ostariophysi, Pisces). *Z. Zellforsch. mikrosk. Anat.* **118**: 203–213.

Rosen, S. & Friedley, N. J. (1973). Carbonic anhydrase activity in *Rana pipiens* skin: biochemical and histochemical analysis. *Histochemie* **36**: 1–4.

Russell, F. E. (1965). Marine toxins and venomous and poisonous marine animals. *Adv. mar. Biol.* **3**: 255–384.

Scheer, B. T., Mumbach, M. W. & Thompson, A. R. (1974). Salt balance and osmoregulation in salientian amphibians. In *Chemical zoology* **9**: 51–65. Florkin, M. & Scheer, B. T. (eds). London and New York: Academic Press.

Schliwa, M. (1975). Cytoarchitecture of surface layer cells of the teleost epidermis. *J. Ultrastruct. Res.* **52**: 377–386.

Spearman, R. I. C. (1973). *The integument*. Cambridge: University Press.

Van Lennep, E. W. & Komnick, H. (1971). Histochemical demonstration of sodium and chloride in the frog epidermis. *Cytobiol.* **3**: 137–151.

Voûte, C. L., Hänni, S. & Ammann, E. (1972). Aldosterone induced morphological changes in amphibian epithelia *in vivo*. *J. ster. Biochem.* **3**: 161–165.

Voûte, C. L., Thummel, J. & Brenner, M. (1975). Aldosterone effect in the epithelium of the frog skin—a new story about an old enzyme. *J. ster. Biochem.* **6**: 1175–1179.

Watlington, C. O. & Huf, E. G. (1971). β-Adrenergic stimulation of frog skin mucous glands: non-specific inhibition by adrenergic blocking agents. *Comp. gen. Pharmacol.* **2**: 295–305.

Whitear, M. (1970). The skin surface of bony fishes. *J. Zool., Lond.* **160**: 437–454.

Whitear, M. (1971a). The free nerve endings in fish epidermis. *J. Zool., Lond.* **163**: 231–236.

Whitear, M. (1971b). Cell specialization and sensory function in fish epidermis. *J. Zool., Lond.* **163**: 237–264.

Whitear, M. (1972). The location of silver in frog epidermis after treatment by Ranvier's method, and possible implication of the flask cells in transport. *Z. Zellforsch. mikrosk. Anat.* **133**: 455–461.

Whitear, M. (1974). The nerves in frog skin, *J. Zool., Lond.* **172**: 503–529.

Whitear, M. (1975). Flask cells and epidermal dynamics in frog skin. *J. Zool., Lond.* **175**: 107–149.

Whitear, M. (1976a). Apical secretion from taste bud and other epithelial cells in amphibians. *Cell Tiss. Res.* **172**: 389–404.

Whitear, M. (1976b). Identification of the epidermal "Stiftchenzellen" of frog tadpoles by electron microscopy. *Cell Tiss. Res.* **175**: 391–402.

Winkelmann, R. K. & Breathnach, A. S. (1973). The Merkel cell. *J. invest. Dermatol.* **60**: 2–15.

Yamada, J. (1966). Fingerprint-like patterns found in the squamous epithelium cells of the epidermis of some teleosts. *Zool. Mag., Tokyo* **75**: 140–144.

Symp. zool. Soc. Lond. (1977) No. 39, 315–316.

CHAIRMAN'S SUMMING UP
ON HIGHER ANIMALS

A. JARRETT

Dermatology Department,
University College Hospital Medical School,
London, England

Dr Collette presented us with a most interesting paper on development of breeding tubercles in fishes. I understand that these organs are dependent upon the photoperiod and are therefore under hormonal influence either directly or indirectly from the pituitary. In this context it is interesting to recall that the skin of adult intact mammals is not responsive to even very large doses of androgenic or oestrogenic hormones. It is only in aged human skin that progesterone, oestrogens and androgens have been shown to have an effect on epidermal thickness, keratinization and metabolic activity. There is of course the exception of the human vaginal mucosa which is highly sensitive to circulating hormones and which undergoes variation in its state of keratinization during the menstrual cycle. There is also possibly some degree of sensitivity of the oral mucosa to the action of sex hormones. The sebaceous glands are also responsive to these hormones especially dihydrotestosterone. This is due to special binding sites for this hormone in human sebaceous glands, and also to the ability of the glands to convert less potent steroids derived from the ovaries and adrenals of females into the more potent androgen by virtue of the presence of the appropriate alpha-reductases, and alpha-hydroxysteroid dehydrogenases.

The high degree of sensitivity of human vaginal mucosa to circulating maternal oestrogens is shown by the fact that baby girls are born with an adult type of vaginal mucosa; about a week after birth when the hormonal stimulation has ceased the mucosa is exfoliated and the vaginal mucosa becomes of the infantile type. This sudden loss of vaginal mucosa has been given the rather colourful name of "vaginal crisis". It would seem from Dr Collette's paper that fish epidermis is also responsive to circulating hormones and it may be relevant to note that this tissue, like the mammalian vaginal mucosa, does not show a high degree of kertinization.

From the comparative aspect Dr Fox's paper is of great interest in that it underlines lysosomal activity and lysosomal enzymes in the normal physiological activity of the skin. There are a normal feature of cell lysis in mammalian epidermis prior to the formation of the horny layer. He also drew attention to the action of leucocytes in phagocytosis of collagen in the larval and adult frog. There is good reason to believe that there is a fairly rapid turnover rate of collagen in human skin, but the mechanism is not yet clearly understood although a comparable involvement of leucocytes does not seem to occur. It is thought that collagenases of the fibroblasts are probably responsible for the breakdown of the connective tissue.

Dr Mary Whitear's review of fish and amphibian epidermis draws our attention to the finding of Merkel cells in the epidermis of amphibians and teleost fishes. These cells are of great interest to those of us who study human and mammalian skin. There are a number of dendritic cells within mammalian epidermis, and these include melanocytes, Langerhans cells, Merkel cells and possibly also Schwann cells. It has also been suggested that macrophages may contribute to the dendritic cell population of the epidermis. The presence of these cells, some of which are derived from the neural crest and thus have some relation to the central nervous system, has been the object of our studies for some time. It appears possible that these cells may play a role in the determination of the type of epidermis and horny layer that is produced over a given dermal site. It is reasonable to suppose that the Merkel cell is performing a sensory function in the skin but it may also have other functions; we suspect that the melanocyte may have additional activities other than that of supplying melanin to the epidermis. It will require a considerable amount of work to elucidate their functions, but now that the attention of zoologists has been drawn to their presence in skin it can be hoped that a clue as to their function may be forthcoming from a study of their distribution at certain skin sites and in particular species.

Symp. zool. Soc. Lond. (1977) No. 39, 317–334.

ASPECTS OF MOULTING IN ANURANS AND ITS CONTROL

POVL E. BUDTZ

August Krogh Institute,
University of Copenhagen,
Copenhagen, Denmark

SYNOPSIS

Studies on anuran skin structure during normal moulting cycles give important information on the differentiation processes and the final, rapid transformation of differentiated cells into keratinized cells, and provide a structural background for investigations on the control of moulting. The events occurring during normal moulting cycles are briefly discussed with special reference to the toad, *Bufo bufo*.

Following hypophysectomy the moulting cycle of toads is arrested in the preparation phase and it is shown that this phase is reached within 16–25 h after hypophysectomy.

The only hormones known to be able to elicit a moult in hypophysectomized toads are ACTH and corticosteroids, but this study shows that these hormones are neither able to inhibit the increased rate of formation of keratinized layers, nor to mimic a normal moult.

By skin homografting experiments it is shown that the moulting rhythm is a result of a rhythm inherent in the skin as well as changing levels of systemic factors.

It is suggested that differentiation and maybe proliferation, although in different ways, are also controlled by interaction of patterns of activity inherent in the skin and systemic factors, the role of the ACTH–corticosteroid system being exclusively permissive.

INTRODUCTION

All amphibians after metamorphosis undergo moulting cycles (Larsen, 1976). Although moulting in amphibians has been known for at least 125 years (Marshall, 1850; Turner, 1850), the processes which lead up to the formation of the stratum corneum and its shedding are poorly understood, as is the control of these processes.

The toad is for several reasons an ideal object for the study of anuran skin dynamics, including moulting and its control. (1) It is possible to determine the phase within the actual moulting process by recording the characteristic behaviour, with a well defined sequence of events, which accompanies the moult. Prior to shedding, gaping and eye movements are seen, followed by adoption of a characteristic moulting posture. By movements of the body and legs, coincident with a copious slime secretion, the detached stratum corneum (the slough) is then pulled into the mouth and eventually swallowed. (For further details on the moulting behaviour, see Bendsen, 1956; and Larsen, 1976) (2) One can record when a moult *has* occurred by marking toads with lipstick, which does not penetrate the stratum corneum and consequently disappears after a moult. By repeated markings the time between individual moults, the so-called intermoult period, can be determined. (3) The time of a new moult may be predicted, although with some uncertainty, because the toad intermoult period is fairly regular for each individual, at 20°C about seven to ten days.

In the following account of the anuran moulting cycle, the toad, *Bufo bufo*, will therefore be used as a model.

THE ANURAN SKIN STRUCTURE
DURING THE NORMAL MOULTING CYCLE

The anuran skin has usually been studied in random skin samples, the layers from the stratum germinativum to the stratum corneum being considered as successive stages in differentiation (light microscopy: Fahrenholz, 1927; Hergersberg, 1957; Porto, 1936; Spannhof, 1959/60; Spearman, 1968; electron microscopy: Bani, 1966; Farquhar & Palade, 1964, 1965; Lavker, 1971, 1973, 1974; Parakkal & Alexander, 1972; Parakkal & Matoltsy, 1964; Voûte, 1963; Whitear, 1974; Yoon, Chang & Choi, 1969). However, only few have compared the skin structure in different phases of the moulting cycle. At the light microscopical level structural changes of the epidermis of the toad *Bufo bufo*, as seen during the normal moulting cycle, have been described by Budtz & Larsen (1973). Certain differences in the ultrastructure of the specialized epidermis of the digital pads of *Hyla cinerea*, related to the phase of the moulting cycle, have been described by Ernst (1973), and recently Whitear (1975) and Budtz & Larsen (1975) have reported on epidermal changes as seen by electron microscopy during normal moulting cycles in the frog, *Rana temporaria*, and in the toad, *Bufo bufo*, respectively.

The epidermis of the normal toad consists of about six layers: a single-layered stratum germinativum, a stratum intermedium three to four cells thick, of which the outermost layer will be termed the replacement layer because after shedding it becomes the new stratum corneum, and finally a single-layered stratum corneum.

On the basis of behaviour and of the macroscopical appearance of the skin, and also by different staining reactions and the morphology of the epidermis, the moulting cycle of the toad may be divided into five phases: *intermoult phase*; *preparation phase*, in which the membranes of the stratum corneum alter (prior to adoption of moulting behaviour); *early shedding phase* with a gradual separation of the stratum corneum from the underlying epidermis, coincident with a swelling of the replacement layer and the stratum corneum and a release of large dense granules into the subcorneal space; and, after the actual shedding, the *late shedding phase*, in which the initial keratinization takes place and the skin appears slimy; and finally the *differentiation phase*, during which the epidermis regains its intermoult appearance by the laying down of a dense matrix in the new stratum corneum and by differentiation of tight junctions in the new replacement layer (Budtz & Larsen, 1973, 1975). It should be stressed, however, that these phases constitute a continuum of events.

Cell proliferation takes place in the stratum germinativum only, and as post-mitotic cells leave the stratum germinativum they differentiate and finally become transformed to keratinized stratum corneum cells. Looking in a little more detail at the processes which lead to formation of the stratum corneum cells, we may begin with the proliferation. Reports on mitotic activity in amphibians are rather conflicting, which may reflect species differences as well as different experimental conditions and methods in estimating the mitotic activity. In toads the slough is usually shed as a continuous sheet. This implies that the loss of cells at moult is rhythmic and discontinuous. Since in any tissue in equilibrium one new cell must be produced for each old one that is lost, the question is whether the pattern of cell production is also rhythmic, or a continuous process. Recently Jørgensen & Levi (1975) have measured the cell production in the epidermis of the toad during a normal moulting cycle as the number of stratum germinativum cells which incorporated tritiated thymidine. These authors showed that labelled cells, i.e. cells in the S-phase, appeared continuously in the stratum germinativum at rates that did not seem to be correlated with the phase of the moulting cycle. This differs from the condition found in, for example, lizards and snakes. These animals, too, moult at regular intervals (Alexander & Parakkal, 1969; Maderson & Licht, 1967; Roth & Jones, 1967), but proliferation of stratum germinativum cells is cyclic (Maderson, Chiu & Philips, 1970; Maderson, Flaxman, Roth & Szabo, 1972).

As the post-mitotic cells move outwards they become further differentiated. According to Lavker (1974), in *Rana pipiens* initial events in horny cell formation are digestion by autolysosomes of those cytoplasmic components which are not necessary constituents of the stratum corneum cells, and release of small mucous granules into the intercellular spaces. The small granules are also present in the toad epidermal cells and especially frequent in the layer below the replacement layer. After shedding, these small granules are frequent also in the new replacement layer where they remain during the differentiation phase, but gradually they disappear from this layer early in the intermoult phase without direct morphological manifestation of release, their fate being obscure (Budtz & Larsen, 1975). However, since this happens several days before a new moult and thus a long time prior to other manifestations of initial keratinization, these granules are, at least in the toad, unlikely to be directly involved in horny cell formation. Following the lytic digestion of cell organelles not retained in the stratum corneum cells, the next stage in the transformation process according to Lavker (1974) is the interfibrillar matrix formation by release of the content of large mucous granules retained by the cells, and the final event in the horny cell formation is a modification of the cell membrane. This does not appear to be the sequence of events in the toad. Figure 1 shows the outermost layer of the epidermis less than 10 min after shedding. The condensation of a peripheral dense band against the intracytoplasmic phase of the plasma membrane and absence of an interfibrillar matrix is obvious. Formation of the dense peripheral layer before matrix formation seems also to take place in *Rana temporaria* as judged from fig. VII (e) and (f) in Whitear (1975). A similar condensation is found by Farbman (1966) to be one of the initial events occurring in mammalian epidermal cells as they pass into the stratum corneum. In toads the laying down of matrix follows the modification of the plasma membrane and may take up to 24 h (Budtz & Larsen, 1975). As seen in Fig. 1, a few granules are present, some of which appear empty. These large granules apparently become dispersed in the cytoplasm when the replacement layer, after shedding, becomes the new stratum corneum, but whether they contribute to the formation of the dense peripheral band and/or the dense interfibrillar matrix cannot be answered at present. However, considering the condensation of the peripheral dense band as an indicator of initial keratinization in the toad, the following statements can be made with regard to the normal toad epidermis. (1) Initial keratinization does not take place until the replacement layer, after shedding, becomes the new stratum corneum. (2) Initial keratinization is a rapid process (within the order of minutes). (3) This process takes place with a high degree of synchrony (Budtz & Larsen, 1975).

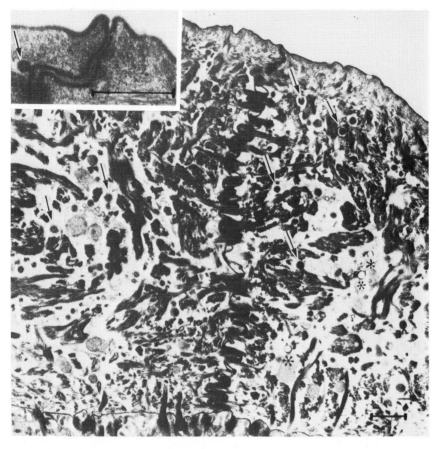

FIG. 1. Electron micrograph of the new stratum corneum less than 10 min after shedding. Note the identical appearance of neighbouring cells, typical of normal late shedding phase. Arrows, dense granules; asterisk, empty granules. For further details, see text. Scale, 1·0 μm. Insert: shows that the dense band is intracellular. Scale, 0·5 μm.

Only little is known about the separation process. We do know that it is gradual (Budtz & Larsen, 1975; Heusser, 1958; Jørgensen & Larsen, 1964; Whitear, 1975). The first signs of detachment are the occurrence of a locally enlarged subcorneal space, especially on top of the flask cells ("lakes", Voûte, Dirix, Nielsen & Ussing, 1969). The separation appears to be accomplished by breaking within the desmosomes themselves, indicating a chemical change within the desmosomes prior to breakage, and/or by rupture of the "pillars" bearing the desmosomal complex between the stratum corneum and the replacement layer, implying rupture of the distal cell membranes of the replacement layer (Budtz & Larsen, 1975; Whitear, 1975). The relative importance, however, of the two modes of separation is not clear, and what causes the desmosomes to break and determines the site of breakage is also unknown.

THE EFFECT OF HYPOPHYSECTOMY ON ANURAN EPIDERMIS

An effect of the endocrine system on the epidermis of amphibians was demonstrated as much as 50 years ago by Giusti and Houssay (see Houssay, 1949). They showed that following hypophysectomy of the toad, *Bufo arenarum*, the surface of the skin became covered by a brown or black hyperkeratinized layer. This effect has since been demonstrated in a number of amphibians, urodeles as well as anurans (see Larsen, 1976). Figures 2 and 3 show in Nomarski technique semi-thin epon sections of toad skin stained with PAS according to Budtz & Larsen (1973). Figure 2 illustrates the condition found in intact controls during the intermoult phase. One notes the single-layered stratum corneum with staining confined to the outer membrane of the cells. Figure 3 shows the epidermis of a toad hypophysectomized 11 days prior to sacrifice. Following this operation shedding is abolished, and the three cornified layers present show that keratinization has taken place at an increased rate, since intact controls during the same period of time produced only one or two sloughs. Note also the staining of all membranes of the keratinized layers, which shows that the skin is in a state similar to that found in the preparation phase of normal toads.

Following hypophysectomy in urodeles (Lodi & Bani, 1971, *Triturus cristatus*), the activity of acid phosphatases and non-specific esterases is strongly increased in the replacement layer and the stratum corneum, and nucleoside triphosphatase activity is increased in the basal layer. So far, however, no reports have been published on the enzymatic activities after hypophysectomy in anurans.

ATTEMPTS AT SUBSTITUTION THERAPY

In a series of papers in the early 1930s Adams and her colleagues were able to show that moulting in the newts *Triturus cristatus* and *Triturus viridescens* is under control of the thyroids, and this later on proved to be the case in all urodeles investigated (for references see Larsen, 1976). In *Bufo arenarum* (Stefano & Donoso, 1964; Ungar, 1932) and *Bufo bufo* (Jørgensen, Larsen & Rosenkilde,

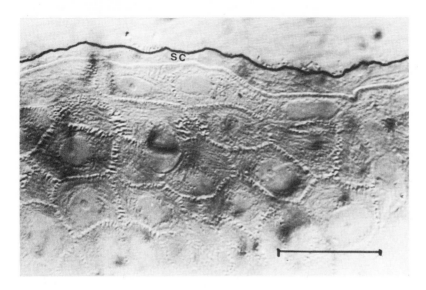

FIG. 2. A 1-μm epon section of the outer epidermis of normal intermoult toad, stained with PAS. SC, single-layered stratum corneum. See text. Scale, 25 μm.

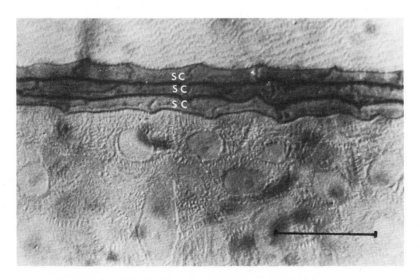

FIG. 3. A 1-μm epon section of the outer epidermis of toad hypophysectomized 11 days prior to sacrifice, stained with PAS. See text. SC, triple-layered stratum corneum. Scale, 25 μm.

1965), however, thyroidectomy has no effect on moulting, but it has been shown that in hypophysectomized toads, moulting can be elicited by ACTH or adrenocorticosteroids (Jørgensen & Larsen, 1964; Stefano & Donoso, 1964). Interestingly, however, these hormones, when injected into intact toads, did not elicit a moult, and it could further be shown that after hypophysectomy of toads, moult can only be elicited after a certain time lapse, usually about 17–24 h (Jørgensen & Larsen, 1964). As shown above, 11 days after hypophysectomy the epidermis from a structural point of view was in a state similar to that found in the preparation phase of intact toads. In a recent experiment the structural changes of the epidermis as a function of time after hypophysectomy were followed by taking skin biopsies from ten toads at intervals from two hours to 14 days after the operation (Budtz, in prep.). Four of the ten toads were still in the intermoult phase 16–17 h after the operation, but biopsies taken 24–25 h after the operation showed in all an epidermis in a state similar to the preparation or very early shedding phase. Thus a close correlation between change of PAS-stainability of the outer epidermis and development of responsiveness of the skin to ACTH or corticosteroids could be demonstrated. We are, however, lacking information on how the hormones exert their action when they elicit a moult, so at present the significance of this correlation cannot be evaluated.

ACTH and corticosteroids are the only hormones which in physiological doses are known to elicit moult in hypophysectomized toads, and it is therefore of great interest to investigate to what extent changes in epidermal structure during induced moult resemble those found during a normal moult. Hypophysectomized toads can be kept alive for more than three weeks if ACTH or corticosteroids are injected three times a week, and almost invariably administration of these hormones in hypophysectomized toads elicits a moult within 6–8 h. The following results are based on 33 toads hypophysectomized 11 days before injecting each toad with 5 μg of the mineralocorticoid aldosterone ("Aldocorten", Ciba). Groups of three were sacrificed at regular intervals from 45 min to 26 h after the injection. Moulting behaviour and macroscopic appearance of the skin were apparently similar to the conditions found during a normal moult, but some differences were found at the level of light and electron microscopy. Typical "lake" formation prior to final separation was not observed. Figure 4 shows a toad skin 5 h after injection of aldosterone. Two sloughs are fully detached and one partly. One notes the absence of

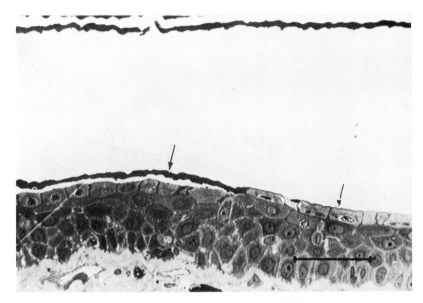

FIG. 4. Abnormal skin structure during shedding elicited with aldosterone in hypophysectomized toad. Arrows point to stratum corneum. See text. A 1-μm epon section, stained with toluidine blue. Scale, 50 μm.

swelling of the detached stratum corneum which indicates that this process is not essential to the process of separation. Shortly after shedding, precipitation of a dense peripheral band had taken place in some new stratum corneum cells, but not in others (Fig. 5). This seems to be the normal condition in *Rana pipiens* (Lavker, 1974) and *Rana temporaria* (Whitear, 1975), but differs from that found in normal toads (Budtz & Larsen, 1975). Thus it appears that initial keratinization in toads is less synchronous during an induced moult than during a normal moult.

One final experiment on the effect of the ACTH/corticosteroid system should be mentioned. Following hypophysectomy and subsequent administration of ACTH three times a week, moulting becomes more frequent than in normal moulting cycles. Under these conditions, epidermal homeostasis is apparently maintained for up to four weeks (H. Levi & C. Ursin, pers. comm.). In long-term experiments, however, this is not the case. Table I shows that after three months (and 52 ACTH injections) the epidermal thickness and the stratum corneum recruitment pool (SCRP) (i.e. the number of cells in stratum germinativum plus stratum intermedium per 100 μm of stratum corneum) were significantly

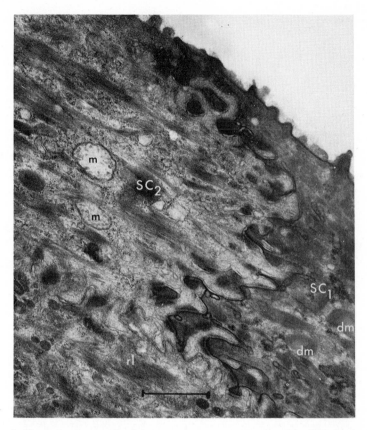

FIG. 5. Electron micrograph of the new stratum corneum less than 30 minutes after induced moult (see text). Different state of keratinization in two neighbouring stratum corneum cells (SC_1 and SC_2). In SC_1 presence of peripheral dense band, filaments and areas with dense interfibrillar matrix (dm). In SC_2 presence of mitochondria (m) and unmodified cell membrane; rl, replacement layer. Scale, $1\cdot0$ μm.

reduced. This shows that proliferation and shedding under these conditions are not dependent on a critical or "quantal" mitosis before terminal differentiation of the keratinocyte (Brown & Jones, 1974).

It thus appears that in toads ACTH or adrenocorticosteroids in the regime offered are neither able to inhibit the increased rate of keratinization following hypophysectomy, nor to mimic a normal moult. It may be suggested that some other pituitary hormone or hormones may act together with ACTH. However, daily injections of pituitary extracts were not better than ACTH in maintaining normal moulting in hypophysectomized toads (Jørgensen & Larsen, 1961, 1964).

TABLE I

Effect of increased moulting rhythm on toad epidermal structure

	Epidermal thickness in μm	SCRP
Controls ($n = 19$)	$53\cdot4 \pm 2\cdot0$	$44\cdot5 \pm 1\cdot1$
Hypophysectomized, 52 ACTH injections ($n = 15$)	$30\cdot3 \pm 2\cdot4$	$30\cdot0 \pm 1\cdot3$

Mean ± SEM. $P < 0\cdot001$.

ARE MOULTING RHYTHMS IN TOADS INDUCED BY CHANGING LEVELS OF HUMORAL FACTORS, OR INHERENT IN THE SKIN?

In order to elucidate this question I have performed some skin homografting experiments, assuming that the moulting rhythm of a skin homograft will coincide with that of the recipient if the moulting rhythm is mainly induced by humoral factors, and with that of the donor if it is mainly inherent in the skin.

In this study 28 male toads in which moults had previously been recorded for at least two months were used. In 24 of these toads, pieces of skin approximately 8×10 mm were interchanged between individuals with a moulting phase differing from one another by half a moulting cycle. Grafting was performed under MS 222 (Sandoz) anaesthesia. The piece of skin removed from one toad to be grafted on the recipient was left in frog Ringer at room temperature while a piece of skin of the same size was removed from the recipient. Now this piece of skin was transferred to frog Ringer and the first piece of skin grafted on the recipient by sewing with 3/8 circle reverse cutting, atraumatic needle and sterile, silicone treated silk (Davis & Geck American Cyanamid Company) (Fig. 6). Finally the second piece of skin was grafted to the site from which the first piece of skin was removed. Thus each toad of a pair acted as donor as well as recipient. Four toads autografted by interchange of pieces of skin between the left and the right antero-lateral parts of the belly served as controls.

Figure 7 shows a homograft six weeks after grafting. The survival of the grafts varied from 17 days to at least three months, when the animals were sacrificed, and altogether 102 moultings of the homografts and 125 moultings of the recipients were recorded

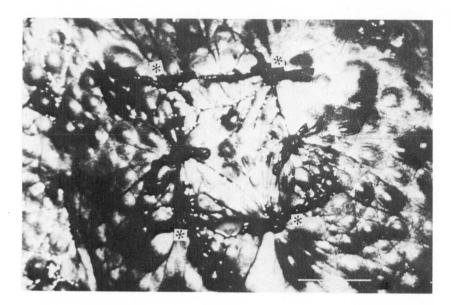

FIG. 6. Toad skin homograft on the day of grafting. Asterisks mark corners of graft. Scale, approx. 5 mm.

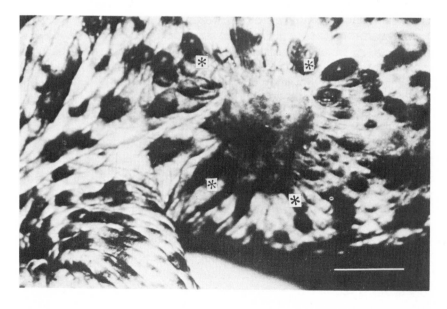

FIG. 7. Toad skin homograft six weeks after grafting. Asterisks mark corners of graft. Scale, approx. 5 mm.

before signs of rejection were observed. "Moulting" does in fact mean separation, because, as previously mentioned, the shedding of the slough in the moult involves a sequence of behaviour. As there are no reasons to believe that "moult" of a graft should elicit moulting behaviour in the recipient, the graft was inspected every day, and fine tweezers were used to test whether a slough of the graft could be removed. In three toads, however, this test was not applied until 29 days (one toad) or 19 days (two toads) after grafting, during which period the lipstick method was used instead. Separations during this period were therefore not recorded in these animals, for the reasons given above.

The first question is whether the skin homografts were responding by separation when shedding was taking place in the recipients. Table II shows that this was only partly the case. At the time of the 125 recorded moults of the recipients, simultaneous "moults" occurred in 60% of the grafts whereas 40% did not respond. When studied as a function of time after grafting there was, however, about a 50-50 chance during the first month of the experiment, and after two months all grafts "moulted" synchronously with the recipients.

One may now ask if the absence of response in such a high percentage of the homografts may express the timing of the shedding cycle found in the donor? When looking at the overall totals of the 102 "moults" of the grafts recorded (Table III) there seems to be very little evidence that the "moulting" rhythm of the graft reflects that of the donor, only about 5% being exclusively correlated with moulting of the donor. However, when the time after grafting is taken into consideration it is interesting to note

TABLE II

The effect of moult of recipient on "moulting" in toad skin homografts

Moults of the recipient	Total no.	%	Days after grafting				
			1–10	11–20	21–30	31–60	61–90
With simultaneous "moult" of the graft	75	60	9	18	14	17	17
Without simultaneous "moult" of the graft	50	40	11	19	13	7	0

TABLE III

Correlation between "moulting" of toad skin homografts and moulting of recipient and donor

"Moults" of grafts coincident with moult of:	Total no.	%	Days after grafting				
			1–10	11–20	21–30	31–60	61–90
Recipient	56	54·9	5	15	10	11	15
Donor	5	4·9	2	3	0	0	0
Recipient + donor	7	6·9	3	3	1	0	0
Neither recipient, nor donor	34	33·3	20	9	5	0	0

that the cases in which the graft "moulted" at the same time as the donor, or "moulted" independently of both donor and recipient, all fell within the first month after grafting, and that "moulting" of the grafts after one month became exclusively synchronous with that of the recipients.

In the controls, the autografts moulted synchronously with the rest of the skin.

These results may be interpreted to mean that the moulting rhythm of the graft has been influenced by an inherent rhythm reminiscent of the donor as well as by an endocrine mechanism found in the recipient. This interpretation supports the hypothesis put forward by Jørgensen & Larsen (1961, 1964), that amphibian moulting is a result of autonomous cyclic processes in the epidermis, sensitive to changes in the level of activity of the endocrine system. This conclusion is consistent with the findings on mammalian hair growth cycles (Ebling, 1965; Johnson, 1965). In snakes, however, moulting rhythms inherent in the skin appear to be absent (Terebey, 1972).

SUMMARY AND CONCLUSIONS

Morphological studies on random skin samples have shown that differentiating cells of the stratum intermedium resemble one another although filaments of the outer part of this stratum are usually more tightly packed than in the basal parts. However, the different structure of the adjacent stratum corneum and the usual absence of intermediate stages indicate a rapid transformation of differentiated cells into terminal horny cells (Lavker, 1974). The investigations on the structure of the toad skin in successive stages of the normal moulting cycle (Budtz & Larsen, 1973, 1975) have mainly been provided to act as a morphological background for studies on control of moulting, but they also have provided useful information on the differentiation processes leading to the final formation of the keratinized stratum corneum cells. It was shown that in toads with an intermoult period of about seven to ten days this final transformation is in fact a rapid process, within the order of 24 h. In *Bufo bufo*, the sequence of events leading to horny cell formation appears to be a break-down of mitochondria, Golgi apparatus and endoplasmic reticulum in the replacement layer during the day prior to shedding, immediately after shedding a rapid initial keratinization of these cells by formation of a peripheral dense band, occurring with a high degree of synchronization, and then the final keratinization by a less synchronous laying down of a central, interfibrillar dense matrix which may last up to 24 h (Budtz & Larsen, 1975). This sequence of events is inconsistent with the findings of Lavker (1974) on *Rana pipiens*. Lysosomes, granules and filaments appear to be important in the keratinization process, but little is known of an eventual role of other parts of the cells since only scattered information is available on the chemistry of the anuran skin in relation to differentiation.

By skin grafting experiments the present investigation has provided evidence that moulting rhythms in toads are the result of rhythms inherent in the skin as well as changing levels of systemic factors.

The increased rate of formation of keratinized layers and abolition of shedding following hypophysectomy of toads, as found by other authors, were confirmed in the present study. It was further shown that the moulting cycle is arrested in the preparation or very early shedding phase and that this condition of the skin is reached after 16–25 h, irrespective of the time of operation in relation to the preceding moult. This correlates with the onset of responsiveness of the skin to ACTH and adrenocorticosteroids after hypophysectomy (Jørgensen & Larsen, 1964). These results may be explained by assuming that not only the moulting rhythm, but also differentiation and maybe proliferation, although in different ways, are results of patterns of activity inherent in the skin, influenced by changes in the level of systemic factors. This suggestion would be consistent with findings on periodically sloughing reptiles (Squamata). Thus in lizards, the length of the resting phase is under hormonal control (Maderson &

Licht, 1967), whereas the control of changing patterns of cell differentiation resides within the epidermis itself (Flaxman, Maderson, Szabo & Roth, 1968).

In conclusion, the failure of ACTH and corticosteroids—although they are the only hormones known that are able to elicit a moult in hypophysectomized toads—to normalize the differentiation processes, and even shedding, makes it likely that their role in the processes occurring during the moulting cycle is exclusively permissive. How the rate of formation of keratinized layers and the separation are controlled are still open questions.

REFERENCES

Alexander, N. J. & Parakkal, P. F. (1969). Formation of α- and β-type keratin in lizard epidermis during the moulting cycle. Z. Zellforsch. mikrosk. Anat. 101: 72–87.

Bani, G. (1966). Osservazioni sulla ultrastruttura della cute di Bufo bufo (L.) e modificazioni a livello dell'epidermide, in relazione a differenti condizioni ambientali. Monitore zool. ital. 74: 93–112.

Bendsen, J. (1956). Shedding of the skin of the common toad, Bufo bufo. Vidensk. Meddr dansk. naturh. Foren. 118: 211–225.

Brown, J. E. & Jones, K. W. (1974). Basic concepts of differentiation and growth of cells. In Differentiation and growth of cells in vertebrate tissues: 1–51. Goldspink, G. (ed.). London: Chapman and Hall.

Budtz, P. E. & Larsen, L. O. (1973). Structure of the toad epidermis during the moulting cycle. I. Light microscopic observations in Bufo bufo. Z. Zellforsch. mikrosk. Anat. 144: 353–365.

Budtz, P. E. & Larsen, L. O. (1975). Structure of the toad epidermis during the moulting cycle. II. Electron microscopic observations in Bufo bufo. Cell Tiss. Res. 159: 459–483.

Ebling, F. J. (1965). Systemic factors affecting the periodicity of hair follicles. In Biology of the skin and hair growth: 507–524. Lyne, A. G. & Short, B. F. (eds). Sidney: Angus and Robertson.

Ernst, V. V. (1973). The digital pads of the tree frog, Hyla cinerea. Tissue & Cell 5: 83–96.

Fahrenholz, C. (1927). Die Flaschenzellen der Amphibienepidermis und ihre Beziehungen zum Häutungsvorgang. Z. mikr.-anat. Forsch. 10: 297–312.

Farbman, A. I. (1966). Plasma membrane changes during keratinization. Anat. Rec. 156: 269–282.

Farquhar, M. G. & Palade, G. E. (1964). Functional organization of amphibian skin. Proc. natn. Acad. Sci. U.S.A. 51: 569–577.

Farquhar, M. G. & Palade, G. E. (1965). Cell junctions in amphibian skin. J. Cell Biol. 26: 263–291.

Flaxman, B. A., Maderson, P. F. A., Szabo, G. & Roth, S. I. (1968). Control of cell differentiation in lizard epidermis in vitro. Devl Biol. 18: 354–374.

Hergersberg, H. (1957). Untersuchungen über den Verhornungsprozess in der Epidermis. Z. Zellforsch. mikrosk. Anat. 45: 569–577.

Heusser, H. (1958). Zum Häutungsverhalten von Amphibien. Rev. suisse Zool. 65: 793–823.

Houssay, B. A. (1949). Hypophyseal functions in the toad *Bufo arenarum* Hensel. *Q. Rev. Biol.* **24**: 1–27.

Johnson, E. (1965). Inherent rhythms of activity in the hair follicle and their control. In *Biology of the skin and hair growth*: 491–505. Lyne, A. G. & Short, B. F. (eds). Sidney: Angus and Robertson.

Jørgensen, C. B. & Larsen, L. O. (1961). Molting and its hormonal control in toads. *Gen. comp. Endocr.* **1**: 145–153.

Jørgensen, C. B. & Larsen, L. O. (1964). Further observations on molting and its hormonal control in *Bufo bufo*. *Gen. comp. Endocr.* **4**: 389–400.

Jørgensen, C. B., Larsen, L. O. & Rosenkilde, P. (1965). Hormonal dependency of molting in amphibians: Effect of radiothyroidectomy in the toad *Bufo bufo* L. *Gen. comp. Endocr.* **5**: 248–251.

Jørgensen, C. B. & Levi, H. (1975). Incorporation of ^{3}H-thymidine in stratum germinativum of epidermis in the toad *Bufo bufo bufo* (L.): An autoradiographic study of moulting cycle and diurnal variations. *Comp. Biochem. Physiol.* **52A**: 55–58.

Larsen, L. O. (1976). Physiology of molting. In *Physiology of amphibians*. **3**: 53–100. Lofts, B. (ed.). New York and London: Academic Press.

Lavker, R. M. (1971). Fine structure of clear cells in frog epidermis. *Tissue & Cell* **3**: 567–578.

Lavker, R. M. (1973). A highly ordered structure in frog epidermis. *J. Ultrastructr. Res.* **45**: 223–230.

Lavker, R. M. (1974). Horny cell formation in the epidermis of *Rana pipiens*. *J. Morph.* **142**: 365–378.

Lodi, G. & Bani, G. (1971). Microscopic, submicroscopic and histoenzymologic features of the epidermis of the normal and hypophysectomized crested newt. *Boll. Zool.* **38**: 111–125.

Maderson, P. F. A., Chiu, K. W. & Philips, J. G. (1970). Endocrine-epidermal relationships in squamate reptiles. *Mem. Soc. Endocr.* **18**: 259–284.

Maderson, P. F. A., Flaxman, B. A., Roth, S. I. & Szabo, G. (1972). Ultrastructural contributions to the identification of cell types in the lizard epidermal generation. *J. Morph.* **136**: 191–209.

Maderson, P. F. A. & Licht, P. J. (1967). Epidermal morphology and sloughing frequency in normal and prolactin treated *Anolis carolinensis* (Iguanidae, Lacertilia). *J. Morph.* **123**: 157–172.

Marshall, W. (1850). Toads and their skins. *The Gardeners' Chronicle and Agricultural Gazette*: 500.

Parakkal, P. F. & Alexander, N. J. (1972). *Keratinization. A survey of vertebrate epithelia*. New York and London: Academic Press.

Parakkal, P. F. & Matoltsy, A. G. (1964). A study of the fine structure of the epidermis of *Rana pipiens*. *J. Cell Biol.* **20**: 85–94.

Porto, J. (1936). *Contribucion al estudio de la histofisiologia del tegumento de los bratrachios*. Thesis: Buenos Aires.

Roth, S. I. & Jones, W. A. (1967). The ultrastructure and enzymatic activity of the boa constrictor (*Constrictor constrictor*) skin during the resting phase. *J. Ultrastr. Res.* **18**: 304–323.

Spannhof, L. (1959/60). Histologische Untersuchungen am Krallenfrosch *Xenopus laevis* Daud. nach Hypophysectomie und Implantation von Hypophysengewebe. II. Untersuchungen an der Epidermis und den Hautdrüsen. *Wiss. Z. Humboldt-Univ. Berl. (Math. Nat.)* **9**: 173–188.

Spearman, R. I. C. (1968). Epidermal keratinization in the salamander and a comparison with other amphibia. *J. Morph.* **125**: 129–144.

Stefano, F. J. E. & Donoso, A. O. (1964). Hypophyso-adrenal regulation of moulting in the toad. *Gen. comp. Endocr.* **4**: 473–480.

Terebey, N. (1972). The effect of shedding on skin homografts in the garter snake, *Thamnophis sirtalis. Am. J. Anat.* **135**: 435–440.

Turner, W. (1850). Way in which toads shed their skins. *The Gardeners' Chronicle and Agricultural Gazette*: 181.

Ungar, I. (1932). La causa de la producción de una pelicula cutánea en el sapo hipofisoprivo o con lesión tuberiana. *Revta Soc. argent. Biol.* **8**: 616.

Voûte, C. L. (1963). An electron microscopic study of the skin of the frog (*Rana pipiens*). *J. Ultrastr. Res.* **9**: 497–510.

Voûte, C. L., Dirix, R., Nielsen, R. & Ussing, H. H. (1969). The effect of aldosterone on the isolated frog skin epithelium (*R. temporaria*). *Expl Cell Res.* **57**: 448–449.

Whitear, M. (1974). The nerves in frog skin. *J. Zool., Lond.* **172**: 503–529.

Whitear, M. (1975). Flask cells and epidermal dynamics in frog skin. *J. Zool., Lond.* **175**: 107–149.

Yoon, J. S., Chang, S. H. & Choi, K. D. (1969). An electron microscopic study on the junctional complex in frog epithelia. *Yonsei Med. J.* **10**: 56–64.

Symp. zool. Soc. Lond. (1977) No. 39, 335–352.

KERATINS AND KERATINIZATION

R. I. C. SPEARMAN

*Dermatology Department, University College Hospital
Medical School, London, England*

SYNOPSIS

Keratin complexes are formed in horny cells by the bonding together of very many different component proteins of various types, some of which are fibrous and others globular proteins. Different horny structures contain different proportions of these components. In addition keratinization involves alteration in the plasma membranes and enzymatic cytolysis of much of the original cell structure, while hard structures show additional calcification. These variables allow wide differences in structure and mechanical properties of horny cells. Because of the many proteins involved in keratin formation keratinization can probably occur only within cells.

INTRODUCTION

Keratin protein complexes are the main constituents of the dead horny cells which form the superficial layer of the epidermis in a few fish, in many amphibians and in all reptiles, birds and mammals. In invertebrates keratin appears to occur only in the intrasyncytial spines and hooks of parasitic platyhelminths (Swiderski, 1972). The best known sources of keratins are mammalian hair and the feathers of birds. The characteristic feature of keratin complexes is the presence of a heterogeneous collection of pure proteins which are bonded together to a large extent by disulphide linkages of cystine. Because of the large number of proteins present in the supermolecule, keratin formation is unlikely to occur outside cells. The cystine-bonded proteins in the extracellular metacercarial cyst and in the cuticle of the hemichordate *Rhabdopleura* (Dilly, 1971) are probably fewer in number and are best termed keratin-like proteins.

The only keratinized structures to have been subjected to thorough chemical and physical analysis are hairs and, to a lesser extent, paired horns, hooves and feathers (Fraser, MacRae & Rogers, 1972; Gillespie, 1965; Gillespie & Frenkel, 1974). Epidermal horny layers are less well understood and analogy to hairs and feathers can be confusing. At the light microscopical level a considerable amount of information has accumulated using cytochemical methods (Jarrett, 1973), but because of the backwardness of ultra-structural cytochemistry this cannot often be related to fine structure (Zelickson, 1967; Breathnach, 1971). Nevertheless there have been several ultrastructural methods for cystine (Pearse, 1972; Spearman & Hardy, 1975a).

Total analyses of keratins in hair samples show quite wide variation in amino acid compositions in different samples from the same species and even breed (Ryder & Stephenson, 1968). This is probably due to the very large number of separate proteins formed, each by a different gene and at individual rates, which make up the keratin supermolecule. This is far more complex than any other protein quaternary structure and the complex is bounded only by the plasma membrane of the cell.

Keratinization of an epidermal cell involves several different variable factors. These are: the proportions of the different pure proteins formed and in the final stage bonded together as the keratin complex, alteration of the plasma membranes which at this stage become thickened and sometimes chemically altered, cell death which occurs suddenly with release of lysosomal hydrolases which degrade cell organelles, and occasionally mineralization by deposition of crystalline calcium salts on chemical nuclei provided by keratin proteins. These factors will now be considered separately.

THE COMPOSITE MOLECULAR STRUCTURE OF KERATINS

Hair keratins

The hair cortical cell is packed with a keratin complex which has a two-phase structure, with cystine-poor fibrous proteins with long alpha-helical segments embedded in a matrix of cystine-rich globular proteins (Spearman, 1977) (Fig. 1). This recalls the two-phase structure in arthropod cuticles and the two-phase arrangement in the collagenous cuticle of nematodes. However, keratins are intracellular and the fibrils in arthropods are formed of chitin. Undoubtedly this two-phase arrangement provides strength with elasticity, as is well known in engineering—fibre glass resin is an example (Slayter, 1962). The hair fibrils are approximately 7 nm in diameter.

In analytical procedures the keratin complex is separated into individual proteins first by reduction of the disulphide linkages which hold the matrix together and then by breaking hydrogen bonds which are important in the alpha-helical fibrils. Polar linkages are also important but are disrupted in alkaline conditions.

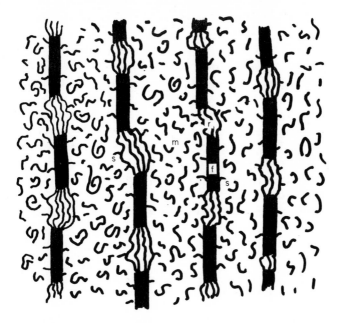

FIG. 1. Diagramatic representation of hair keratin molecular complex. Abbreviations: f, packed alpha-helical fibrils; r, randomly oriented segments; m, matrix globular proteins of various kinds; s, side chains. Cross-linkages between matrix proteins are not shown.

These linkages, which are formed in the final stage of keratinization, are shown in Fig. 2. Complete separation of pure proteins has not yet been achieved and involves electrophoresis followed by chromatography of separated bands and gel filtration. Three main groups of proteins occur in mammalian keratin complexes; fibrous alpha-helical sulphur-poor proteins, tyrosine- and glycine-rich matrix proteins and the important sulphur-rich matrix proteins which are the most heterogeneous (Gillespie & Frenkel, 1974). Proteins can be further subdivided into families and subfamilies. Finally, small groups of proteins are found which differ in only one or two amino acid sequences (Fraser et al., 1972). The few pure proteins which have been isolated in the subfamilies all have the peculiarity of acetylated N-terminal amino acids; serine for fibrous proteins and alanine for sulphur-rich matrix proteins, while the tyrosine- and glycine-rich proteins are not acetylated but always have glycine at the N-terminus. These markers make it unlikely that separated proteins are degradation products. The multiplicity of proteins in groups already separated suggest that the entire hair keratin complex probably contains between 80 and 100 different proteins, but there could be many more. That such a large number of different proteins should be formed in a cell with only limited numbers of ribosomes available is probably explained by sequential synthesis. This is suggested by isotope studies (Fukuyama & Epstein, 1969; Fukuyama & Bernstein, 1963; Fukuyama, Nakamura & Bernstein, 1965) and by the fact that only very small quantities of individual proteins are required. Long amino acid sequences have been examined in a few hair keratin proteins (Fraser et al., 1972). The amino acid compositions of the three main groups of hair proteins are shown in Table I. Gillespie & Frenkel (1974) believe from analyses of hairs, horns and hooves in a variety of species, that differences in proportions of the main constituents formed in different sites are responsible for keratin variation. Thus

TABLE I

Amino acid analyses of different keratins expressed as residues per 100 residues

Residue	Feather rachis[a]	Wool low-sulphur fraction[b]	Wool high-sulphur fraction[c]	Wool high-glycine–tyrosine fraction[d]
Alanine	8·7	6·4	2·9	0·5
Arginine	3·8	7·3	6·7	4·8
Aspartic acid + asparagine	5·6	8·1	4·1	1·9
Half-cystine*	7·8	6·8	17·9	12·4
Glutamic acid + glutamine	6·9	14·1	6·4	1·2
Glycine	13·7	8·8	5·4	33·0
Histidine	0·2	0·7	0·9	0·1
Isoleucine	3·2	3·7	3·0	0·5
Leucine	8·3	10·3	5·0	5·7
Lysine	0·6	4·1	0·7	0·1
Methionine	0·1	0·6	0	0
Phenylalanine	3·1	3·0	2·4	2·7
Proline	9·8	4·2	13·6	3·2
Serine	14·1	7·3	11·9	11·3
Threonine	4·1	4·4	10·4	2·0
Tyrosine	1·4	4·3	1·9	19·4
Valine	7·8	5·9	6·7	1·1

Some figures rounded to nearest 0·1.
Data: [a]From Harrap & Woods (1964). [b]From Thompson & O'Donnell (1962). [c]From Lindley et al. (1971). [d]From Gillespie & Darskus (1971).
* Content of cysteine + reduced cystine expressed as half-cystine residues.

hooves, nails and claws contain more tyrosine- and glycine-rich proteins than hairs (Fig. 3). Variation in half-cystine content is shown in Fig. 4. Differences in keratin proteins formed from site to site in an individual are readily explained in terms of gene restriction during development.

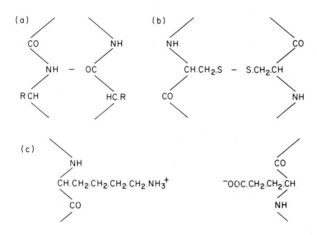

FIG. 2. Important cross-linkages in the keratin molecule. (a) Hydrogen bond; (b) cystine link; (c) polar link.

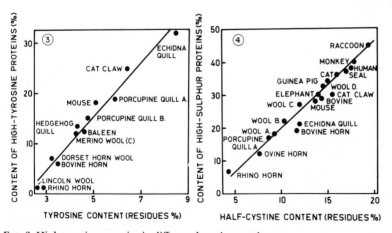

FIG. 3. High tyrosine proteins in different keratin complexes.

FIG. 4. High-sulphur proteins in different keratin complexes. Reduced cystine is shown as half-cystine residues.

(Both Figs 3 and 4 courtesy of J. M. Gillespie & M. J. Frenkel (1974). *Comp. Biochem. Physiol.* **47B**: 339.)

Feather keratins

Feather keratins (see Table I) are not so well understood as hair keratins (Brush, 1974). Fibrils which are ~4 nm in diameter and largely composed of beta pleated chains are embedded in a protein matrix, but unlike in hair the latter appears to be derived as side chains from the fibrils while the N-terminals are acetylated (Filshie & Rogers, 1962; Fraser & MacRae, 1963). The whole super-molecule is rich in cystine in comparison with the differential arrangement in hair (Harrap & Woods, 1967). This may be the reason why the outer beta-keratin region of the lizard scale is richer in cystine than the alpha zone underneath (Spearman & Riley, 1969).

Other keratinized structures

The horny layer of the epidermis in vertebrates contains randomly oriented filaments, except in birds in which only matrix proteins appear to be formed (Matoltsy, 1969), also found by the present author in the adult fowl. As in hairs and feathers there is a general correlation between the presence of a predominantly alpha-helical X-ray diffraction picture and cells containing approximately 7 nm keratin fibrils, and a beta pattern and approximately 4 nm fibrils (Fraser et al., 1972). This has suggested keratin structures in horny layer cells which have been much less adequately studied by chemical analysis than these keratinized appendages. Often the analogy has gone too far and Jarrett (1973) has emphasized how speculation has exceeded the actual knowledge of even the mammalian horny layer, and its relation to skin disorders in man. In fact more is known about the horny scales in lizards and snakes (Fraser et al., 1972). The most useful work on horny layer composition has been in cytochemistry (Jarrett, 1973; Cane & Spearman, 1967; Spearman, 1966, 1973).

The most important division in the vertebrate horny layers is between fish, amphibians, reptiles and birds on the one hand and mammals on the other. This is because in the former the cytoplasm is filled with the keratin complex, but in mammalian hairy skin matrix keratin occurs only as a thin shell around the cell periphery and while weak keratin fibrils form a random meshwork in the interior the intervening cytoplasm is lysed to a soup of degradation products.

The matrix keratin just beneath the plasma membrane frequently forms a denser shell in electron micrographs (Farbman, 1966) in a variety of vertebrate horny layers and this region appears richest in cystine (Spearman, 1973). Except for the horny scales of reptiles, vertebrate horny layer cells contain relatively little cystine. Again mammals are peculiar, for in the hairy skin of the guinea-pig the horny layer when first keratinized contains more cystine than later when the cells have been pushed upward and subjected to cytolysis. This suggests that the disulphide bonds which normally protect keratins from proteolytic hydrolysis are possibly present here not as cross-linkages but as intrachain linkages (Spearman & Hardy, 1975a).

In mammals matrix keratin is retained throughout the cytoplasm in mouse tail scales and in palmar and plantar horny cells (Spearman & Hardy, 1975b), as well as in the abnormal condition of parakeratosis in which horny scales are formed. This retrogressive change to a type of cornification seen mainly in non-mammals occurs in many different skin disorders of man and domestic animals, including psoriasis (Jarrett, 1973). Normal parakeratosis occurs in whales (Spearman, 1972) and on the snouts of some terrestrial mammals.

THE PLASMA MEMBRANES

While all keratinized cells have thickened membranes, the stability of the protein structure varies widely from site to site. Some increase in thickness is due to deposition of material outside the cells, and matrix keratin just beneath the membrane, which appears to increase its cystine content in hair, is sometimes included in chemical analyses. However, there is also actual swelling of the unit membrane, and at least in the frog and in mammalian horny layer cystine is incorporated in the membrane protein (Figs 5 and 6) (Matoltsy & Matoltsy, 1966; Spearman & Hardy, 1975a). This renders the membranes particularly stable and tough. The amino acid composition is similar to the high-sulphur matrix proteins (Fraser *et al.*, 1972) but the proteins are different in that unlike keratin they are highly resistant to alkali (Matoltsy & Matoltsy, 1966). Guinea-pig plantar horny cells have much weaker membranes which are disrupted by chloroform (Spearman & Hardy, 1975b) and some other sites have weak membranes (Farbman, 1966). Hair cell membranes do not contain cystine (Alexander, Hudson & Earland, 1963).

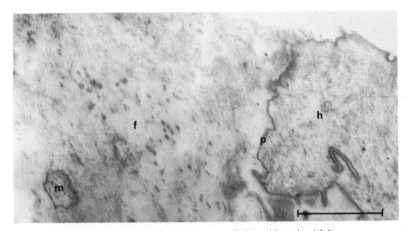

FIG. 5. Electron micrograph of frog *Rana* superficial epidermis with h, stratum corneum cell, and f, flask cell, with m, mitochondrion. The horny cell membrane, p, stains darkly for cystine but the flask cell membrane is unstained. Tissue glutaraldehyde fixed followed by peracetic acid oxidation and staining in uranyl acetate to demonstrate cystine-rich sites. Scale 1 μm.

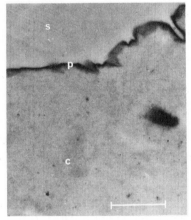

FIG. 6. Guinea-pig stratum corneum cell from hairy back skin. Electron micrograph after method for cystine used in Fig. 5. Abbreviations: s, intercellular space; p, cystine-bonded membrane and peripheral matrix keratin; c, autolysed cytoplasmic contents with no cystine. Scale 1·5 μm.

KERATIN BIOSYNTHESIS

Derivation of the keratin complex

The possibility has been suggested by Jarrett (1973) that keratin in the broad sense is not a true secretion like, for example, insulin formed by the pancreatic islet cells, but instead is probably made up of normal cytoplasmic proteins which become bonded together. The reason for this view is the very large number of different proteins which form the keratin complex, a much greater number than in any other complex quaternary protein structure. It is probable that keratins are derived in this way from cytoplasmic structural proteins analogous to the contractile proteins of muscle, which are not considered to be a secretion but normal cytoplasmic constituents. As in muscle, protein organization can occur in the living epidermal cell, and this would explain the appearance of prekeratin protein fibrils similar to those in keratin in the still living cells. Nevertheless, developmental stages in cytoplasmic protein organization occur in epidermis; but this is no different to developmental changes in non-keratinized epithelia. The component proteins of keratinized epidermis as a result of evolutionary selection have sequential arrangements of amino acids which permit the requisite cross-linkages to form in the superficial cells that undergo keratinization. Without this the keratin complex would not be formed although the cells would contain keratin-like proteins. There are several instances which support this concept.

Thus, in the guinea-pig horny layer, matrix proteins are poorly cross-bonded (Spearman & Hardy, 1975a); in the cyclical keratinization which occurs in lizards and snakes the epidermal cells fail to form a keratin complex at one stage which is autolysed and functions as a fission plane in sloughing (Spearman & Riley, 1969); keratinization can occur at any level of epidermal cell development, in the basal cells of warts and in isolated prickle cells in human and animal skin disorders (Jarrett, 1973) as well as in abnormal frog epidermis (M. Whitear, pers. comm.). Sloughing of the horny layer in amphibians is by breakdown of cell junctions and not as in reptiles (Spearman, 1973). The phylogenetic implication of this concept is that the unkeratinized epidermis of species such as many fish and aquatic urodele amphibians may only require amino acid rearrangement with the addition of the sulphydryl amino acid cysteine for formation of cystine, for keratinization to occur. Indeed, keratin formation does occur, in isolated instances, in cyclostomes and in fish (Spearman, 1966; Mittal & Banerjee, 1974).

Normal sequences of keratin formation

Above the germinal basal layer in mammalian epidermis intense ribonucleic acid synthesis occurs (Fukuyama & Bernstein, 1963; Sims, 1967) and cell volume increases as proteins are formed on polyribosomes (Baden & Cohen, 1965; Jarrett, 1973). Later nucleoli shrink as protein synthesis slows down but superficial living cells can still be stimulated to renewed synthesis by the virus of human warts. In feather formation ribonucleic acid is retained up to the zone of keratin bonding (Spearman, 1966: Cane & Spearman, 1967). Sequential protein synthesis in epidermal cell development is suggested in mammals by uptake of various injected labelled amino acids into cells at different levels (Fukuyama & Epstein, 1969; Fukuyama, Nakamura & Bernstein, 1965).

A unique cyclical switch in the type of keratin complex formed occurs during horny scale formation in snakes and lizards. The sloughing cycle requires re-formation of the horny layer at frequent intervals. First beta-keratin is formed but in the cells underneath there is a switch to alpha-keratin so that the scale is a two-layered structure (Baden, Roth & Bonar, 1966; Spearman & Riley, 1969).

The zone of keratin bonding

In the outermost living epidermal cells the component proteins are bonded together by formation of cross-linkages including the important disulphide bond (Fraser et al., 1972; Jarrett, 1973). This does not require outside energy and the proteins arrange themselves through the whirl of activity which occurs in living cells. Sequential protein synthesis is quite usual in formation of complex proteins (Schultze & Heremans, 1966). Cytoplasmic water is lost as the keratin complex shrinks. Heat is released in the exergonic formation of cystine from two molecules of cysteine. Peripheral increased cystine concentration and presence of unoxidized cysteine in many horny layer cells such as in amphibians and in mammalian palms and soles may be related to atmospheric oxygen tension (Spearman, 1966; Jarrett, 1973). Keratinization normally occurs synchronously in epidermal cells of reptiles and higher vertebrates but it is asynchronous in most amphibians (Spearman, 1966, 1968). Biochemists no longer believe that keratin fibrils are derived from tonofilaments which are associated with desmosome cell junctional complexes in all epithelia whether they are keratinized or not. It so happens that mammalian epidermal tonofilaments are approximately the same diameter as the alpha-microfibrils of hair cortex, and the idea has lingered on among a few electron microscopists that one is derived from the other. This would in any case be difficult to prove and from the viewpoint of protein chemistry it would be very odd for one type of fibril to take on another function. There is as much reason to believe that all man-made fibres of the same diameter and colour are made of the same substance. Certainly prekeratin fibrils in the hair follicle grade into those seen in the hair cortex, and sulphur-rich matrix keratin appears between them at a higher level (Birkbeck, 1964; Mercer, 1961); but the constituent proteins are formed sequentially on polyribosomes (Fraser et al., 1972). However, analysis of ultrastructural change in epidermis is more difficult to elucidate as it is composed of fewer cell layers.

Relationship to mucogenesis

Mucoproteins are formed in amphibian epidermal cells (Parakkal & Matoltsy, 1964) but do not occur in mammalian epidermis to the same extent, although they occur in the intercellular spaces. In mammals mucogenesis and keratinization occur in different cells in the oral epithelium (Jarrett, 1973; Cane & Spearman, 1969) and in different phases of the rat vaginal cycle (Kahn, 1954). Retinol does not inhibit keratinization in adult mammalian epidermis (Spearman & Jarrett, 1974) although it does so, and promotes mucogenesis, in chick embryos (Fell & Mellanby, 1953). Clearly there is some relationship between the two processes but what it is is not obvious.

Membrane proteins

In rodent epidermis the unit membrane swells suddenly and cysteine is incorporated in the membrane protein beforehand (Fukuyama & Epstein, 1969). Oxidation with formation of cystine occurs first in desmosomal sites and spreads thence to the intervening membrane (Spearman & Hardy, 1975a). Cytoplasmic oxidation of prekeratin with cystine formation occurs later at a higher level and the two processes are therefore different.

ORGANIZED CELL DEATH

Site of cell death

The death of a cell as it undergoes keratinization is sudden and occurs between two cell layers, and is synchronous in higher animals although not in most amphibians (Spearman, 1968, 1973). Because of its apparent organization it has been termed controlled and organized cell death by Jarrett (1973), to distinguish it from the quite different slow death of cells encountered in pathology.

Control of cell death

Probably several factors influence the time at which an epidermal cell dies but distance from the dermal vasculature is probably unimportant. In fact, fluid circulation in the intercellular space provides adequate nutrients for the human wart virus which resides in the superficial living cells. Also, atmospheric exchange of respiratory gases can probably take place near the skin surface. Epidermal thickness varies widely: the whale epidermis is 3 mm in depth but that of the mouse is less than 15 μm (Spearman, 1972). Individual variation also occurs because of cyclical changes in epidermal mitosis which affects the thickness of living epidermis (Spearman, 1973). Death is not closely programmed to a certain depth of cells but in different sites and in different species the average depth of living epidermis is constant, suggesting an underlying ageing mechanism. The known final factors involved in epidermal cell death are: first, loss of plasma membrane function in ionic regulation; second, release of hydrolases from lysosomes, probably the Odland bodies which leave some of their enzymes in the cytoplasm (Jarrett, 1973), while others of these bodies traverse the plasma membrane into the intercellular space as membrane coating granules (Matoltsy & Parakkal, 1965), with further release of hydrolases. The inactive enzymes are formed much earlier in the region of protein synthesis (Jarrett, 1973). These enzymes, which include acid phosphatase, a useful marker, degrade the original cell structure and continue to function in the keratinized cells. Third, cross-bonding of the keratin super molecule intimately associated with cytoplasmic structure upsets normal cell function. Rapid loss of water leads to cell shrinkage but at this stage the cells are dead. These various processes are closely interconnected in keratinization but cell death is more primitive than keratin formation for it also occurs in unkeratinized epithelia.

One of the first changes to occur is mitochondrial degradation with a switch from mitochondrial citric acid respiratory cycle dehydrogenases to cytoplasmic pentose pathway dehydrogenases (Jarrett, 1973). Later a variable amount of nuclear degradation occurs in which both specific nucleases and acid phosphatase are implicated.

Extent of cytolysis

The extent of cellular breakdown varies widely in keratinized structures (Figs 7–10) but is normally constant for each tissue although it can alter in pathological states (Spearman, 1964, 1966).

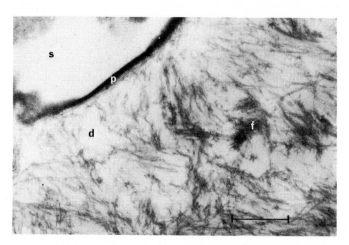

FIG. 7. Guinea-pig back stratum corneum cell. Electron micrograph after glutaraldehyde, pyridine, osmium method. Abbreviations: s, intercellular space; p, thickened darkly stained plasma membrane, with peripheral cytoplasmic matrix keratin. f, Cytoplasmic keratin fibrils are left in a soup of degradation products, d; which fills the cell. Scale 1·5 μm.

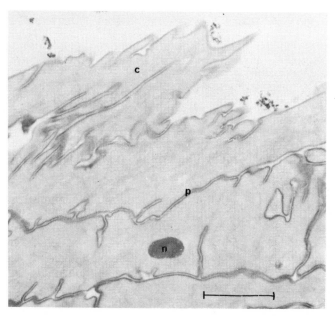

FIG. 8. Guinea-pig back stratum corneum. Electron micrograph after glutaraldehyde, chloroform, osmium method. Less material is extracted than by pyridine. Abbreviations: c, superficial cell; p, plasma membrane; n, nuclear remnant. Scale 4·0 μm. (From R. I. C. Spearman & J. A. Hardy, Br. J. Derm. 89: 265.)

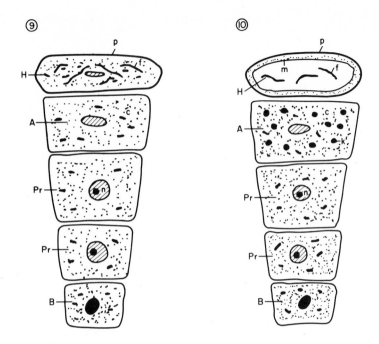

FIG. 9. Diagram showing segment of epidermis in parakeratotic condition with retention of pyknotic nuclei in the stratum corneum and little cytolysis. B, Basal germinal cell; Pr, protein synthesizing cells; A, cells in which autolysis predominates; H, dead stratum corneum; n, nucleus; c, cytoplasm with organelles; f, keratin fibrils; p, thickened plasma membrane.

FIG. 10. Diagram of mammalian epidermal segment from a hairy site showing orthokeratosis with massive autolysis in keratinized cells. k, Keratohyalin granules; m, peripheral matrix keratin. Other labels as in Fig. 9.

Parakeratotic cells (Fig. 9) with nuclear remnants containing some nucleoprotein are retained in the frog *Rana* horny layer (Spearman, 1968) and in the mouse *Mus musculus* tail scales (Jarrett & Spearman, 1964; Jarrett, 1973). In hair cells membranous ghosts of nuclei without any nucleoprotein are retained (Fraser *et al.*, 1972) but there are no cytoplasmic organelles. In most non-mammals some cytoplasmic structure is left, or the keratin·complex fills the space beneath the plasma membrane as in the hair. The only site where cytoplasmic destruction is complete (except for keratin fibrils, but with loss of matrix keratin) is the horny layer of mammalian hairy skin, including human skin (Figs 7 and 10). Soluble products of cytolysis, mainly lipids and free amino acids, are left in the horny cells, but are extracted leaving empty spaces during histological processing (Spearman, 1970; Spearman & Hardy, 1973, 1974).

CALCIFICATION

While many keratinized cells contain calcium, this is usually bound to phospholipid which is associated with the keratin complex (Cane & Spearman, 1967; Spearman, 1970). Examples are calcium in reptilian horny scales (Spearman & Riley, 1969) and in the mouse tail scales. A few hard and brittle keratinized structures contain crystals of hydroxyapatite which play an important part in their mechanical properties. Examples are claws, whale baleen and the beaks of birds (Pautard, 1964). Mineralization occurs in the keratinizing cells by precipitation on chemical nuclei probably provided by keratin proteins.

CONCLUSIONS

There is considerable inbuilt variation in keratinization which operates both under normal and pathological conditions. The possible variables are: (a) proportions of the different keratin protein components present, (b) whether or not the plasma membranes are cystine-bonded, (c) the degree of cytolysis and (d) whether or not separate mineralization with calcium salts occurs.

Keratinized structures serve two main functions: as tough appendages, for instance in breeding tubercles of fish, and in feathers and hairs which serve various purposes; and as a passive barrier to water movement through the skin. Water movement is slowed probably by complexes of keratin and phospholipid in the horny layer (Spearman, 1970). Because of the complexity of the processes involved true keratinization can occur probably only within cells.

These interrelated factors in keratinization determine the mechanical properties of horny structures and the use of the archaic terms hard and soft keratins is best avoided.

The keratin spines of platyhelminths (Swiderski, 1972) differ from vertebrate keratins in that they are laid down in a still-living syncytium. The cytoplasmic changes of keratinization are therefore localized to the spines and hooks which are covered with a thickened plasma membrane as in vertebrates (Jha & Smyth, 1969). Elsewhere the plasma membrane is of normal thickness.

REFERENCES

Alexander, P., Hudson, R. F. & Earland, C. (1963). *Wool. Its chemistry and physics.* London: Chapman & Hall.

Baden, H. P. & Cohen, J. (1965). Protein synthesis in epidermal cells. *Biochim. Biophys. Acta* **108**: 143–146.

Baden, H. P., Roth, S. I. & Bonar, L. C. (1966). Fibrous proteins of snake scale. *Nature, Lond.* **212**: 498–499.

Birkbeck, M. S. C. (1964). Keratin an ultrastructural review. In *Progress in the biological sciences in relation to dermatology.* **2**: 193–203. Rook, A. & Champion, R. H. (eds). London: Cambridge University Press.

Breathnach, A. S. (1971). *An atlas of the ultrastructure of human skin.* London: Churchill.

Brush, A. H. (1974). Feather keratin—analysis of subunit heterogeneity. *Comp. Biochem. Physiol.* **45B**: 661–670.

Cane, A. K. & Spearman, R. I. C. (1967). A histochemical study of keratinization in the domestic fowl *Gallus gallus. J. Zool., Lond.* **153**: 337–352.

Cane, A. K. & Spearman, R. I. C. (1969). The keratinized epithelium of the house mouse *Mus musculus* tongue. Its structure and histochemistry. *Arch. Oral Biol.* **14**: 829–841.

Dilly, P. N. (1971). Keratin like fibres in the hemichordate *Rhabdopleura compacta. Z. Zellforsch. mikrosk. Anat.* **117**: 502–515.

Farbman, A. (1966). Plasma membrane changes during keratinization. *Anat. Rec.* **156**: 269–281.

Fell, H. B. & Mellanby, E. (1953). Metaplasia produced in chick ectoderm by vitamin A. *J. Physiol., Lond.* **119**: 470–488.

Filshie, B. K. & Rogers, G. E. (1962). An electron microscope study of the fine structure of feather keratin. *J. Cell Biol.* **13**: 1–12.

Fraser, R. D. B. & MacRae, T. P. (1963). Structural organisation in feather keratin. *J. molec. Biol.* **7**: 272–280.

Fraser, R. D. B., MacRae, T. P. & Rogers, G. E. (1972). *Keratins, their composition structure and biosynthesis.* Springfield Ill.: Thomas.

Fukuyama, K. & Bernstein, I. A. (1963). Site of synthesis of ribonucleic acid in mammalian epidermis. *J. invest. Derm.* **41**: 47–52.

Fukuyama, K. & Epstein, W. L. (1969). Sulphur containing proteins and epidermal keratinization. *J. Cell Biol.* **40**: 830–838.

Fukuyama, K., Nakamura, T. & Bernstein, I. A. (1965). Differentially localised incorporation of amino acids in relation to epidermal keratinization in the newborn rat. *Anat. Rec.* **152**: 525–536.

Gillespie, J. M. (1965). The high sulphur proteins of normal and aberrant keratins. In *Biology of skin and hair growth*: 377–398. Lyne, A. G. & Short, B. F. (eds). Sydney: Angus & Robertson.

Gillespie, J. M. & Darskus, R. L. (1971). The relation between tyrosine content of various wools and their content of a class of proteins rich in tyrosine and glycine. *Aust. J. Biol. Sci.* **24**: 1189–1197.

Gillespie, J. M. & Frenkel, M. J. (1974). The diversity of keratins. *Comp. Biochem. Physiol.* **47B**: 339–346.

Harrap, B. S. & Woods, E. F. (1964). Soluble derivatives of feather keratins 1. Isolation fractionation and amino acid composition. *Biochem. J.* **92**: 8–18.

Harrap, B. S. & Woods, E. F. (1967). Species differences in the proteins of feathers. *Comp. Biochem. Physiol.* **20**: 449–460.

Jarrett, A. (1973). *The physiology and pathophysiology of the skin.* **1**. The epidermis. London and New York: Academic Press.
Jarrett, A. & Spearman, R. I. C. (1964). *Histochemistry of the skin psoriasis.* London: English Universities Press.
Jha, R. K. & Smyth, J. D. (1969). *Echinococcus granulosus,* ultrastructure of microtriches. *Expl Parasit.* **25**: 232–244.
Kahn, R. H. (1954). Effect of locally applied vitamin A and oestrogen on the rat vagina. *Am. J. Anat.* **95**: 309–328.
Lindley, H., Broad, A., Damaglou, A. P., Darskus, R. L., Elleman, T. C., Gillespie, J. M. & Moore, C. H. (1971). The high sulphur protein fraction of keratins. *Appl. Poly. Symp.* **18**: 21–35. New York: Interscience Publishers.
Matoltsy, A. G. (1969). Keratinization of the avian epidermis. An ultrastructural study of new born chick skin. *J. Ultrastruct. Res.* **29**: 438–458.
Matoltsy, A. G. & Matoltsy, M. N. (1966). The membrane proteins of horny cells. *J. Invest. Derm.* **46**: 127–129.
Matoltsy, A. G. & Parakkal, P. F. (1965). Membrane coating granules of keratinizing epithelia. *J. Cell Biol.* **24**: 297–307.
Mercer, E. H. (1961). *Keratins and keratinization.* Oxford: Pergamon Press.
Mittal, A. K. & Banerjee, T. K. (1974). Structure and keratinization of the skin of a freshwater teleost *Notopterus notopterus* (Notopteridae, Pisces). *J. Zool., Lond.* **174**: 341–355.
Parakkal, P. F. & Matoltsy, A. G. (1964). A study of the fine structure of the epidermis of *Rana pipiens. J. Cell Biol.* **20**: 85–94.
Pautard, S. G. E. (1964). Calcification of keratin. In *Progress in the biological sciences in relation to dermatology.* **2**: 227–240. Rook, A. & Champion, R. H. (eds). London: Cambridge University Press.
Pearse, A. G. E. (1972). *Histochemistry theoretical and applied.* **2**: 3rd edn. London: Churchill.
Ryder, M. L. & Stephenson, S. K. (1968). *Wool growth.* London and New York: Academic Press.
Schultze, H. E. & Heremans, J. F. (1966). *Molecular biology of human proteins.* **1**. Amsterdam: Elsevier.
Sims, R. T. (1967). Synthesis of nucleic acids in hair. *Nature, Lond.* **213**: 387–388.
Slayter, G. (1962). Two-phase materials. *Scient. Am.* **206**: 124–134.
Spearman, R. I. C. (1964). The evolution of mammalian keratinized structures. *Symp. zool. Soc. Lond.* No. 12: 67–81.
Spearman, R. I. C. (1966). The keratinization of epidermal scales feathers and hairs. *Biol. Rev.* **41**: 59–96.
Spearman, R. I. C. (1968). Epidermal keratinization in the salamander and a comparison with other amphibia. *J. Morph.* **125**: 129–144.
Spearman, R. I. C. (1970). Some light microscopical observations on the stratum corneum of the guinea pig, man, and the common seal. *Br. J. Derm.* **83**: 582–590.
Spearman, R. I. C. (1972). The epidermal stratum corneum of the whale. *J. Anat.* **113**: 373–381.
Spearman, R. I. C. (1973). *The integument. A textbook of skin biology.* London: Cambridge University Press.
Spearman, R. I. C. (1977). The biochemistry of hair formation and the chemistry of hair keratins. In *Physiology and pathophysiology of the skin.* **4**: 1417–1456. Jarrett, A. (ed.). London and New York: Academic Press.

Spearman, R. I. C. & Hardy, J. A. (1973). The action of solvents on the ultrastructural appearance of keratohyalin and the horny layer in guinea pig back epidermis. *Br. J. Derm.* **89**: 265–276.

Spearman, R. I. C. & Hardy, J. A. (1974). Some ultrastructural observations on keratohyalin granules of guinea pig back epidermis. *Arch. Derm. Forsch.* **250**: 149–158.

Spearman, R. I. C. & Hardy, J. A. (1975a). Ultrastructural demonstration of cystine in guinea pig back stratum corneum. *Arch. Derm. Forsch.* **251**: 289–294.

Spearman, R. I. C. & Hardy J. A. (1975b). Plantar epidermis of the guinea pig and characteristics of the stratum corneum. *Acta anat.* **91**: 196–204.

Spearman, R. I. C. & Jarrett, A. (1974). Biological comparison of isomers and chemical forms of vitamin A (retinol). *Br. J. Derm.* **90**: 553–560.

Spearman, R. I. C. & Riley, P. A. (1969). A comparison of the epidermis and pigment cells of the crocodile with those in two lizard species. *J. Linn. Soc. (Zool).* **48**: 453–466.

Swiderski, Z. (1972). La structure fine de l'onchosphère du cestode *Catenotaenia pusilla* (Groeze). *Cellule* **69**: 207–237.

Thompson, E. O. P. & O'Donnell, I. J. (1962). Studies on reduced wool. 1: The extent of reduction of wool with increasing concentrations of thiol and the extraction of proteins from reduced and alkylated wool. *Aust. J. Biol. Sci.* **15**: 757–768.

Zelickson, A.S. (1967). *Ultrastructure of normal and abnormal skin.* London: Kimpton.

Symp. zool. Soc. Lond. (1977) No. 39, 353–372.

CHANGES IN MOUSE TAIL EPIDERMAL KERATINIZATION INDUCED BY TAR DERIVATIVES

ROSANNE WRENCH

Department of Dermatology, University College Hospital Medical School, London, England

SYNOPSIS

Mouse tail epidermis undergoes two distinct types of keratinization. In the scale areas a parakeratotic horny layer is associated with the failure of a granular layer to form, whereas a flexible orthokeratotic horny layer is found above a well formed granular layer which occurs only in areas of hair production. The latter type of keratinization is also found in the majority of the fur-covered body skin of the mouse and in man. Man can also display the scale-type keratinization in the pathological condition psoriasis. In this common skin disease, an increased epidermal mitotic rate and the possibly associated lack of a granular layer result in parakeratosis—characterized by the conservation of nuclear material in the horny layer.

Using antipsoriatic drugs, which have a primary effect on keratinization, it is also possible to change parakeratotic areas of the mouse tail to the orthokeratinizing type. In these experiments, the mouse tail epidermis provided a standardized model for the assay of tar fractions for use in chronic psoriasis. The screening demonstrated a far greater specificity on the part of high boiling phenols to induce a granular layer in mouse tail scales than other tar constituents. The subsequent change to orthokeratinization, revealed by characteristic keratin fluorescence changes, suggested that these phenols may be valuable for the treatment of chronic psoriasis. In addition, the scale areas having a flat dermo-epidermal junction provided a simple means of assessing epidermal thickening actions of the topical treatments. The revelation that basic and neutral mixtures served only to thicken both the scale and follicular epidermis sugested that the antipsoriatic properties of coal tar preparation may be increased further by their omission.

ORTHOKERATINIZATION AND PARAKERATINIZATION IN MICE AND MAN

Mouse tail skin (Mus musculus)

Mouse tail skin is readily identified from the rest of the body skin by its scaly appearance. The production of the horny layer of the fur-covered body skin involves the development of a granular layer prior to the horny layer. The granular layer of mammalian epidermis is a region of cells containing basophilic cytoplasmic granules, sometimes referred to as keratohyalin (Spearman & Hardy, 1974). Jarrett & Spearman (1964) have suggested that the multitude of hydrolytic enzymes released in this region are responsible for the destruction of the epidermal cell contents (including nuclear material) whilst keratin polymers are being formed. The keratin is thus laid down in a cell relatively empty of organelles, the cells together forming a flexible horny layer. This process is referred to

353

as orthokeratinization. The work of Spearman (1970) suggests that routine processing for microscopic visualization leads to dissolution of lysed cell contents by histological agents, leaving the resistant keratin network which then has the typical "basket-weave" appearance of mammalian orthokeratinization.

Mouse tail horny layer is, however, formed without the development of this zone of rich enzyme activity (Fig. 1). Cytoplasmic and nuclear contents remain, so that keratin is thus laid down in a fairly intact cell structure and the keratinized cells form the relatively inflexible horny layer (parakeratinization). Basophilic nuclear remnants are visible in the horny layer, and it is possible to demonstrate the presence of certain hydrolytic enzymes such as acid phosphatase (Jarrett & Spearman, 1964). These workers suggest that the release of the hydrolytic enzymes has been somewhat retarded, perhaps by overstabilized lysosomal membranes, and orthokeratinization cannot occur without granular layer formation.

Spearman (1964) has traced how the establishment of a true granular layer is a consequence of the evolution of orthokeratinizing hairy skin in mammals. Such areas of orthokeratinization, i.e. horny layer similar to the previously described fur-covered skin, can be seen in the mouse tail confined to areas of hair production (Spearman, 1973), (Fig. 1). This is clearly demonstrated in very

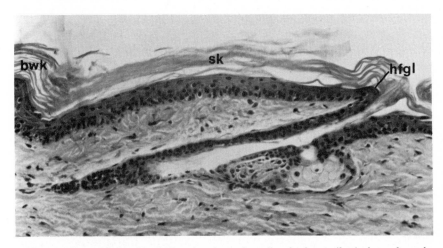

FIG. 1. Mouse tail skin. Vertical section through a tail scale along tail axis shows the scale keratin (sk) produced without granular layer formation. A keratohyalin granular layer (hfgl) is found surrounding the hair follicle; the flexible "basket-weave" keratin (bwk) is evident above this layer.

young mice—up to five days old—when the tail hair follicles are crowded together. Figure 2 shows that the granular layers associated with the closely packed hair follicles form a continuous granular layer along the length of the tail and indeed the outer horny layer appears smooth. Within one or two days, the interfollicular scale regions expand as the whole tail rapidly lengthens. The absence of a granular layer in these developing regions is apparent (Fig. 3), and the consequent parakeratotic horny layer is evidence that the adult keratinization pattern is established.

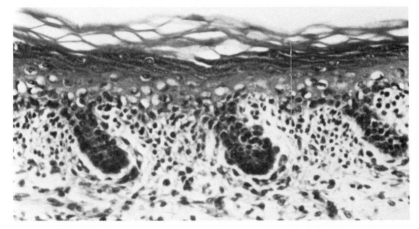

FIG. 2. Young mouse tail skin—two days old. The granular layers associated with the closely packed hair follicles form a continuous layer along the length of the tail. The resultant "basket-weave" keratin gives the skin an outer smooth appearance.

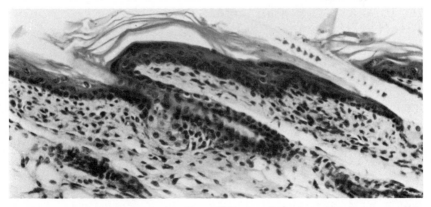

FIG. 3. Young mouse tail skin—six days old. The interfollicular scale regions are rapidly appearing. Lacking a granular layer, horny layers of these regions are developing the characteristic scaly appearance of the adult mice.

The importance of a granular layer for the characteristically mammalian orthokeratinization is established (Jarrett, 1973) and it is also exemplified by the use of external stimuli which influence keratinization by changing the activity of this layer. For instance, follicular-type orthokeratinization can be induced in former scale regions following granular layer induction. This has been achieved by vitamin A (retinol). Applications of vitamin A to mouse tail skin results in granular layer formation in previously scaly areas and an increase in epidermal mitotic rate (Bern, Elias, Pickett, Powers & Harkness, 1955; Lawrence & Bern, 1958; Jarrett & Spearman, 1964). Vitamin A is also capable of inducing granular layer formation and therefore orthokeratinization in the parakeratotic areas of psoriasis in man.

Psoriasis

Psoriasis is a chronic scaling skin disease which has been said to affect about 2% of the Caucasian population (Ingram, 1954; Kidd & Meenan, 1961). The prevalence varies amongst different races and it is most infrequent in full-blooded negroes (J. H. Lewis, 1943; Clarke, 1962). Lesions may occur in small plaques causing little disturbance, or there may be extensive body involvement, which can severely disturb the working and social life of the patient.

The dermis shows inflammatory changes of vasodilatation and infiltration of polymorphonucleocytes and lymphocytes which sometimes aggregate to form Munro abscesses. The epidermal changes are characterized by a sevenfold increase in mitotic rate of the basal layer cells with mitoses also visible in the cells above (Goodwin, Hamilton & Fry, 1974), increased epidermal thickness, and the failure of a granular layer to form. As in mouse tail skin, cell contents are not lysed and basophilic nuclear remnants are obvious in the horny layer.

Jarrett & Spearman (1964) consider that the failure of a granular layer to develop may be in part the result of the rapid transit time of the keratinocytes through the epidermis, leaving insufficient time for full differentiation. The lack of hydrolysis of cell contents in the granular region, whilst keratin formation continues, results in abnormal horny layer cells, which are inflexible and stick together to form unsightly scales. Hydrolytic enzymes which were not released in the granular layer region can be demonstrated in the now parakeratotic horny layer of psoriatic lesions as in mouse tail scales. The plaques have a silvery-white appearance due to air spaces between the scales (Burks & Montgomery, 1943), and the redness is due to the dilated tortuous superficial dermal blood vessels.

Psoriasis is an incurable disease, owing to its hereditary and recurrent nature (Novotny, 1966; Kimberling & Dobson, 1973). However it is possible to alleviate the suffering of patients by encouraging a return of orthokeratinization. This can be achieved by reducing the elevated mitotic rate and reinducing a granular layer. Similarly, scale regions of mouse tail epidermis can be changed to the follicular orthokeratotic type by the same agents. Jarrett & Spearman (1964) first used the mouse tail skin model to show that the antipsoriatic drug combination of vitamin A and triamcinolone also produced orthokeratinization in formerly scaly areas by induction of a granular layer and suppression of mitotic rate. The ability to parallel both histologically and histochemically the changes occurring in the healing psoriatic lesion in a simple animal model is an invaluable tool in antipsoriatic drug assay.

Mouse tail scale epidermis as a model for psoriasis

The continuing need for antipsoriatic drug assay

Restoration of the psoriatic epidermis to an orthokeratinizing state is at present achieved with varying degrees of safety and success. A look at the range of treatments which have been employed is perplexing (Champion, 1966). In the main, tar preparations, dithranol (1, 8, 9-trihydroxyanthracene) and corticosteroids are used. The synthetic halogenated corticosteroids have been extremely popular for their potent general anti-inflammatory and anti-mitotic properties. At first, resolution of the plaques is remarkable, but the skin soon becomes tolerant. Greater amounts are required leading to increasing systemic absorption and gross interference with endogenous corticosteroids, causing muscular weakness and osteoporosis from excessive protein breakdown, carbohydrate and electrolyte disturbances. Effects on the skin are collagen atrophy, sometimes causing scarring (striae), and telangiectasia (redness due to capillary dilatation). Sudden withdrawal of the treament, be it topical or systematic, leads to severe rebound conditions, which are often intractable to treatment (Burry, 1973; Leyden, Thew & Kligman, 1974).

Dithranol is a compound irritant to the surrounding clinically normal skin and must be applied under medical supervision. Dithranol stains the plaques, but is an effective and safe treatment.

However as the staining of the skin is finally fading, the lesion is often starting to relapse.

Coal tar preparations are widely used as safe and effective treatments for many cases of chronic psoriasis. However they are very messy and smelly and in some cases irritant. The preparations are very variable and unpredictable in their efficiency. This can be due to both a poor choice of vehicle and the lack of specification of the type of tar necessary to treat the various stages of psoriasis. It is essential to state the type of tar to be used in terms of its parent coal and temperature of formation (Downing & Bauer, 1948; Wrench & Britten, 1975a).

Mode of action of antipsoriatic drugs

There are many ideas on the modes of action of the above treatments. In the case of corticosteroids, the known suppression of the carbohydrate metabolising enzymes has suggested that the energy available for the greatly increased mitotic rate is reduced (Belsan, Neumann & Blazkova, 1965; Halprin, Fukui & Ohkawara, 1969). The fall in epidermal mitotic count after treatment with topical corticosteroids (Spearman & Jarrett, 1975; Fry & McMinn, 1968) is accompanied by induction of a granular layer and the consequent return of flexible horny layer production, orthokeratosis. Jarrett & Spearman (1964) suggest that by reducing the mitotic rate, the increased transit time of the epidermal cell through the epidermis may be sufficiently lengthened to allow full differentiation into the granular layer stage. Although corticosteroids are well known for their anti-inflammatory action of lysome stabilization, at higher doses they can cause rupture of lysosomal membranes (Lewis & Day, 1972). It is possible that the high local concentration of a topical corticosteroid on the psoriatic plaque initiates release of hydrolytic enzymes "locked" in the lysosomes of the parakeratotic horny layer so that orthokeratinization can ensue.

Dithranol also interferes with the enzymes of carbohydrate metabolism (Hammar, 1970) and this may be important in its anti-mitotic actions (Swanbeck & Lundquist, 1972). Dithranol may also be capable of directly inducing a granular layer before exerting its anti-mitotic effect (Raab & Patermann, 1966; Fry & McMinn, 1968), although this was not seen when dithranol was applied to mouse tail skin at 10% concentrations (Wrench & Britten, 1975d).

In the case of coal tar, it is impractical to suggest a common mode of action for all the tar preparations which have been used. Coal tar itself is a complex mixture of hydrocarbons, phenols and bases, the relative proportions varying widely with the mode of tar production. Coal tars have been used in many different vehicles, some of which are certain to have retarded release of coal tar constituents into the skin and these probably afforded only occlusive treatment. However, following coal tar treatment of psoriatic lesions, a granular layer does reform; but Fry & McMinn (1968) found it impossible to determine whether this was the primary effect. Coal tar in cotton seed oil was shown to inhibit incorporation of labelled amino acids into the epidermis (Freedberg, 1965). Ruzicka, Novotna-Kasparkova & Burda (1969) found that tar pastes inhibited the pentose phosphate pathway, which has been shown to be elevated in psoriatic plaques (Jarrett, 1971).

To date there is no treatment for psoriasis effective and safe in the long term and also cosmetically acceptable. Considering the proven safety of coal tar preparations, it would be desirable to isolate the active principles and formulate them into cosmetically aesthetic treatments.

The experimental model

The many previous attempts to identify components of coal tar which may be beneficial in treating psoriasiform diseases have met with little success. In many cases, fractions and vehicles seem to have been chosen at random (Kerr & Plein, 1953; Lloyd & King, 1959), and the experimental situations have consisted only of clinical observations of their effects on psoriatic lesions, which can tend to be subjective. There has been virtually no histological nor histochemical monitoring of the resultant changes in keratinization. In fact the use of psoriatic lesions for what must be in the first instance a large scale assay is not feasible, since it is necessary to classify the test lesions. This would mean taking an unacceptably large number of biopsies to determine the stage of the disease, and psoriasis is certainly a disorder which requires distinctly different types of therapies throughout the life of the lesion. Also interpretation of results from clinical situations is difficult, because of the high incidence of spontaneous remissions occurring especially under hospitalization and trial conditions (Samitz, 1958). To locate compounds with specific effects on keratinization, an animal model of similar parakeratinization tendencies is required which allows standardization by species, strain, age, sex and weight. The choice of mouse tail skin was prompted by the work of Jarrett & Spearman (1964) on the screening of antipsoriatic drug combinations for their effects prior to clinical use. Mouse tail skin provides follicular orthokeratinizing regions to monitor for possible irritant effects on surrounding clinically normal skin, and extensive parakeratotic scale areas to observe for signs of conversion to an orthokeratotic state with induction of a granular layer. The flat dermo-epidermal junction facilitates quick and easy measurements of epidermal thickness, enabling statistical evaluation. The induction of a granular layer in formerly parakeratotic regions is considered a suitable parameter in assaying for a specific antipsoriatic effect for the following reasons.

(a) Although it is not yet agreed whether the primary psoriatic stimulus is dermal or epidermal in origin (Pinkus & Mehregan, 1966), there is much data to implicate the epidermis as the initial site of the developing lesion (Paslin & Sprague, 1975).

(b) It has been frequently observed that the re-formation of the granular layer is the primary event in a healing psoriatic lesion. This has been noted during drug trials in psoriatics—with corticosteroids (Komisaruk, Kosek & Schuster, 1962; Freedman, Reed & Becker, 1963), dithranol and the anti-mitotic agent, methotrexate (Fry & McMinn, 1968).

TAR DERIVATIVES AND EPIDERMAL KERATINIZATION

Toxic actions of coal tar

Coal tar is probably more renowned for its ability to cause skin disease than for its dermatologically therapeutic effects. One of the many actions of tar is to stimulate epidermal mitosis and promote the development of many types of tar tumours (Fisher, 1953). Its irritant actions lead to various dermatoses including folliculitis, acute and chronic erythemas and pruritis. Systemic toxicity in animals due to percutaneous absorption of coal tar constituents has also been reported (Davidson, 1925; Babes & Lazaresco-Pantzu, 1928; Grigor'ev, 1959).

Tar in psoriasis

Coal tars have been used for many years to treat psoriasis and other skin diseases including eczema (Nelson & Osterberg, 1927), atopic dermatitis (Clyman, 1957) and even ringworm of the feet (Pardo-Castello, 1944). Crude coal tar and various fractions have been formulated in a multitude of vehicles. It became apparent that the majority of psoriatics benefited from ultraviolet light therapy and especially in conjuction with a coal tar regimen. Goeckerman

(1925) described such a treatment routine which is still used in its original and in modified forms (Perry, Soderstrom & Schulze, 1968; Young, 1972). Even with extensive body coverage, Goeckerman reported no systemic toxicity.

Coal tar has certainly stood the test of time as a dermatologic therapy, but its unwanted side-effects still remain. It has an unpleasant and lingering smell, and many preparations are immiscible with water and therefore difficult to remove from the skin and clothes (Combes, 1947). The irritant effects can also be a problem for some patients (Carney & Zopf, 1955). Previous work on the improvement of the therapeutic and cosmetic properies of tar preparations has ranged from the screening of various fractions alone (Nelson & Osterberg, 1927; Jaffrey, 1928) or in combination with substances like allantoin (Bleiberg, 1958; Singer, 1962) and corticosteroids (Orris, 1966) to the testing of individual components of tar (Obermayer & Becker, 1935) and the formulation of tar constituents into "synthetic tar" preparations (Guy, Jacob & Weber, 1939; Simon & Brandt, 1953; Kinmont & Jowett, 1958). However, in his review of antipsoriatic drugs, Champion (1966) stated that the active constituents of coal tar had still not been isolated, and that commercial tar preparations seemed to differ more in cost than efficacy. Consequently the use of crude coal tar is still recommended despite its undesirable properties. Now for the first time, an animal model was employed to monitor for specific antipsoriatic tar fractions.

Tar and mouse tail skin

Methods

Two types of tar were tested—a low temperature tar formed at about 500°C, and a high temperature tar produced at temperatures in excess of 1200°C (see Wrench & Britten, 1975a). These were split into acidic, neutral and basic fractions and were formulated with both cream and ointment bases. These were applied daily to the proximal half of the mouse tail. At first, treatments lasted up to one month but later when very active granular layer inducers were isolated, the effects were produced within a few days (Wrench & Britten, 1975c). At the end of each experiment, the mice were killed and their tail skin was removed for qualitative histological examination and measurement of epidermal thickness. (Epidermal thickness was measured from the basal layer to the beginning of the horny layer.)

Results

Granular layer induction. A granular layer was induced in the scale regions of the mouse tail by the acidic (phenolic) fractions of coal tar only. These acids are most conveniently discussed in terms of their boiling ranges. The predominant effects of the low boiling acids (boiling between 175–210°C and containing phenol, the cresols and xylenols) was to thicken the epidermis. However, higher boiling xylenols caused granular layer formation in the formerly parakeratotic regions surrounding the hair follicles, so that the hair follicle granular layer extended into the scale regions. The greatest induction of a granular layer was produced by the ranges 290–340°C, maximizing in the range 330–340°C (Fig. 4.). Less activity was shown by acids boiling over 340°C and between 225–290°C and virtually none by acids below 225°C. It was concluded that acids boiling in the range 330–340°C had a more specific action in inducing layers than did the parent tars at similar concentrations. The acids were still causing epidermal thickening and in some cases induced extensive peeling of the epidermis. However, these effects seemed to follow an initial induction of a granular layer, as evidenced by experiments in which mice were removed daily from a treated group and killed to monitor the events with time. In some mice, granular layers were obvious after four treatments, this effect maximizing after six to nine treatments.

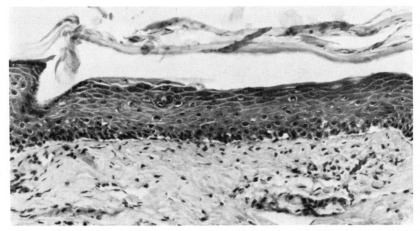

FIG. 4. Phenol-treated mouse tail skin. The phenolic fraction boiling between 330–340°C has induced a granular layer in formerly parakeratotic regions. Note also epidermal cell hypertrophy and hyperplasia.

Further applications caused extensive peeling and epidermal cell death, as the phenols were, presumably, absorbed to greater depths (Wrench, 1973: 135).

Epidermal thickening. Neutral and basic fractions and their parent tars failed to induce granular layers in the tail scales, but caused highly significant thickening of the epidermis (see Table I). This was first observed when the neutral compounds were being applied in an oil-in-water cream, which was also shown to thicken the epidermis. This vehicle was abandoned in favour of an inert yellow soft paraffin/wool fat base. Spearman & Garretts (1966) pointed out that rubbing can alter keratinization by stimulating mitosis. However, experiments to show whether mere application of the preparations was sufficient to cause thickening revealed that rubbing with cotton wool for about 30 seconds each day was not an adequate stimulus (Wrench, 1973: 171), and any epidermal thickening was thus attributed to the actions of the tar constituents.

TABLE I

Effects of tar on mouse tail skin

	Days treated	e.t.	s.e.	n	t	P
Control	(28)	23·6	1·20	7		
40% Avenue tar	28	53·2	3·09	7	8·95	0·001
40% Avenue oils (A.O.)	28	33·8	2·51	7	3·67	0·005
40% Avenue oil acids	9	40·3	1·24	9	9·54	0·001
40% A.O. bases + neutrals	28	31·8	2·66	7	2·81	0·05
40% A.O. neutrals	28	37·5	1·65	8	6·68	0·001
40% Coalite tar (C.T.)	28	54·4	3·72	9	7·08	0·001
40% C.T. acids	28	64·0	3·92	6	10·58	0·001
40% C.T. bases + neutrals	28	42·6	3·61	7	5·02	0·001
40% C.T. neutrals	28	41·6	2·39	10	5·92	0·001
40% Coalite oils (C.O.)	28	40·1	1·79	10	6·97	0·001
40% C.O. acids	11	Not measureable				
40% C.O. bases + neutrals	28	39·3	0·96	10	10·34	0·001
40% C.O. neutrals	21	35·1	1·40	6	6·27	0·001

Initial no. mice/group = 10; weight range = 23–27g.
Avenue tar: high temperature tar (National Coal Board).
Coalite tar: low temperature tar (Coalite and Chemical Products Ltd).
e.t. Epidermal thickness (μm); s.e. standard error; n number of mice at termination; t Student's t test; P probability.
(By courtesy of the Editor, *British Journal of Dermatology*.)

The propensity for neutral tar constituents (hydrocarbons) to increase epidermal thickness was again demonstrated by experiments involving daily application of a commercial "synthetic tar", "Psorox" (Fisons Pharmaceuticals Ltd). The hydrocarbon content is over 75%—notably phenanthrene, anthracene and naphthalene. The preparation only caused highly significant epidermal thickening without any formation of a granular layer in the mouse scales (Wrench & Britten, 1975d). Young (1970) showed clinically that this type of preparation was of little value in the treatment of psoriasis. Also the tar acid content comprises about 8%, and consists of the low boiling phenols—phenol and the cresols—which failed to induce granular layers in the mouse scale regions (Wrench & Britten, 1975b).

Although the granular layer-inducing acidic fractions caused epidermal thickening, it would seem that the thickening properties of coal tar preparations may be reduced by omitting these fractions, and that by the use of higher phenols alone, the ratio of granular layer–inducing properties to epidermal thickening effects has increased to that produced by the parent tars.

Skin staining. One of the major objections to the use of tars in dermatologic therapy has been the propensity to stain the skin and clothing. The acidic fractions unfortunately seem to possess these properties. Many former attemps to "clean up" coal tar formulations have lead to a decrease in efficacy (Champion, 1966). The well-known phenolic antipsoriatic drug dithranol also causes skin staining. The non-phenolic analogue triacetoxyanthracene is said to reduce staining, but there is also a great drop in antiparakeratotic actions. However, as with the epidermal thickening, skin staining seems to be reduced in comparison to possible therapeutic effects by the use of high-boiling tar acids only.

Irritant actions. A preparation was judged irritant when the mice scattered when approached for treatment, and displayed burrowing behaviour after tar applications. At this point the experiment was terminated. Irritation was caused by extensive and rapid peeling of epidermal layers leaving exposed sensitive surfaces, and also by the direct irritant effects of the acids on the eroded skin.

Although again the most promising fractions, boiling between 330–340°C, caused peeling, this fraction was well tolerated even on peeling skin. The lower boiling phenols were far more irritant, and since they appear to be therapeutically inferior, tar preparations may be improved by their omission.

Vehicle effects. After abandonment of the oil-in-water emulsion cream, which promoted epidermal thickening, the yellow soft paraffin-based ointment was used for the majority of the tar screening. Later a penetration enhancing vehicle "Plastibase" (Squibb & Sons Ltd) was used. This vehicle comprises liquid paraffin in a polyethylene network.

Ideally, all fractions and constituents should be screened in a large number of different vehicles since some compounds may have been missed because of lack of dissolution in, or release from, the vehicle. However, it is unlikely that very active granular layer inducers were overlooked, as other experiments suggest that granular layer induction is one of the primary events occurring in the uppermost levels of the parakeratotic epidermis, and this most important event in this case does not seem to require deep percutaneous penetration of the inducers.

Histochemical demonstrations of effects of tar acids. (a) Acid phosphatase. In both psoriatic and mouse tail scale epidermis, lysosomal enzymes fail to be released in the transitional region beneath the horny layer. Their presence can be demonstrated in the parakeratotic horny layer only (Jarrett & Spearman, 1964). In the orthokeratotic areas surrounding the hair follicles, acid phosphatase activity is obvious in the granular layer and is absent from the basket-weave horny layer above (Fig. 5).

In the experimental alteration of keratinization described, acid phosphatase activity was induced in the newly formed granular layer and there was no activity then in the horny layer. This is in

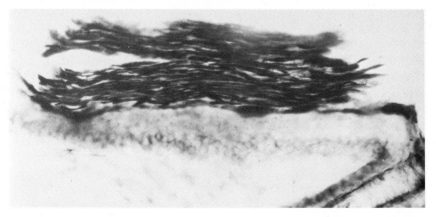

FIG. 5. Acid phosphatase—normal mouse tail skin. The activity is confined to the granular layer of the hair follicle and to the parakeratotic scale horny layer.

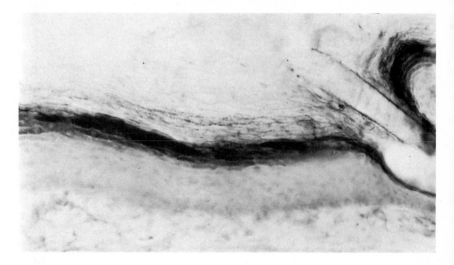

FIG. 6. Acid phosphatase—phenol treated tail. Activity has been induced in the newly-formed granular layer, and is also present in the peripheries of the lower "basket-weave" horny layer cells.

agreement with the findings of Jarrett & Spearman (1964) after applications of vitamin A and triamcinolone to mouse tail skin. These workers have described similar shifts in distribution of this and other hydrolytic enzymes in chronic psoriatic lesions and in clinically normal skin.

Figure 6 illustrates the induced acid phosphatase in the granular layer. Activity is also present in the peripheries of the orthokeratinized cells above; this has previously been described in human plantar and palmar skin (Jarrett & Spearman, 1964: 12).

(b) Horny layer fluorescence. Jarrett & Spearman (1964) have evolved a fluorescent microscopic method which differentiates orthokeratinized and parakeratinized sites. By staining with Congo red and thioflavine T, and visualizing with ultraviolet light, the parakeratotic horny layer of both mouse tail scales and of psoriatic plaques fluoresce blue and the orthokeratotic follicular regions of mouse tail skin and normal human back skin fluoresce red. In these particular experiments, using slightly different filters, parakeratin fluoresced green. After treatment with vitamin A and triamcinolone, mouse tail scale epidermis fluoresces completely red (Jarrett & Spearman, 1964). However, none of the tar fractions completely changed the fluorescence of the scale horny layer to red. The maximum change caused by the highest boiling phenols was to produce strands of red fluorescing orthokeratinized cells with other green parakeratinized cells. Similar effects were obtained after treating mouse tail skin with 0·1% triamcinolone in a cream base for 18 days (Jarrett & Spearman, 1964: 47). Spearman & Garretts (1966) describe this "sandwich" effect of alternating orthokeratinized cells and parakeratinized cells in mouse tail scales following subcutaneous saline injections, which caused both granular layer induction and mitotic stimulation. These workers proposed that the two types of keratinization produced were due to the daily periodicity of treatments, parakeratosis being the result of a process which includes the formation of a granular layer. The two types of keratinization are manifestations of the increased mitotic rate and also of granular layer induction. A similar sequence of events is postulated for the variable effects on keratinization produced by the tar acids.

Duration of tar treatments. It appears that tar fractions which only caused epidermal thickening with no granular layer induction produced increases in thickness which did not vary significantly with the duration of treatment (Wrench & Britten, 1975a). However, substances which caused granular layer induction caused inflammatory reactions when they penetrated deeper into the epidermis and the manifestations of the multitude of sequelae of course varied greatly with treatment time. The effects on the skin may produce a confused record of events after several days treatment, i.e. granular layer induction, peeling and mitotic stimulation and a resultant parakeratosis. If early sections are not taken, (within the first week), the initial granular layer may not be observed, and the epidermal thickening effects may appear to be the predominant actions of the fraction under test.

Suggested modes of action of tar on mouse tail skin

Epidermal thickening. Since mitotic counts were not made, it is not possible to determine how much mitotic stimulation and epidermal cell hypertrophy contributed to the observed increased epidermal thickness. It was obvious though that all tar fraction treatments caused an increase in both the number and size of the epidermal cells. Stimulation of mitotic rate may have occurred by a direct action of the phenols and/or as a reaction to the peeling initiated by these compounds at higher levels in the epidermis. Loss of keratinized cells by sellotape stripping is a well known potent stimulus of epidermal cell proliferation (Pinkus, 1952; Allenby, Palmer & Weddell, 1966), and the trauma of stripping off cell layers can result in oedema and hypertrophy of the cells (Pinkus, 1970). It is most unlikely that the primary action of the phenols was one of direct mitotic stimulation, since differentiation into the granular layer phase is not favoured in conditions of rapid cell proliferation (cf. in psoriasis) (Jarrett & Spearman, 1964).

Granular layer induction. Previous work with topical administration of granular layer-inducing agents in both animals (Bern *et al.*, 1955) and in man (Fry & McMinn, 1968) suggests, from the speed at which a granular layer reforms, that this is one of the first events in the conversion from a parakeratotic to an orthokeratotic state. Vitamin A injected subcutaneously does not induce granular layers nor increase epidermal thickness (Bern *et al.*, 1955). Similarly, it appears that the phenols initially produced granular layer formation. However, when these acids permeated into a milieu of sensitive highly viable living keratinocytes, they may have constituted an inflammatory stimulus (Lazarus, Hatcher & Levine, 1975). Jarrett & Spearman (1970) proposed this idea in terms of lysosome rupture, which in the uppermost layers of the epidermis would release the enzymes necessary for orthokeratinization to proceed, but in the lower epidermis would stimulate mitosis. This was suggested from the observations that vitamin A could induce granular layers despite a seemingly contradictory increase in epidermal cell turnover.

The extensive peeling often observed may be the result of the phenols causing a too rapid and lethal hydrolysis of epidermal cells by lysosomal hydrolase release; in some cases the whole epidermis was being shed.

CONCLUSIONS

Because an animal model is never identical in all respects to a pathological state in man, findings from the use of such a model to assay drugs for use in a human skin disorder must always be interpreted with caution. Thus, for example, the mouse tail dermis is not in an erythematous state with dilated capillaries as is found in the psoriatic lesion, but the important processes of keratinization are certainly very closely paralleled. Initial screening on an animal model is of paramount value in that it cuts down the number of clinical tests required.

In mouse tail skin experiments, high boiling tar acids appear to be most specific in inducing a granular layer in formerly parakeratotic epidermis, and hence may provide a basis for a more specific approach to therapy in chronic psoriasis. In 1928 Jaffrey reported from clinical findings that the acids in the range 170–300°C were more beneficial; these included both low and high boiling acids. The possible beneficial effects of high boiling tar acids were also suggested by Obermayer & Becker (1935). Hellier & Whitefield (1967) in their work on dithranol suggested that polyhydric phenols may constitute the therapeutic fraction of tar, and that their high volatility causes their inevitable removal in some of the "purification" procedures adopted in the past. This could account for the great loss in efficacy reported from the use of refined tar preparations.

Further work requires screening of individual high boiling tar acids and their synthetic analogues in this animal model, leading to trials of promising compounds in patients suffering with chronic psoriasis. From the above work, it appears that these higher phenols should be incorporated into a vehicle which does not significantly penetrate the epidermis, i.e. the phenols are released only into the parakeratotic horny layer where hydrolytic enzymes can be released so that orthokeratinization can be restored.

REFERENCES

Allenby, C. F., Palmer, E. & Weddell, G. (1966). Changes in dermis of human hairy skin resulting from stripping the keratinized layer off the epidermis. *Z. Zellforsch. mikrosk. Anat.* **69**: 566–572.

Babes, A. & Lazaresco-Pantzu, Mme (1928). [Lesions of the spleen produced in the rabbit by painting with tar]. *C. r. Séanc. Soc. Biol.* **99**: 1077–1079. [In French.]

Belsan, I., Neumann, E. & Blazkova, B. (1965). Kinetics of glycolysis after fluocinolone acetonide in psoriasis. *Acta derm.-venereol.* **45**: 297–301.

Bern, H. A., Elias, J. J., Pickett, P. B., Powers, T. R. & Harkness, M. N. (1955). The influence of Vitamin A on epidermis. *Am. J. Anat.* **96**: 419–441.

Bleiberg, J. (1958). Clinical experience with a new preparation for the treatment of psoriasis. *Ann. N.Y. Acad. Sci.* **73**: 1028–1031.

Burks, J. W. & Montgomery, H. (1943). Histopathologic study of psoriasis. *Arch. Derm. Syph.* **48**: 479–493.

Burry, J. N. (1973). Topical drug addiction: Adverse effects of fluorinated corticosteroid creams and ointments. *Med. J. Aust.* **1**: 393–396.

Carney, R. & Zopf, L. C. (1955). An improved coal tar ointment using a surfactant. *Arch. Derm.* **72**: 266–271.

Champion, R. H. (1966). Treatment of psoriasis. *Br. med. J.* **1966 2**: 993–995.

Clarke, G. H. V. (1962). Skin disease in a developing tropical country. *Br. J. Derm.* **74**: 123–126.

Clyman, S. G. (1957). Comparative effects of hydrocortisone and hydro-cortisone—coal tar extract creams in cases of atopic dermatitis. *Postgrad. Med.* **21**: 309–313.

Combes, F. C. (1947). Coal tar in dermatology. *Arch. Derm. Syph.* **56**: 583–588.

Davidson, J. (1925). On liver necrosis and cirrhosis produced experimentally by coal tar. *J. Path. Bact.* **28**: 621–626.

Downing, J. G. & Bauer, C. W. (1948). Low and high temperature coal tars in the treatment of eczema and psoriasis. *Arch. Derm. Syph.* **57**: 985–990.

Fisher, R. E. W. (1953). Occupational skin cancer in a group of tar workers. *Arch. Ind. Hyg. Occupational Med.* **7**: 12–18.

Freedberg, I. M. (1965). Effects of local therapeutic agents upon epidermal macromolecular metabolism. *J. Invest. Derm.* **45**: 529–538.

Freedman, R. I., Reed, W. B. & Becker, S. W. (1963). Effects of local corticosteroids on psoriasis. *Arch. Derm.* **87**: 701–705.

Fry, L. & McMinn, R. M. H. (1968). The action of chemotherapeutic agents on psoriatic epidermis. *Br. J. Derm.* **80**: 373–383.

Goeckerman, W. H. (1925). The treatment of psoriasis. *N.W. Med., Seattle* **24**: 229–231.

Goodwin, P., Hamilton, S. & Fry, L. (1974). The cell cycle in psoriasis. *Br. J. Derm.* **90**: 517–524.

Grigor'ev, Z. E. (1959). [Toxicity of so-called heavy tar obtained from Cheremkhovo coal.] *Gig. Sanit.* **24**: 33–37. [In Russian.]

Guy, W. H., Jacob, F. M. & Weber, F. (1939). Synthetic tar paste. *Arch. Derm. Syph.* **40**: 90–91.

Halprin, K. M., Fukui, K. & Ohkawara, A. (1969). Flurandrenolone (Cordran) tape and carbohydrate metabolising enzymes. Use in the epidermis of people with psoriasis. *Arch. Derm.* **100**: 336–341.

Hammar, H. (1970). Glyceraldehydephosphate dehydrogenase and glucose-6-dehydrogenase activities in psoriasis and neurodermatitis and the effect of dithranol. *J. Invest. Derm.* **54**: 121–125.

Hellier, F. F. & Whitefield, M. (1967). The treatment of psoriasis with triacetoxyanthracene. *Br. J. Derm.* **79**: 491–496.

Ingram, J. T. (1954). The significance and management of psoriasis. *Br. med. J.* **1954(2)**: 823–828.

Jaffrey, W. R. (1928). A report on the therapeutically active principle fraction of crude coal tar. *Can. med. Ass. J.* **18**: 680–681.

Jarrett, A. (1971). The pentose phosphate pathway in human and animal skin. *Br. J. Derm.* **84**: 545–553.

Jarrett, A. (1973). Normal epidermal keratinization. In *The physiology and pathophysiology of the skin* **1**: 161–212. Jarrett, A. (ed.). London and New York: Academic Press.

Jarrett, A. & Spearman, R. I. C. (1964). *Histochemistry of the skin—psoriasis.* London: English Universities Press.

Jarrett, A. & Spearman, R. I. C. (1970). Vitamin A and the skin. *Br. J. Derm.* **82**: 197–199.

Kerr, G. R. & Plein, E. M. (1953). Coal tar and coal tar ointment. *Drug Standards* **21**: 10–25.

Kidd, C. B. & Meenan, J. C. (1961). A dermatological survey of long-stay mental patients. *Br. J. Derm.* **73**: 129–133.

Kimberling, W. & Dobson, R. L. (1973). The inheritance of psoriasis. *J. Invest. Derm.* **60**: 538–540.

Kinmont, P. D. C. & Jowett, G. H. (1958). Clinical trial. *Arch. Derm.* **77**: 635–641.

Komisaruk, E., Kosek, J. C. & Schuster, D. S. (1962). Histology of psoriasis injected with triamcinolone. *Arch. Derm.* **86**: 422–425.

Lawrence, D. J. & Bern, H. A. (1958). On the specificity of the response of mouse epidermis to Vitamin A. *J. Invest. Derm.* **31**: 313–325.

Lazarus, G. S., Hatcher, V. B. & Levine, N. (1975). Lysosomes and the skin. *J. Invest. Derm.* **65**: 259–271.

Lewis, D. A. & Day, E. H. (1972). Biochemical factors in the action of steroids on diseased joints in rheumatoid arthritis. *Ann. rheum. Dis.* **31**: 374–378.

Lewis, J. H. (1943). *The biology of the negro.* Cambridge: University Press.

Leyden, J. J., Thew, M. & Kligman, A. M. (1974). Steroid Rosacea. *Arch. Derm.* **110**: 619–622.

Lloyd, W. R. & King, J. C. (1959). Development and formulation of coal tar ointments. *Am. Perfum. Aromat.* **73**: 37–40.

Nelson, O. & Osterberg, A. E. (1927). A purified coal tar ointment for the treatment of infantile eczema. *Arch. Derm. Syph.* **15**: 669–671.

Novotny, F. (1966). [The changes in healthy skin of psoriatic persons.] *Cesk. Derm.* **41**: 168–181. [In Czech.]

Obermayer, M. E. & Becker, S. W. (1935). A study of crude coal tar and allied substances. *Arch. Derm. Syph.* **31**: 796–810.

Orris, L. (1966). Treatment of psoriasis with tar-steroid cream under occlusive dressing. *Clin. Med.* **73**: 63–64.

Pardo-Castello, V. (1944). Rational pharmaceutic treatment of diseases of the skin. *Arch. Der. Syph.* **49**: 223.

Paslin, D. A. & Sprague, E. A. (1975). Psoriasis on tumour. *Arch. Derm.* **111**: 622–624.

Perry, H. O., Soderstrom, C. W. & Schulze, R. W. (1968). The Goeckerman treatment of psoriasis. *Arch. Derm.* **98**: 178–182.

Pinkus, H. (1952). Examination of the epidermis by the strip method. II. Biometric data on regeneration of the human epidermis. *J. invest. Derm.* **19**: 431–447.

Pinkus, H. (1970). The direction of growth of human epidermis. *Br. J. Derm.* **83**: 556–564.

Pinkus, H. & Mehregan, A. H. (1966). The primary histologic lesion of seborrheic dermatitis and psoriasis. *J. Invest. Derm.* **46**: 109–116.

Raab, W. & Patermann, F. (1966). Die Wirkung externa antipsoriatica auf die Zellatmung. *Arch. Klin. exp. Derm.* **226**: 144–152.

Ruzicka, J., Novotna-Kasparkova, V. & Burda, V. (1969). Effect of coal tar and yperite ointments on the oxidative metabolism of glucose in psoriatic skin. *Arch. Klin. exp. Derm.* **234**: 175–181.

Samitz, M. H. (1958). Therapeutic approaches in psoriasis. *Ann. N.Y. Acad. Sci.* **73**: 1020–1027.

Simon, C. R. & Brandt, R. (1953). Eczematous hypersensitivity to coal tar. *Arch. Derm. Syph.* **68**: 584–586.

Singer, A. J. (1962). *Allantoin and coal tar extract composition and treatment of psoriasis.* U.S. Patent Office. No. 3,043,745. 10th July 1962.

Spearman, R. I. C. (1964). The evolution of mammalian keratinized structures. *Symp. zool. Soc. Lond.* No. 12: 67–81.

Spearman, R. I. C. (1970). Some light microscopical observations on the stratum corneum of the guinea-pig, man and common seal. *Br. J. Derm.* **83**: 582–590.

Spearman, R. I. C. (1973). *The integument.* Cambridge: University Press.

Spearman, R. I. C. & Garretts, M. (1966). The effects of subcutaneous saline injections on growth and keratinization of mouse tail epidermis. *J. Invest. Derm.* **46**: 245–250.

Spearman, R. I. C. & Hardy, J. A. (1974). Some ultrastructural observations on keratohyalin granules of guinea pig epidermis. *Arch. Derm. Forsch.* **250**: 149–158.

Spearman, R. I. C. & Jarrett, A. (1975). Bio-assay of steroids for topical application. *Br. J. Derm.* **92**: 581–584.

Swanbeck, G. & Lundquist, P. G. (1972). Ultrastructural changes of mitochondria in dithranol-treated psoriatic epidermis. *Acta derm.-venereol.* **52**: 94–98.

Wrench, R. (1973). *The isolation, production and development of dermatologically active constituents in coal tar.* Ph.D. Thesis: Aston University.

Wrench, R. & Britten, A. Z. (1975a). Evaluation of coal tar fractions for use in psoriasiform diseases using the mouse tail test. Part I: High and low temperature tars and their constituents. *Br. J. Derm.* **92**: 569–574.

Wrench, R. & Britten, A. Z. (1975b). Evaluation of coal tar fractions for use in psoriasiform diseases using the mouse tail test. Part II: Tar oil acids. *Br. J. Derm.* **92**: 575–579.

Wrench, R. & Britten, A. Z. (1975c). Evaluation of coal tar fractions for use in psoriasiform diseases using the mouse tail test. Part III: High boiling tar oil acids. *Br. J. Derm.* **93**: 67–74.

Wrench, R. & Britten, A. Z. (1975d). Evaluation of dithranol and a "synthetic tar" as anti-psoriatic treatments using the mouse tail test. *Br. J. Derm.* **93**: 75–78.

Young, E. (1970). The external treatment of psoriasis; a controlled investigation of the effects of coal tar. *Br. J. Derm.* **82**: 510–515.

Young, E. (1972). Ultraviolet therapy of psoriasis: a critical study. *Br. J. Derm.* **87**: 379–382.

Symp. zool. Soc. Lond. (1977) No. 39, 373–404.

SEASONAL CHANGES IN THE SKIN OF MAMMALS

ELIZABETH JOHNSON

Department of Zoology, The University,
Whiteknights, Reading, England

SYNOPSIS

Seasonal changes in the skin of non-domesticated field mammals are described and possible controlling mechanisms discussed, using the field vole (*Microtus agrestis*) and the roe deer (*Capreolus capreolus*) as particular examples.

Changes in insulation are achieved by the cyclic growth and replacement of hair being regulated by the endocrine system in such a way that it is geared to seasonal changes in the environment. In the vole a spring hair replacement produces a sparse pelage with coarse hairs through which air will easily circulate; an autumn replacement produces a dense pelage with fine hairs which trap warm air between them. In the roe deer insulation depends upon air contained within the guard hairs and is not dependent on hair density; winter hairs are a more efficient insulator because they contain more air in the enlarged medullary spaces.

All mammals have sebaceous glands which coat the skin and hair with a waterproof layer. In addition, larger field mammals develop apocrine glands over the general body surface which are important in thermoregulation. The size and activity of both the sebaceous and apocrine sweat glands vary seasonally and in male mammals appear to be dependent on the output of androgens. Specialized regions of skin with enlarged skin glands, such as the caudal gland of the male vole and the forehead gland of the roe buck are also androgen-dependent and fluctuate in size with the testicular cycle. The roe forehead gland metabolizes testosterone with androstenedione as the major product, and the amount of testosterone metabolized varies over the period of the rut.

INTRODUCTION

Mammalian skin is covered by a keratinized epidermis which is much more pliable than that of reptiles and which gives rise to various epidermal derivatives such as hair follicles, sebaceous glands and sweat glands (Fig. 1). Hairs are an exclusively mammalian feature which gave rise to the old name for the class, Pilifera. The current view is that hairs were completely new epidermal derivatives, although their initial trio arrangement suggests that they originally developed in the interscale hinge region of mammal-like reptiles; an arrangement which persists on the tails of rodents (Spearman, 1964).

Primitively hairs may have been primarily tactile and being well supplied with nerves they still serve this function. However, their main function in present day terrestrial mammals is undoubtedly one of insulation, and without such a device for conserving heat, shared with the feathers of birds, it is unlikely that homeothermy

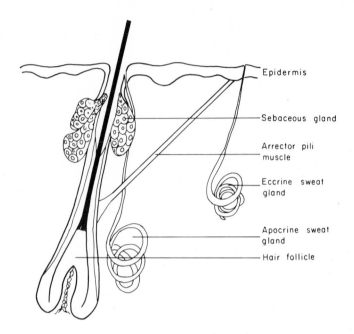

Epidermis

Sebaceous gland

Arrector pili muscle

Eccrine sweat gland

Apocrine sweat gland

Hair follicle

FIG. 1. Generalized diagram of epidermal derivatives in mammalian skin.

could have evolved. The insulative efficiency of the coat may be enhanced by piloerection, although arrector pili muscles are absent in some mammals. For the majority of mammals a seasonally variable insulative layer is required and this seems to have been achieved by hair growth being regulated by the endocrine system in such a way that it is geared to changes in the environment.

For effective insulation it is important that the hair is kept dry and this is achieved by coating the outer surface of the hairs with an oily secretion from the sebaceous glands which accompany every hair follicle group. The size of the sebaceous glands varies seasonally, as does that of the sweat glands. The majority of mammals have apocrine sweat glands associated with hair follicles rather than eccrine sweat glands, which seem to require a relatively naked skin for the efficient dispersal of their watery secretions to be useful in thermoregulation. In a number of mammalian species the sebaceous and apocrine glands in certain regions of the body produce special secretions with particular social functions.

I propose to examine the seasonal changes in these epidermal derivatives in non-domesticated field mammals and to discuss the possible controlling mechanisms. I shall use as particular examples the field vole (*Microtus agrestis*) and the roe deer (*Capreolus capreolus*) which we have studied both in the field and in the laboratory.

SEASONAL ADAPTIVE COAT CHANGES

Although mammals can tolerate only a narrow range of body temperatures, they occupy a wide and fluctuating range of environmental temperatures. Well adapted arctic mammals maintain their body temperature in winter not by metabolic adjustment but by insulation; for example the arctic fox (*Alopex*) is able to withstand a temperature of −50°C without altering its metabolism (Scholander, Hock, Walters, & Irving, 1950). The arctic summer may have temperatures some 80°C different from those of winter so that seasonal adjustment in insulation is important. Thus one finds, for example, that the summer fur of the arctic black bear (*Euarctos*) provides 52% less insulation than the winter fur. Other examples are shown in Table I. Similar changes in insulation occur in temperate mammals in the field. By a similar method to that of Hart, using cured pelts as insulators and measuring the power input required to maintain a hotplate at body temperature, it was shown that the insulating property of roe deer fur in winter was 2·5 times greater than the summer fur (Table II).

The low thermal conductivity and hence the insulating power of animal fur is dependent upon the amount of air trapped within the coat and is correlated with fur depth. In the majority of mammals the coat is made up of coarse guard hairs or overhairs

TABLE I

Seasonal changes in insulation of the pelage

	Insulation °C/cal/m²/h		
	Summer	Winter	% Change in insulation
Black bear	0·583	1·21	52
Polar bear	0·655	0·965	32
Wolf	0·612	1·05	41
Red fox	0·631	0·944	33
Deermouse	0·180	0·229	21
Muskrat	0·534	0·606	12

Data from Hart (1956).

TABLE II

Power input required to maintain a hotplate at thermal equilibrium
at 39–40°C in a cold room at 11°C with a wind speed of 1·8 m/sec

	Power input joules sec^{-1}
Winter pelt in position	1·25
Summer pelt in position	3·13
Winter skin with fur removed	7·8
Summer skin with fur removed	7·8

Data from Johnson & Hornby (1975).

and an undercoat of fine hairs or wool. In such a coat the insulation depends upon the density of fine hairs which trap warm air between them. The arctic muskrat which spends much of the time each day swimming in water at near freezing temperatures has a dense non-wettable fur which holds a large volume of air. If this air is removed by wetting the fur with lauryl sulphate the animals are unable to maintain their body temperature when immersed in water at 2°C (Johansen, 1962).

In a small rodent such as the vole (*Microtus agrestis*) the number of hairs per unit area is greater in winter than in summer (Khateeb & Johnson, 1971a) (Figs 2 and 3) and this is largely due to an increase in the number of fine hairs (Figs 4 and 5). The summer hairs are also coarser than winter hairs. In summer air will easily circulate into the sparse coat with coarse hairs. In winter the dense coat with fine hairs will act as a good insulator. A similar seasonal change has been described for a variety of other mammals, such as deer mice (*Peromyscus*; Sealander, 1951), shrews (*Sorex*; Borowski, 1958), field mice (*Apodemus*; Haitlinger, 1968) and mink (*Mustela vison*; Stevenson, 1962) as well as larger species such as moorland ponies (Speed, 1960) and Scottish wild goats (Ryder, 1970) in which underfur is completely lacking in summer.

The Southern elephant seal (*Mirounga leonina*) lacks underfur and this may be regarded as an aquatic adaptation which requires streamlining of the body. There is also an absence of arrector pili muscles so that the hairs lie completely flat when the seal enters the water (Ling, 1970). In the completely aquatic Cetacea insulation is provided by a thick layer of subcutaneous blubber instead of fur. Reduction or complete absence of hair follicles together with the presence of abundant apocrine glands is a feature of the tropical

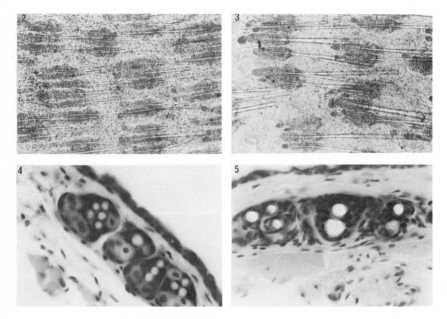

FIG. 2. Whole mount of dorsal skin of the vole (*Microtus agrestis*) with resting follicles in winter (×54).
FIG. 3. Whole mount of dorsal skin of the vole with resting follicles in summer (×54).
FIG. 4. Transverse section of dorsal vole skin in winter. Hair follicle group has a central overhair and a number of fine hairs (×330).
FIG. 5. Transverse section of dorsal vole skin in summer. The hairs are coarser than in winter and there are fewer fine hairs (×330).
From Khateeb & Johnson, 1971a.

Rhinocerotidae (Cave, 1969). In these species the skin is adapted for losing heat in a tropical environment and this is supplemented by wallowing in mud or water. On the other hand, in a desert mammal such as the camel the insulative woolly coat serves to prevent heat gain from the environment (Schmidt-Nielsen, Schmidt-Nielsen, Jarnum & Houpt, 1957).

In some mammals, notably the Cervidae, insulation depends on air contained within the enlarged medullary spaces of the guard hairs. It is suggested that such hairs provide both insulation and buoyancy in the seasonal migrations of reindeer across lakes and rivers (Flerov, 1952). In the roe deer (*Capreolus capreolus*) the winter guard hairs (Fig. 6) are twice the width of the summer guard hairs (Fig. 8) because of the larger medullary air spaces within the winter hairs (Figs 7 and 9). Although there is no difference in number of hairs per unit area of skin the pelt depth in winter is

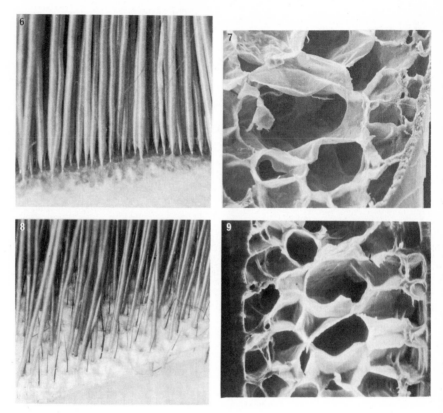

FIG. 6. Winter pelt of roe deer (*Capreolus capreolus*) in February (×6).
FIG. 7. Scanning EM of cross-section of winter hair (×306).
FIG. 8. Summer pelt of roe deer in June (×6).
FIG. 9. Scanning EM of cross-section of summer hair (×306).
From Johnson & Hornby, 1975.

twice that of summer because the wider winter hairs are piled up (Fig. 10) whereas the narrow summer hairs lie flat (Fig. 11).

Thus, insulation in deer again depends upon air trapped within the coat but is unusual in that the air is trapped within the guard hairs rather than between the fine hairs. In the roe deer the extremely fine non-medullated underhairs probably play only a minor role in insulation except at the time of the moult, which is the only time that fine hairs are present in large numbers.

The most obvious seasonal changes of coat involve a change in colour. There is no doubt that coat colour has a role in concealment and camouflage (Cott, 1940), but it may also have a role in thermoregulation. For example, the resumption of a dappled summer

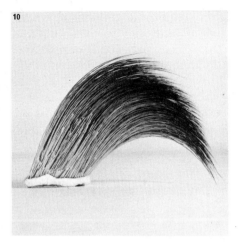
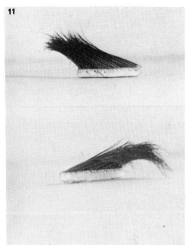

FIG. 10. Piece of winter dorsal skin of a roe deer (*Capreolus capreolus*) (×0·75).
FIG. 11. Piece of summer dorsal skin of a roe deer photographed from left and right (×0·75).
From Johnson & Hornby, 1975.

coat by the European fallow deer (*Dama dama*) provides effective camouflage amongst the trees in summer. However, the resumption of a bright russet glossy summer coat by the roe deer is certainly no aid to concealment—but it may aid the reflection of sunlight from the body, as seems to occur in some tropical breeds of cattle with similarly coloured coats (Bonsma & Pretorius, 1943). A change from a brown or grey summer coat to a white winter coat occurs in many arctic and northern species. Because the change to winter whiteness is linked to the presence of snow so that the mountain hare (*Lepus timidus*) has a complete change to winter whiteness in northern Scandinavia, but seldom changes to white in Ireland, it seems likely that one adaptive function of the change is camouflage. However, it has also been suggested that a white winter coat is an aid to thermoregulation by reducing the radiation of heat (Severaid, 1945).

Seasonal activity of the hair follicle

Changes in the character of the coat such as hair density and hair length or thickness are possible because growth and replacement of hair is a cyclic phenomenon which for mammals in the wild is geared to seasonal changes in the environment.

Primary hair follicles develop as epidermal inpushings which grow downwards through the dermis and enclose mesenchymal cells to form a dermal papilla at their base. Sebaceous glands and apocrine sweat glands, if present, arise as outgrowths from the developing hair follicle. From the mitotically active base thus formed a growing hair is established which emerges at the skin surface and grows to a definitive length. Mitoses then cease and the growing hair is transformed to a resting club hair. The first formed follicles are usually arranged in groups of three with later formed

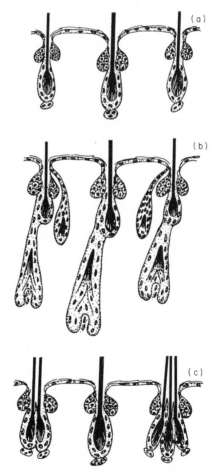

FIG. 12. Growth of the juvenile coat in the vole (*Microtus agrestis*): (a) trio group of follicles, (b) growth of secondary follicles as branches, (c) adult complement of hair follicles established. (From Khateeb & Johnson, 1971a.)

follicles arising in the vicinity of these trio groups. The central first formed follicles of the trio group produce a coarse guard hair whilst the later formed lateral follicles may produce coarse hairs or fine hairs. The birth coat of many mammals including the vole is a sparse coat consisting of groups of trio follicles with single or paired follicles arranged between the trio groups. In the majority of field mammals the birth coat is replaced by a second or juvenile coat in which secondary follicles develop as branches from the primary follicles to establish the adult complement of hair follicles (Fig. 12). Many young field mammals are unable to regulate their body temperature until this second coat is achieved. The secondary follicles which arise by branching always produce fine hair and in domestic sheep which are bred for wool production these are the most important component of the coat.

Subsequently, the hair follicles continue to have periods of activity when new hairs are produced and periods of rest when the hairs are moulted or retained. At the start of the hair cycle (Fig. 13) cells at the base of the resting follicle become mitotically active and extend downwards to enclose the dermal papilla (a). From the

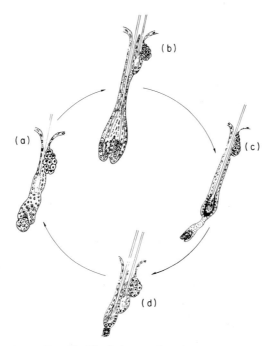

Fig. 13. The hair growth cycle.

active bulb thus formed cells divide, move upwards and become keratinized to form the growing hair (b) which emerges alongside the resting hair. At the end of this growing stage or *anagen* mitoses cease, and the growing hair is transformed to a "club" hair with a characteristic brush-like end formed of incompletely keratinized cells (c). During this intermediate or *catagen* stage the follicle migrates upwards through the skin leaving behind an epithelial strand of cells which subsequently shortens and exposes the dermal papilla (d). During the resting or *telogen* stage thereby achieved the resting hair is firmly anchored in the follicle and for fur bearers the pelt is diagnosed as "prime". Whilst the new hair is growing, or at subsequent stages, the old resting hair may be moulted or it may be retained in the follicle and so increase the density of the coat.

Variations in the hair cycle may occur in the initiation of activity, thus determining when the hairs grow and how many hairs grow; in the amount of hair produced by each active follicle and in the loss or retention of club hairs. In the vole fewer of the follicles which produce fine hairs become active at the spring moult than at the autumn moult (Figs 14 and 15). The growing follicles produce thicker guard hairs during the spring growing period and more club hairs are lost at the spring moult than at the autumn moult. The summer coat thus has fewer fine hairs and coarser guard hairs than the winter coat.

Very little is known about the changes occurring in follicles which produce hairs with a seasonal colour change (Billingham & Silvers, 1960). Follicles which produce pigmented hairs have melanocytes in the active matrix which supply pigment granules to the dividing cells contributing to the growing hair. It is only during anagen that it is possible to detect dopa and tyrosine oxidase activity in the hair follicle and the fate of melanocytes during telogen remains unresolved. What happens to the melanocytes in a seasonal change from pigmented to white hairs is not known. The melanocytes might migrate from the follicle or they might stop synthesizing melanin.

The majority of field mammals achieve their seasonal change of coat in a similar way to the vole by having two moults a year, in spring and autumn. A smaller number of mammals investigated achieve a change in coat by having only one moult a year. For example the wild ass (Mazak, 1962), the moorland pony (Speed, 1960) and the silver fox (Bassett & Llewellyn, 1948) shed the heavy winter coat in spring whilst new hairs are short and still growing, and these new hairs continue to grow throughout the summer

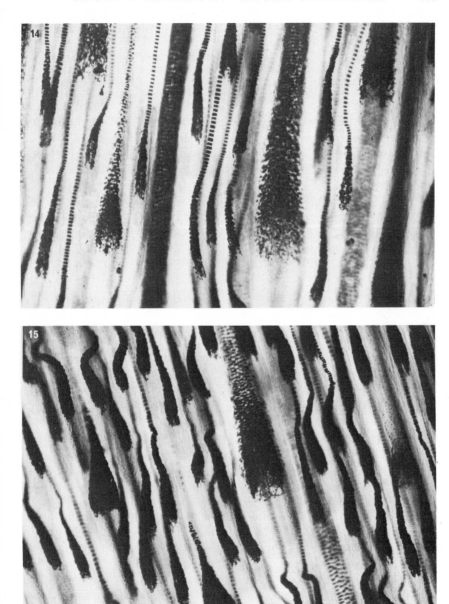

FIG. 14. Whole mount of dorsal skin of the vole (*Microtus agrestis*) with active follicles in spring (×107).

FIG. 15. Whole mount of dorsal skin of the vole with active follicles in autumn (×107). From Khateeb & Johnson, 1971a.

together with further generations of new hairs so that a prime thick coat is achieved by winter.

The majority of field mammals replace their coat in a wave-like pattern, either starting on the belly and spreading over the flanks to the back or starting on the head and spreading from the back to the belly. Such a pattern of replacement will avoid any abrupt change in insulation. In old mammals hair replacement may become diffuse as described for the meadow mouse (*Microtus californicus*; Ecke & Kinney, 1956), the muskrat (*Ondatra*; Shanks, 1948) as well as for the vole (*Microtus agrestis*). The diffuse hair replacement which occurs at the second autumn moult of the vole results in an incomplete change from summer to winter coat, which may be one of the reasons why voles usually do not survive a second winter in the field, although they may have a much longer life span in captivity.

Environmental factors influencing the pelage changes

Although fewer studies have been made on the effects of environmental factors on hair growth in wild species of mammals compared with domesticated species such as sheep and cattle, there is evidence that daylength, temperature and nutrition do affect the moult progression and type of pelage produced.

Light

Bissonnette (1935) was the first to show that the timing of the hair cycle and the sexual cycle in ferrets was related to daylength. These studies and further studies by Harvey & MacFarlane (1958) have shown that with increasing daylength female ferrets come into oestrus and grow a sparse, coarse summer coat. On the other hand decreasing daylength leads to the assumption of a dense winter coat together with the onset of anoestrus. Experimental alteration of the daylength results in the growth of a summer coat and active gonads when ferrets are maintained on long days in winter and the growth of a winter coat and anoestrus on short days in summer. Similarly, voles kept on long days in autumn did not regress sexually and grew a summer-type coat with low density of hairs and coarse guard hairs, whereas short days in summer advanced the onset of anoestrus and the growth of a dense, fine winter coat (Khateeb & Johnson, 1971b). Artificial shortening of the daylength similarly advanced the autumn moult of the mink (Bassett & Llewellyn, 1949), whereas extended daylength through the spring and summer encouraged the single annual moult of the silver fox to proceed faster (Bassett, Pearson & Wilkie, 1944). Extending the hours of daylight during winter caused the varying hare (*Lepus americanus*) to remain brown, whereas short days in summer induced a change to winter whiteness (Lyman, 1943). The white-tailed buck (*Odocoileus virginianus*) responded to extended day-length during winter over a three-year period by an earlier rut and an advancement of the spring and autumn moult (French, McEwen, Magruder, Rader, Long & Swift, 1960).

Temperature

Although light appears to be the principal factor affecting seasonal changes of pelage there is evidence that temperature has a modifying role. When weasels (*Mustela*) were kept on long days in winter at warm or cold temperatures all the animals changed from a white to a brown coat. However, the change to brown pelage proceeded more slowly in the cold because of a delay in shedding of the white hair (Rust, 1962). It is generally agreed that the colour change of the Scottish mountain hare (*Lepus timidus scoticus*) is initiated by changes of daylength, but the rate of progression of the moult either to white in winter or to brown in summer appears to depend upon the temperature (Hewson, 1958; Watson, 1963; Flux, 1970; Jackes & Watson, 1975). The deermouse (*Peromyscus*) showed an increase in pelage density when kept at low temperatures in the summer and a decrease in density at high temperatures in winter (Sealander, 1951). It has also been suggested that the increased density and finer hair of three species of chinchilla (*Chinchilla*) living at increasingly higher altitudes in the Andes may be related to the temperature differences at different heights (Seele, 1968).

Nutrition

The rate of mitoses in the growing hair follicle is one of the highest in the mammalian body, with a consequent high metabolic requirement for the growing follicle. It is not surprising, therefore, that hair growth should be affected by nutrition. Subjecting mink to a low protein diet whilst the juvenile coat was developing resulted in a marked reduction in the number of secondary follicles formed compared with mink fed a high protein diet (Dolnick, Warner & Bassett, 1960). An exactly similar respose to adverse nutrition occurs in the fleece of sheep (Short, 1955). Voles born and reared under long or short days and two planes of nutrition completed their juvenile moults earlier on long days than short days and the well fed groups moulted earlier than the low fed groups (Pinter, 1968).

It seems likely that the seasonal changes in light, temperature and available food act together to influence the seasonal changes of pelage.

Control of the seasonal pelage changes

Since it is well established that the environmental factors which influence hair growth also influence seasonal breeding, it is not surprising that there is a correlation between the moulting cycles and the sexual cycles of many mammals. Seasonal changes in endocrine glands other than the gonads are less well documented.

In the vole there is evidence that the pituitary, thyroid and adrenal cortex as well as the gonads are more actively secreting hormones in spring and summer than during autumn and winter (Khateeb & Johnson, 1971a). The increase in hormone output by the pituitary relates to the sexual maturation of the gonads (Clarke & Forsyth, 1964) and the seasonal variation in thyroid activity is supported by other studies on *Microtus agrestis* (Forsyth, 1962) and *Microtus arvalis* (Delost, 1951). The adrenal cortex of the shrew (*Sorex araneus*) has also been shown to vary seasonally (Siuda, 1964).

Seasonal changes in the endocrine glands of mammals in the wild cannot be inferred from the changes induced in laboratory animals subjected to changes of temperature. Field mammals do not respond to cold by an increase in thyroid activity such as occurs in laboratory rats (Rand, Riggs & Talbot, 1952) and guinea-pigs (Stevens, D'Angelo, Paschkis, Cantarrow & Sunderman, 1955). It seems likely that in the laboratory experiments the animals were provided with unlimited food; in the wild it is obviously more efficient for a mammal to adapt to cold by changing its insulation rather than by increasing its metabolism when food is scarce.

In the field vole (*M. agrestis*) the spring moult occurs when the pituitary, gonads, thyroid and adrenal cortex are actively secreting hormones, whereas the autumn moult coincides with regression of these endocrine glands. It seemed likely, therefore, that the pelage changes are mediated through the endocrine system rather than directly controlled by environmental factors. An attempt has been made to separate the effects of the various hormones (Khateeb & Johnson, 1971c).

Castration of male voles before the onset of the spring pelage change resulted in a more rapid change of coat and the density of hairs in the new coat was high, similar to that of winter field voles. However, the guard hairs grown were coarse as in the normal spring replacement. Castration in August advanced the onset of the autumn hair replacement and the voles grew a coat with high density of hairs whether they were kept on long or short days. However, castrated voles kept on long days in autumn produced coarse guard hairs of the summer type, whereas castrates on short days produced hairs of fine winter type. It may therefore be suggested that male sex hormone inhibits the growth of hairs since its removal allowed more hairs to grow, but the amount of hair produced during the growing stage must depend upon some other factor which is stimulated by light. Thyroid hormone appears to be involved since treatment of castrates with thyroxine whilst keeping them on short days produced an autumn coat of winter type density but with guard hairs of coarse, summer type. The spring hair replacement was completely inhibited in voles which had the thyroid gland inhibited with propyl thiouracil, although a single vole which survived until September did replace its coat in autumn. Stimulation of the adrenals with ACTH completely inhibited the autumn hair replacement. Treatment with ACTH for one month after the winter coat had grown resulted in a pelage with low summer-type density which suggests that adrenal hormones encourage the loss of club hairs. Thus, the seasonal moult in the vole appears to be influenced in the following way. In spring, thyroid hormone initiates follicular activity but the increased output of sex hormones inhibits the follicles so that fewer hairs grow. Increased secretion of thyroid hormone results in the production of coarse hairs and increased secretion of adrenal cortical hormones encourages loss of club hairs. In spring, therefore, the voles grow a sparse pelage with coarse hair. In autumn the reduced output of sex hormones allows more hairs to grow, whilst lowered amounts of adrenal cortical hormones allow retention of club hairs. The hairs produced are finer because thyroid secretion is low. In autumn, therefore, the voles grow a dense pelage with fine hairs.

Reineke, Travis & Dolnick (1962) similarly found that the thyroid gland was essential for the growth of the spring pelage in the mink (*Mustela vison*) and the stimulating effect of thyroid hormone on the amount of wool grown in sheep is well known (Labban, 1957).

Lyman (1943) was the first to demonstrate that the pituitary gland was involved in seasonal colour change. He was able to induce the varying hare to change from its white winter coat to a brown summer coat by feeding whole sheep pituitaries. Lyman concluded that gonadotropic hormones were responsible but it is now known that pituitary melanocyte-stimulating hormone (MSH) is responsible for the colour change although not for stimulating the hair replacement. Thus hypophysectomized weasels grew a white coat regardless of the photoperiod, whereas hypophysectomized animals treated with MSH grew brown hair from follicles stimulated to grow by plucking, even though a spontaneous pelage change did not occur (Rust, 1965). After injection of α-MSH laboratory agouti mice will grow black hairs from follicles stimulated by plucking. The black hairs result from an increased deposition of melanin in the hair follicle with the loss of the yellow terminal band (Geschwind, 1966).

One may conclude that the seasonal changes of coat are adjusted to environmental changes by way of the endocrine system. The moult cycle appears to be linked with cycles of activity in the gonads, adrenals and thyroid glands as well as being influenced by a changing output of MSH in animals with a seasonal colour change. Adjustments to the environment presumably occur by way of the hypothalamus and adenohypophysis in the same way that control of the sexual cycles is mediated (Donovan & Harris, 1954).

There is increasing evidence that the pineal gland mediates information about light received by a nervous route into an endocrine output of melatonin (Axelrod, 1970). The output of melatonin depends upon the activity of a pineal enzyme, hydroxyindole-O-methyl transferase (HIOMT) which converts the stored amine, serotonin (5HT) to melatonin. Melatonin has an inhibitory effect on the gonads, probably by inhibition of the hypothalamus (Martini, Carraro, Caviezal & Fochi, 1968). The pineal enzyme activity is inhibited by light and consequently less melatonin is produced thereby allowing seasonal gonad enlargement.

Implantation of melatonin into male weasels in the spring caused them to become reproductively quiescent and to grow a white coat (Rust & Meyer, 1969), whereas control animals developed large testes and grew a brown coat. This provides further support for the control of the seasonal pelage cycle being mediated via the endocrine system.

As a result of natural selection the environmental cycle will be linked with both the endocrine cycle and the moult cycle. On the other hand, domestication tends to disengage the cycles. Thus, in animals such as laboratory rodents there are no seasonal changes in the endocrine glands and no seasonal moult, but hair growth is still influenced by hormones (Mohn, 1958; Johnson, 1958 a,b; Davis, 1963). Even in humans there are seasonal differences in hair growth (Table III) and the post-partum hair loss which occurs in women (Lynfield, 1960) may indicate a former synchrony of the hair cycle and the sexual cycle; in other mammals a similar post-partum loss of hair is used in nest building.

TABLE III

Seasonal differences in the amount of hair grown in normal human males
$(mg/10 \; cm^2/week)$

Forearm		Thigh	
Winter	Summer	Winter	Summer
0·15	0·58	0·11	0·28
0·20	0·59	0·13	0·31
0·30	0·66	0·12	0·35

Data from Casey, Burger, Kent, Kellie, Moxham, Nabarro & Nabarro (1966).

STRUCTURE AND FUNCTION OF SKIN GLANDS

Skin glands of the general body surface

Sebaceous glands

Over the general body surface sebaceous glands develop in association with hair follicles. The secretion is holocrine, thus maintenance of a particular gland size depends upon cell replacement. The secretion, which is mainly lipid, passes into the hair canal and flows out to coat the hair and the skin surface with a waterproof layer. The lipid layer is important in waterproofing the hair and in aquatic forms such as seals, which show a progressive loss of hair, the sebaceous secretion becomes more important in waterproofing the skin (Ling, 1965). The sebaceous secretion of seals has a different composition to that of terrestrial mammals, lacking the water-soluble cholesterol and containing a greater proportion of wax esters (Ling, 1968).

Sweat glands

It seems reasonable to suggest that the eccrine and apocrine sweat glands are basically thermoregulatory in function. Cooling by evaporative sweating requires the loss of quantities of water which small mammals cannot afford and sweat glands are usually not developed over the general body surface of small mammals. Such small mammals rely on evaporative cooling by panting, or by licking the fur with subsequent evaporation of the saliva, and many small mammals find it necessary to stay out of the hot sun.

Eccrine sweat glands develop directly from the epidermis. They are found all over the general body surface in primates and are most numerous in man. In non-primates eccrine sweat glands are found only on the hairless foot pads and in specialized regions such as the rabbit's muzzle and the pig's snout (Weiner & Hellman, 1960). Eccrine sweat consists of a hypotonic salt solution containing 200–400 mg% sodium chloride, which seems to require a relatively naked skin for its effective evaporation. The secretion is truly merocrine, involving no cell breakdown in its release.

Apocrine sweat glands develop from the epithelium of the hair follicle and open by a straight duct into the hair canal usually just above the sebaceous gland (Fig. 1). The classical description of apocrine secretion was that it was mid-way between holocrine and merocrine in that the free edge of the cell ruptured to release the secretion but was then able to repair. The fine details of apocrine secretion are still not fully worked out; it involves the discharge of large secretory blebs via microvilli and in the process of active secretion cell integrity is lost and cell renewal occurs. The evidence on the composition of apocrine sweat is incomplete; it is probably highly variable as the secretion may vary from sparse and oily to profuse and watery.

The temperature regulating function of apocrine glands has not always been accepted. Weiner & Hellman (1960) quote Schumacher saying in 1935 that "neither the hare, the fox nor the deer sweat when chased for hours by the dog, nor does the dog who chases them". We now know that this is not true. For example, the dog does have functional sweat glands present all over the body surface (Aoki & Wadia, 1951) and there is good evidence for evaporative cooling by sweating in sheep (Lee, 1950; Riek, Hardy, Lee & Carter, 1950), the horse (Lovatt Evans & Smith, 1956), the donkey (Maloiy, 1971), the camel (Schmidt-Nielsen et al., 1957) and cattle (Ferguson & Dowling, 1955). The latter authors have shown that the number of sweat glands varies from $600/cm^2$ in shorthorn cattle to $1600/cm^2$ in zebu cattle and suggest that this is linked with the greater ability of zebu to regulate their body temperature in hot conditions. Adolph & Dill (1938) were probably the first authors to record the heat tolerance of the desert donkey as being due to its sweat output and as Schmidt-Nielsen (1975) has pointed out, in hot conditions the fur will not impede the evaporation of sweat. In true seals in which thermoregulation is achieved by an insulating layer of blubber sweat glands are insignificant (Ling, 1965).

Specialized regions of skin glands

The majority of mammals studied have skin glands in particular regions of the body which are larger than those of the general body surface and which produce special odoriferous secretions important in intraspecific communication. In small mammals the scent is usually produced by modified sebaceous glands. In larger mammals apocrine glands form an important component of scent-producing regions and many authors regard scent production as the main function of apocrine glands.

The preputial glands of rodents are composed of specialized sebaceous glands whose secretions may be important as a sex attractant (Bronson & Caroom, 1971) as well as eliciting aggression between males (Mugford & Nowell, 1971). Many rodents have other specialized areas of skin with enlarged sebaceous glands, producing secretions which may be important in recognition, sex attraction and other unidentified functions. Examples of such regions are the caudal, rump or flank glands of microtine rodents (Quay, 1968), the supracaudal gland of the guinea-pig (*Cavia*; Martan, 1962), the ventral gland of the gerbil (*Meriones unguiculatus*; Mitchell, 1965; Glenn & Gray, 1965), and the flank gland of the hamster (*Cricetus*; Montagna & Hamilton, 1949). The glands at the angle of the jaw in a number of microtine rodents are unusual in containing apocrine sweat glands, which are otherwise restricted to the foot pads (Quay, 1962). Another small mammal with apocrine tubules as a component of its scent glands is the shrew (*Sorex*; Eadie, 1938; Pearson, 1946; Dryden & Conaway, 1967). It is suggested that the apocrine glands in the head region produce a highly volatile scent which is trapped by the sebaceous secretions of the large side glands as these are rubbed over objects. The odour may be partly protective in function as it is repulsive to certain carnivores.

Enlarged apocrine glands form the chin glands in the rabbit (*Oryctolagus*; Lyne, Molyneux, Mykytowycz & Parakkal, 1964), which are used for marking territory. The majority of scent-producing skin glands of larger mammals comprise a mixture of enlarged apocrine and sebaceous glands, both of which contribute to the secretion. Examples are the anal glands of many species, extracts from which are used in the perfume industry (Kingston,

1964), the inguinal glands of rabbits (Mykytowycz & Goodrich, 1974) and the forehead, tarsal and interdigital glands of deer (Quay & Müller-Schwarze, 1970).

SEASONAL CHANGES IN SKIN GLANDS

In the field vole, the sebaceous glands over the general body surface are larger in summer than in winter. In addition, the coat appears greasier during the summer months, so that hairs tend to mat together. A rough measure of sebum secretion was obtained by shaving the fur from the whole body of groups of male and female voles in summer (July) and winter (November) and weighing the sample before and after removal of the fat with acetone. More fat was removed from the hair of males than females and approximately ten times as much fat was removed from the hair of either sex in summer than in winter (Khateeb & Johnson, unpublished observations).

The difference in sebum secretion between males and females can be partly accounted for by the enormous development during the summer breeding season of male voles, of sebaceous glands in an area encircling the anus and extending anterior dorsal to the tail: the caudal gland (Figs 16 and 17). In the winter non-breeding season the sebaceous glands of this region are only slightly larger than those of the general body skin.

In the roe deer the sebaceous glands and the apocrine glands of the general body surface are larger in summer than in winter (Figs 18 and 19). The increased sebaceous secretion during the summer months is presumably responsible for the extreme glossiness of the summer coat compared with the dull winter coat. Such a glossy summer coat may benefit the roe deer in the same way as it does glossy coated cattle, which have been shown to reflect more heat from their glossy surface and thereby suffer less in hot conditions when their body temperature pulse rate and respiration rate is compared with dull-coated cattle (Bonsma & Pretorius, 1943). If, as seems likely, apocrine secretion in roe deer does have a thermoregulatory role, the seasonal changes in size of these glands could also be of adaptive significance.

The roe deer has several specialized skin regions with enlarged sebaceous and apocrine glands, which also undergo seasonal changes. One such region is a triangular area on the forehead of the roe buck with its base between the antlers and its apex between the eyes: the forehead gland. Seasonal changes in this region were first outlined by Schumacher (1936).

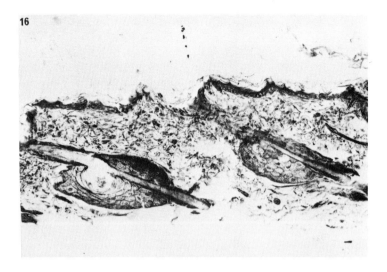

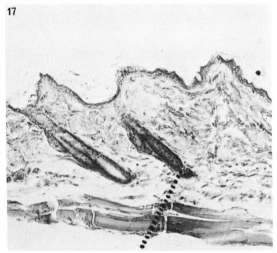

FIG. 16. Sagittal section of caudal gland region of vole (*Microtus agrestis*) skin in summer with enlarged sebaceous glands (×160).

FIG. 17. Sagittal section of dorsal body skin of vole in summer with much smaller sebaceous glands (×160).

Our observations (Adams & Johnson, in prep.) show that in January the sebaceous and apocrine glands of this region are only slightly larger than winter glands of the general body skin (Fig. 20). By May the glands of this region have enlarged considerably and remain large throughout the summer. Figure 21 shows a section of skin from this region in June, in which the sebaceous glands are large and actively secreting sebum and the apocrine gland area is much increased. Apocrine gland activity as judged by epithelial cell height is also much increased. Secretion from these tubules is much greater than from the glands of the general body skin and leads to the eventual loss of whole cells together with phagocytic invasion of the tubule at around August (Fig. 22). The cell debris passes out of the tubule with the final copious secretion and the tubules then regress to the winter size.

The increase in size of the forehead gland exactly parallels the increase in size of the testes and the regression of the glands occurs at the same time as regression of the testes (Fig. 23).

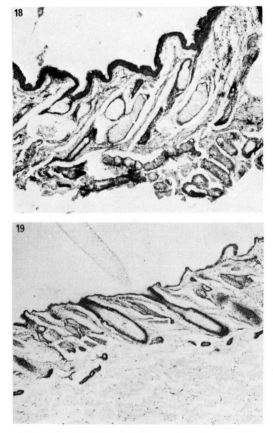

FIG. 18. Sagittal section of dorsal body skin of a roe buck (*Capreolus capreolus*) in summer. The sebaceous glands and apocrine sweat glands are large (×40).

FIG. 19. Sagittal section of dorsal body skin of a roe buck in winter. The sebaceous glands and apocrine sweat glands are reduced in size (×40).

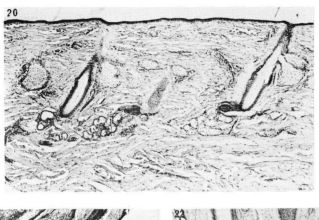

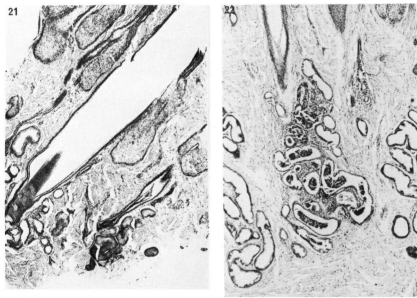

FIG. 20. Sagittal section of forehead skin of a roe buck (*Capreolus capreolus*) in January (×40). (Photograph by Martin Adams.)

FIG. 21. Sagittal section of forehead skin of a roe buck in June. Most of the hair follicle has been removed by plucking (×40). (From Johnson & Leask, in prep.)

FIG. 22. Sagittal section of forehead skin in August. The lower portion of the apocrine tubule contains phagocytes and cell debris (×40). (Photograph by Martin Adams).

The secretions from the forehead gland are used for marking the territory and this activity increases in intensity towards the rut. At the time of the rut (mid July to mid August in southern England), a copious red secretion is produced which has a rancid type of odour detectable by humans. The peaks obtained when the

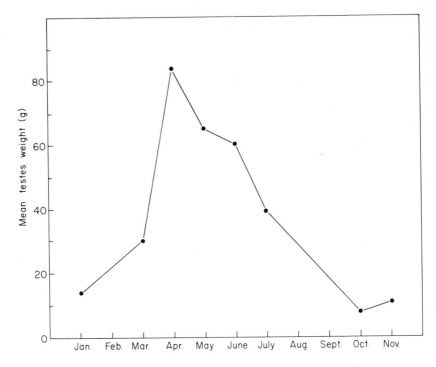

FIG. 23. Seasonal changes in weight of the testes in roe bucks (*Capreolus capreolus*).

forehead secretion is separated on a gas chromatogram are different from those produced by the secretions of the general body skin.
They also vary over the period of the rut, indicating that different
compounds are being synthesized at this time, although the components have not, as yet, been identified (Adams & Johnson,
unpublished observations). Observations by foresters suggest that
the fraying of trees, which causes considerable economic damage,
may occur at sites where one roe buck meets the odour of another.
Of the identified chemicals used as mammalian pheromones, many
have macrocyclic ketones as the active component (Kingston,
1964). In the black-tailed deer (*Odocoileus hemionus columbrans*) the
active component of the scent from the tarsal gland is an unsatu-
rated γ-lactone (Brownlee, Silverstein, Müller-Schwarze & Singer,
1969). The structurally similar musk odoured sterols such as 5α-
androst-16-en-3-one produced by the boar testis can be synthesized from progesterone (Katkov & Gower, 1968) and this raises
the possibility of hormone metabolism and scent production being
interrelated.

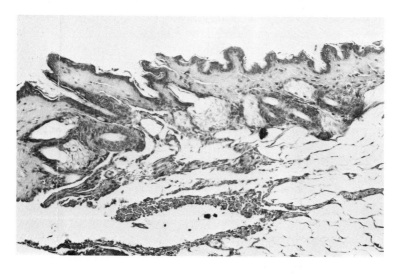

FIG. 24. Sagittal section of caudal gland region of a castrated male vole (*Microtus agrestis*) in summer (compare with Figs 16 and 17) (×160).

Control of the seasonal changes in skin glands

The fact that the skin glands of the male vole and the roe buck enlarge during the breeding season and regress during the non-breeding season suggests that they are androgen dependent. The androgen dependence of the sebaceous glands in man and laboratory rodents is well established (Strauss & Ebling, 1970). Similar experimental evidence for reduction in size of sebaceous glands after castration and hypertrophy after treatment with testosterone has been obtained for the flank gland of hamsters (Hamilton & Montagna, 1950) the supracaudal gland of the guinea-pig (Martan, 1962), the ventral gland of the gerbil (Mitchell, 1965; Glenn & Gray, 1965; Thiessen, Friend & Lindzey, 1968), and the side glands of the shrew (Dryden & Conaway, 1967). Castration of male voles during the breeding season reduced the size of the sebaceous glands in the caudal gland (Fig. 24), although they remained larger than winter glands suggesting that hormones other than testosterone are involved in their control. Laboratory-bred male voles maintained in constant conditions develop much larger sebaceous glands in the caudal region than field voles and there is no seasonal variation (Clarke & Frearson, 1972). These authors suggest that it is the high and constant androgen level in these laboratory-maintained voles which is responsible for the large and constant size of the specialized sebaceous glands. The glands of this laboratory stock are similarly reduced by castration and restored with testosterone. The side glands of the shrew, which are predominantly sebaceous, are stimulated by progesterone (Dryden & Conaway, 1967) and the ventral gland of the gerbil is stimulated by both progesterone and oestrogen (Glenn & Gray, 1965). The effect of progesterone on the unspecialized sebaceous glands of laboratory rats is controversial. Lorincz & Lancaster (1957) claim that progresterone stimulates sebaceous glands in the presence of a sebotropic factor from the pituitary, whereas Ebling (1961) found that progesterone had no effect. It is generally agreed that progesterone does stimulate the specialized preputial glands of laboratory rodents. The stimulation of the gerbil ventral gland with oestrogen is surprising since there is general agreement that oestrogens cause atrophy of sebaceous glands in laboratory rodents.

Evidence that apocrine glands are androgen-dependent has been obtained for the chin gland, inguinal gland and anal gland of wild rabbits, which are larger in males than females, reduced in castrates and restored by treatment with testosterone (Mykytowycz & Goodrich, 1974). The specialized glands of the throat region in the shrew, which are responsible for the musk odour, fluctuate in size with the sexual cycle, atrophy after castration and are restored by testosterone. These apocrine musk glands, which are present in both males and females, are also stimulated by progesterone or oestradiol (Dryden & Conaway, 1967).

The stimulation of the specialized skin glands by testosterone is often greater than that observed in skin glands of the general body surface. One possible reason for this differential response could be a difference in the metabolism of testosterone by the glands.

The metabolism of ^{3}H-testosterone by the forehead gland and dorsal skin of two young captive roe bucks is currently being investigated (Johnson & Leask, in prep.).

The major metabolite over the period so far investigated, from May to September, is $^4\Delta$-androstenedione, with 5α-dihydrotestosterone and 5α-androstanedione produced in smaller amounts. Very small amounts of androstanediols and polar products were also detected. From the results so far obtained there appear to be no marked differences in the proportions of the different metabolites produced by the dorsal skin and the forehead gland. However, the percentage of testosterone metabolized by the different monthly samples did vary between the regions, as shown in Fig. 25. Between May and June there was an increase in the

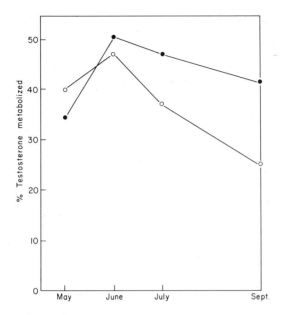

FIG. 25. Testosterone metabolized by skin samples of a roe buck (*Capreolus capreolus*). Closed circles: dorsal skin; open circles: forehead gland.

percentage testosterone metabolized by both the forehead gland and dorsal skin. From June to September the metabolism of testosterone by the forehead gland fell sharply, whereas metabolism by the dorsal skin remained relatively steady. It may therefore be suggested that the androgens available to these specialized skin glands are regulated not only by the circulating levels of testosterone but also by the metabolism of the tissue. Androstenedione appears to be a major product of testosterone metabolism in the skin of various species (Rampini, Voigt, Davis, Moretti & Hsia, 1971) and Ebling (1974) has presented evidence that it is an active androgen-stimulating sebaceous secretion in rat skin.

Evidence for the seasonal variation of skin glands and their hormonal control is incomplete. In particular there is a lack of information about skin glands in female field mammals. It seems possible that in female mammals progesterone could be responsible for a fluctuation in size of the skin glands. In the male the size of the sebaceous and apocrine sweat glands fluctuates with the testicular cycle so that the glands are large in summer and small in winter. The fluctuation in size of the glands of the general body surface may be of adaptive significance in thermoregulation. If this is true, it may be suggested that the specialized regions of skin glands developed by exploiting this hormonal dependence to produce secretions important in social interaction. Differences in metabolism of androgens could account for both the differential sensitivity of the specialized skin glands and for the production of pheromones.

ACKNOWLEDGEMENTS

I wish to thank Amal Al Khateeb, Martin Adams and James Leask for allowing me to present as yet unpublished material; Lyn Millar and Andrew McDouall for technical assistance and Pat Hawkins for the photographs.

REFERENCES

Adams, M. & Johnson, E. (in prep). *Seasonal changes in the skin glands of roe bucks* (Capreolus capreolus).

Adolph, E. F. & Dill, D. B. (1938). Observations on water metabolism in the desert. *Am. J. Physiol.* **123**: 369–378.

Aoki, T. & Wadia, M. (1951). Functional activity of the sweat glands in the hairy skin of the dog. *Science, N.Y.* **114**: 123–124.

Axelrod, J. (1970). The pineal gland. *Endeavour* **108**: 144–148.

Bassett, C. F. & Llewellyn, L. M. (1948). The molting and fur growth pattern in the adult silver fox. *Am. Midl. Nat.* **39**: 597–601.

Bassett, C. F. & Llewellyn, L. M. (1949). The molting and fur growth pattern in adult mink. *Am. Midl. Nat.* **42**: 751.

Bassett, C. F., Pearson, O. P. & Wilkie, F. (1944). The effect of artificially increased length of day on molt, growth and priming of silver fox pelts. *J. exp. Zool.* **96**: 77–83.

Billingham, R. E. & Silvers, W. K. (1960). The melanocytes of mammals. *Q. Rev. Biol.* **35**: 1–40.

Bissonnette, T. H. (1935). Relations of hair cycles in ferrets to changes in the anterior hypophysis and to light cycles. *Anat. Rec.* **63**: 159–168.

Bonsma, J. C. & Pretorius, A. J. (1943). Influence of colour and coat cover on adaptability in cattle. *Fmg S. Afr.* **18**: 101–120.

Borowski, S. (1958). Variations in the density of coat during the life cycle of *Sorex araneus*. *Acta theriol.* **2**: 286–289.

Bronson, F. H. & Caroom, D. (1971). Preputial gland of the male mouse; attractant function. *J. Reprod. Fert.* **25**: 279–282.

Brownlee, R. G., Silverstein, R. M., Müller-Schwarze, D. & Singer, A. G. (1969). Isolation, identification and function of the chief component of the male tarsal scent in black-tailed deer. *Nature, Lond.* **221**: 284–285.

Casey, J. H., Burger, H. G., Kent, J. R., Kellie, A. E., Moxham, A., Nabarro, J. & Nabarro, J. D. N. (1966). Treatment of hirsutism by adrenal and ovarian suppression. *J. clin. Endocr.* **26**: 1370–1374.

Cave, A. J. E. (1969). Hairs and vibrissae in the Rhinocerotidae. *J. Zool., Lond.* **157**: 247–257.

Clarke, J. R. & Forsyth, I. A. (1964). Seasonal changes in the adenohypophysis of the vole (*Microtus agrestis*). *Gen. comp. Endocr.* **4**: 243–252.

Clarke, J. R. & Frearson, S. (1972). Sebaceous glands on the hindquarters of the vole, *Microtus agrestis*. *J. Reprod. Fert.* **31**: 477–481.

Cott, H. B. (1940). *Adaptive coloration in animals*. London: Methuen.

Davis, B. K. (1963). Quantitative morphological studies upon the influence of the endocrine system on the growth of hair by white mice. *Acta endocr. Copenh.* ·Suppl. **85**: 9–102.

Delost, P. (1951). Variations saisonnières de l'activité thyroidienne du campagnol des champs (*Microtus arvalis*). *C. r. Séanc. Soc. Biol.* **145**: 377–380.

Dolnick, E. H., Warner, R. G. & Bassett, C. F. (1960). Influence of diet on fur growth. *Natl Fur News* **32**: 12–13.

Donovan, B. T. & Harris, G. W. (1954). Effect of pituitary stalk section on light induced oestrus in the ferret. *Nature, Lond.* **174**: 503–504.

Dryden, G. L. & Conaway, C. H. (1967). The origin and hormonal control of scent production in *Suncus murinus*. *J. Mammal.* **48**: 420–428.

Eadie, W. R. (1938). The dermal glands of shrews. *J. Mammal.* **19**: 171–174.

Ebling, F. J. (1961). Failure of progesterone to enlarge sebaceous glands in the female rat. *Br. J. Derm.* **73**: 65–68.

Ebling, F. J. (1974). Hormonal control and methods of measuring sebaceous gland activity. *J. invest. Derm.* **62**: 161–171.

Ecke, D. & Kinney, A. (1956). Aging meadow mice (*Microtus californicus*) by observation of molt progression. *J. Mammal.* **37**: 249–254.

Ferguson, K. A. & Dowling, D. F. (1955). The function of cattle sweat glands. *Austr. J. agric. Res.* **6**: 640–644.

Flerov, K. K. (1952). Mammals. **1**. Musk deer and Deer. *Fauna U.S.S.R.* National Science Foundation, Washington. (Translation, 1960).

Flux, J. E. (1970). Colour change of Mountain hares (*Lepus timidus scoticus*) in North-east Scotland. *J. Zool., Lond.* **162**: 345–358.

Forsyth, I. A. (1962). *Seasonal changes in some endocrine organs of the vole* (Microtus agrestis). Thesis: University of Oxford.

French, C. E., McEwen, L. C., Magruder, N. D., Rader, T., Long, T. A. & Swift, R. W. (1960). Responses of white-tailed bucks to added artificial light. *J. Mammal.* **41**: 23–29.

Geschwind, I. I. (1966). Change in hair color in mice induced by injection of α-M.S.H. *Endocrinology* **79**: 1165–1167.

Glenn, E. M. & Gray, J. (1965). Effect of various hormones on the growth and histology of the gerbil (*Meriones unguicalatus*) abdominal sebaceous gland pad. *Endocrinology* **76**: 1115–1123.

Haitlinger, R. (1968). Seasonal variation of pelage in representatives of *Apodemus* found in Poland. *Zoologica pol.* **18**: 330–345.

Hamilton, J. B. & Montagna, W. (1950). The sebaceous glands of the hamster. 1. Morphological effects of androgens on integumentary structures. *Am. J. Anat.* **86**: 191–233.

Hart, J. S. (1956). Seasonal changes in insulation of the fur. *Can. J. Zool.* **34**: 53–57.

Harvey, N. E. & MacFarlane, W. V. (1958). The effects of day length on the coat shedding cycles, body weight, and reproduction of the ferret. *Aust. J. biol. Sci.* **11**: 187–199.

Hewson, R. (1958). Moults and winter whitening in the mountain hare (*Lepus timidus scoticus*). *Proc. zool. Soc. Lond.* **131**: 99–108.

Jackes, A. D. & Watson, A. (1975). Winter whitening of Scottish Mountain hares (*Lepus timidus scoticus*) in relation to day-length, temperature and snow lie. *J. Zool., Lond.* **176**: 403–409.

Johansen, K. (1962). Buoyancy and insulation in the muskrat. *J. Mammal.* **43**: 64–68.

Johnson, E. (1958a). Quantitative studies on hair growth in the albino rat II. The effect of sex hormones. *J. Endocr.* **16**: 351–359.

Johnson, E. (1958b). Quantitative studies on hair growth in the albino rat III. The role of the adrenal glands. *J. Endocr.* **16**: 360–368.

Johnson, E. & Hornby, J. (1975). Seasonal changes of pelage in the roe deer (*Capreolus capreolus*) and its role in thermoregulation. *J. nat. Hist.* **9**: 619–628.

Johnson, E. & Leask, J. (in prep.). *Metabolism of testosterone by forehead skin of the roe buck* (Capreolus capreolus).

Katkov, T. & Gower, P. B. (1968). The biosynthesis of 5α-androst-16 en-3-one from progesterone by boar testis. *Acta Biochim. Biophys.* **164**: 134–136.

Khateeb, A. A. & Johnson, E. (1971a). Seasonal changes of pelage in the vole (*Microtus agrestis*) I. Correlation with changes in the endocrine glands. *Gen. comp. Endocr.* **16**: 217–228.

Khateeb, A. A. & Johnson, E. (1971b). Seasonal changes of pelage in the vole (*Microtus agrestis*) II. The effect of day length. *Gen. comp. Endocr.* **16**: 229–235.

Khateeb, A. A. & Johnson, E. (1971c). Seasonal changes of pelage in the vole (*Microtus agrestis*) III. The role of the endocrine system. *Gen. comp. Endocr.* **16**: 236–240.

Kingston, H. (1964). The chemistry and olfactory properties of musk, civet and castoreum. *Int. Congr. Endocr.* **2** (Excerpta Medica Series 83): 209–214.

Labban, F. M. (1957). The effects of L-thyroxine on sheep and wool production. *J. agr. Sci.* **49**: 26–50.

Lee, D. H. K. (1950). Studies of heat regulation in the sheep with special reference to the merino. *Aust. J. agric. Res.* **1**: 200–216.

Ling, J. K. (1965). Functional significance of sweat glands and sebaceous glands in seals. *Nature, Lond.* **208**: 560–562.

Ling, J. K. (1968). The skin and hair of the Southern elephant seal III. Morphology of the adult integument. *Aust. J. Zool.* **16**: 629–645.

Ling, J. K. (1970). Pelage and molting in wild mammals with special reference to aquatic forms. *Q. Rev. Biol.* **45**: 16–54.

Lorincz, A. L. & Lancaster, G. (1957). Anterior pituitary preparation with tropic activity for sebaceous preputial and harderian glands. *Science, N.Y.* **126**: 124–125.

Lovatt Evans, C. & Smith, D. F. G. (1956). Sweating responses in the horse. *Proc. R. Soc.* (B.) **145**: 61–83.

Lyman, C. P. (1943). Control of coat color in the varying hare *Lepus americanus*. *Bull. Mus. comp. Zool. Harv.* **93**: 393–461.

Lyne, A. G., Molyneux, G. S., Mykytowycz, R. & Parakkal, P. F. (1964). The development, structure and function of the submandibular cutaneous (chin) glands in the rabbit. *Aust. J. Zool.* **12**: 340–348.

Lynfield, Y. L. (1960). Effect of pregnancy on the human hair cycle. *J. invest. Derm.* **35**: 323.

Maloiy, G. M. O. (1971). Temperature regulation in the donkey (*Equus asinus*). *Biochem. Physiol.* **39A**: 403–412.

Martan, J. (1962). Effect of castration and androgen replacement on the supracaudal gland of the male guinea pig. *J. Morph.* **110**: 285–293.

Martini, L., Carraro, A., Caviezal, F. & Fochi, M. (1968). Factors affecting hypothalamic function. In *Pharmacology of reproduction*: 13–30. Diczfalusy, E. (ed.). Oxford: Pergamon Press.

Mazak, V. (1962). Spring moult in *Equus hermionus kiang* and a contribution to the phylogenesis of moulting in the subfamily Equinae. *Zool. Anz.* **168**: 164–170.

Mitchell, O. G. (1965). Effect of castration and transplantation on ventral gland of the gerbil. *Proc. Soc. exp. Biol. Med.* **119**: 953–955.

Mohn, M. P. (1958). The effects of different hormonal states on the growth of hair in rats. In *The biology of hair growth*: 335–398. Montagna, W. & Ellis, R. A. (eds). New York and London: Academic Press.

Montagna, W. & Hamilton, J. B. (1949). The sebaceous glands of the hamster. II. Some cytochemical studies in normal and experimental animals. *Am. J. Anat.* **84**: 365–395.

Mugford, R. A. & Nowell, N. W. (1971). The preputial glands as a source of aggression-promoting odors in mice. *Physiol. & Behav.* **6**: 247–249.

Mykytowycz, R. & Goodrich, B. S. (1974). Skin glands as organs of communication in mammals. *J. invest. Derm.* **62**: 124–131.

Pearson, O. P. (1946). Scent glands of the short tailed shrew. *Anat. Rec.* **94**: 615–629.

Pinter, A. J. (1968). Hair growth responses to nutrition and photoperiod in the vole, *Microtus montanus. Am. J. Physiol.* **215**: 828–832.

Quay, W. B. (1962). Apocrine sweat glands in the angular oris of microtine rodents. *J. Mammal.* **43**: 303–310.

Quay, W. B. (1968). The specialized posterolateral sebaceous glandular regions in microtine rodents. *J. Mammal.* **49**: 427–445.

Quay, W. B. & Müller-Schwarze, D. (1970). Functional histology of integumentary glandular regions in Black-tailed deer (*Odocoileus hemionus*). *J. Mammal.* **51**: 675–694.

Rampini, E., Voigt, W., Davis, B. P., Moretti, G. & Hsia, S. L. (1971). Metabolism of testosterone-4-^{14}C by rat skin: Variations during the hair cycle. *Endocrinology* **89**: 1506–1514.

Rand, C. G., Riggs, D. S. & Talbot, N. B. (1952). The influence of environmental temperature in the metabolism of the thyroid hormone in the rat. *Endocrinology* **51**: 562–569.

Reineke, E. P., Travis, H. F. & Dolnick, E. H. (1962). The effects of thyroid gland destruction and replacement therapy on fur growth in mink (*Mustela vison*) given a thyroxine free diet. *Am. J. vet. Res.* **23**: 121–127.

Riek, R. F., Hardy, M. H., Lee, D. H. K. & Carter, H. B. (1950). The effect of the dietary plane upon the reactions of two breeds of sheep during short exposures to hot environments. *Aust. J. agric. Res.* **1**: 217–230.

Rust, C. C. (1962). Temperature as a modifying factor in the spring pelage change of short-tailed weasels. *J. Mammal.* **43**: 323–328.

Rust, C. C. (1965). Hormonal control of pelage cycles in the short-tailed weasel. *Gen. comp. Endocr.* **5**: 222–231.

Rust, C. C. & Meyer, R. K. (1969). Hair colour, moult and testis size in male, short-tailed weasels treated with melatonin. *Science, N.Y.* **165**: 921–922.

Ryder, M. L. (1970). Structure and seasonal change of coat in Scottish wild goats. *J. Zool., Lond.* **161**: 355–362.

Schmidt-Nielsen, K. (1975). *Animal physiology: Adaptation and environment.* Cambridge: University Press.

Schmidt-Nielsen, K., Schmidt-Nielsen, B., Jarnum, S. A. & Houpt, T. R. (1957). Temperature of the camel and its relation to water economy. *Am. J. Physiol.* **188**: 103–112.

Scholander, P. F., Hock, R., Walters, V. & Irving, I. (1950). Heat regulation in some arctic and tropical mammals and birds. *Biol. Bull. mar. biol. Lab. Woods Hole* **99**: 237–258.

Schumacher, S. (1936). Das Stirnorgan des Rehbockes (*Capreolus capreolus*) ein bisher unbekanntes Duftorgan. *Z. mikrosk. anat. Forsch.* **39**: 215–230.

Sealander, J. A. (1951). Survival of *Peromyscus* in relation to environmental temperature and acclimation at high and low temperatures. *Am. Midl. Nat.* **46**· 257–309.

Seele, E. (1968). Haut und Haar der Chinchillidae. *Zool. Anz.* **181**: 60–75.

Severaid, J. H. S. (1945). Pelage changes in the snowshoe hare, *Lepus americanus*. *J. Mammal.* **26**: 41–63.

Shanks, C. E. (1948). The pelt-primeness method of aging muskrats. *Am. Midl. Nat.* **39**: 179–187.

Short, B. F. (1955). Developmental modification of fleece structure by adverse maternal nutrition. *Aust. J. agric. Res.* **6**: 863–872.

Siuda, S. (1964). Morphology of the adrenal cortex of *Sorex araneus* during the life cycle. *Acta theriol.* **8**:115–124.

Spearman, R. I. C. (1964). The evolution of mammalian keratinized structures. *Symp. zool. Soc. Lond. No.* 12: 67–81.

Speed, J. G. (1960). The importance of the coat in Exmoor and other mountain and moorland ponies living out of doors. *Br. Vet. J.* **116**: 91–98.

Stevens, C. E., D'Angelo, S. A., Paschkis, K. E., Cantarrow, A. & Sunderman, F. W. (1955). The response of the pituitary thyroid system of the guinea-pig to low environmental temperature. *Endocrinology* **56**: 143–155.

Stevenson, J. M. J. (1962). Moult in mink and silver fox. *Bull. Mammal Soc. Br. Isl.* **17**: 13–14.

Strauss, J. S. & Ebling, F. J. (1970). Control and function of skin glands in mammals. *Mem. Soc. endocr.* **18**: 341–372.

Thiessen, D. D., Friend, H. D. & Lindzey, G. (1968). Androgen control of territorial marking in the Mongolian gerbil. *Science, N.Y.* **160**: 432–434.

Watson, A. (1963). The effect of climate on the colour change of Mountain hares in Scotland. *Proc. zool. Soc. Lond.* **141**: 823–835.

Weiner, J. S. & Hellman, K. (1960). The sweat glands. *Biol. Rev.* **35**: 141–186.

Symp. zool. Soc. Lond. (1977) No. 39, 405–407.

CONCLUSIONS FROM THE DISCUSSION

R. I. C. SPEARMAN

*Dermatology Department, University College Hospital
Medical School, London, England*

The recorded discussion extended for over three hours and only a few subjects which came up continually can be summarized here.

Certainly one of the most important functions of the epidermis in the animal kingdom considered as a whole is secretion of mucus, even though it does not occur in mammalian skin although it remains important in the oral mucosa and in ciliated respiratory epithelia. Variation in the viscosity of mucus at different times is important for its functions and is perhaps generally achieved by having different types of secretory cells. Different types of cells were found in oligochaetes by S. K. Richards (Keele), and gamete transport in snails involves a chemically different mucus to that generally produced for other functions. Here one is reminded of the serous and mucous secretory cells of mammalian mucous epithelia responsible for watery and more viscous secretions. The extensive study of molluscan mucus by K. Simkiss (Reading) and K. M. Wilbur (Duke) indicates peculiar physical properties with such rapid changes in consistency that it has been likened to a thixotrophic effect. How far this is applicable to other groups in uncertain but it is interesting that mucus from widely different species can be transferred from one to another and will function perfectly well.

The functions of mucus can be summarized as follows. It is a transporting vehicle in ciliated epithelia for movement of detritus, silt, dead cells, food particles, waste matter and gametes, while parasites are dislodged if they have not got a hold. In species without epidermal cilia, such as fish, particulate matter is removed after being trapped in mucus and the mucus of *Lepidosiren* has been used to clean drinking water. Mucus may also act as an ion trap and in consequence indirectly influences water diffusion into and out of the skin. Viscous mucus gives physical protection to underlying cells and an antimicrobial action has now been shown. In mammalian surface secretions bacterial inhibition is probably mainly due to unfavourable pH as well as to competition with the resident commensal flora. However, removal of mucus from fish skin leaves it more prone to infection. Unusual uses of mucus are as a surface for terrestrial locomotion in land snails and the mucus used for tunnelling into limestone by some molluscs. These various functions depend mainly on the visco-elastic and hygroscopic properties of mucus.

Other participants in the discussion of this subject were M. Whitear (London), T. E. Weis-Fogh (Cambridge), K. M. Lyons (Bryanston), R. D. Harkness (London), M. D. Hainsworth (Isleworth) and members of the audience.

In most groups of animals a toughened outer layer of the skin contains substances with a two-phase composite molecular structure which provides both tensile strength and elasticity. Always a fibrous component is interspersed with a non-fibrous filler. In arthropod hard cuticle the fibrous element is chitin and globular proteins are the filler. Chitin in other invertebrates such as in annelid setae and in pogonophores probably has a similar function. In both arthropod hard cuticle and in annelid setae the proteins are quinone tanned but this type of cross-bonding is rare in collagenous cuticles; it occurs in the outer region of the nematode cuticle but does not occur in annelid cuticle. There is therefore an association between chitin-associated proteins and predominance of quinone sclerotization. The nematode cuticle composed of polymerized collagen fibres interspersed with non-fibrous mucopolysaccharides has a two-phase arrangement (and differs from the supple human dermis in which there is little collagen aggregation and it exists as a hydrated gel with mucopolysaccharides). The arthropod hard cuticle is more rigid than nematode cuticle and rubber-like resilin takes its place in the joints. Abductin in the hinge of a bivalve mollusc is similar in function. The hard arthropod cuticle is used for muscle attachments but the nematode cuticle functions more like the fabric covering of a balloon acting as a restraining envelope to the high pressure within the body. For this purpose a slightly elastic cuticle is required.

This also enables nematode larvae to increase in size between ecdyses which is not possible in an insect larva except during the short period when the new cuticle is still soft immediately following moult.

Vertebrates have adopted neither the chitin type nor the collagen type of composite material for their surface coverings. The disulphide bonded cuticle of *Rhabdopleura* and the similar extra cellular cyst material in platyhelminths is best termed keratin-like protein as there is no evidence that true keratin formation with its multiplicity of proteins can occur outside cells. The keratin complexes of higher vertebrates have a two-phase structure with both fibrous and globular protein components. It is of interest that the only firm evidence of keratin formation in invertebrates is in the spines of the platyhelminth tegument and yet this layer appears not to be homologous with the vertebrate epidermis. Secretion of mucus and keratinization appear mutually opposed and in mammals keratinization is the sole function of the surface epidermis.

The subject was discussed by S. O. Andersen (Copenhagen), T. E. Weis-Fogh (Cambridge), D. L. Lee (Leeds), P. A. Riley (London), S. K. Richards (Keele), R. T. Tregear (Oxford), R. D. Harkness (London), M. Abercrombie (Cambridge), R. I. C. Spearman (London) and others.

Although hormones have minimal effects on the surface epidermis of mammals, hair growth and sebaceous gland activity are influenced by sex hormones as is feather growth in birds and cyclical changes in keratinized breeding tubercles in fish. Seasonal changes in the pelage of wild mammals include differences in hair form in winter and summer, and the hormonal control is more complex than a growth stimulus or inhibition. One possible mechanism which would diversify possible effects of a hormone on the skin in different seasons would be if a variety of active derivatives were produced in the target skin cells as a result of cyclical changes in metabolism. Thus F. J. G. Ebling (Sheffield) suggested that, since the action of an androgen involves its metabolism in the target cells, different androgenic derivatives of testosterone might perhaps have different activities. It was possible that the control of male hormone action through the pituitary was exercised not only by stimulation of the gonads but also by a direct effect on testosterone conversion in the skin, which might show cyclical variation. In comparison, the action of mineralocorticoid hormone on moult in toads is essentially permissive since moult will not occur in its absence, while the hormone will not cause moult during an inter-phase period.

The subject was also discussed by E. Johnson (Reading), P. Budtz (Copenhagen), B. Collette (Washington DC) and members of the audience.

AUTHOR INDEX

Numbers in italics refer to pages in the References at the end of each article.

420   AUTHOR INDEX

Shelton, P. M. J., 274, 288
Shepherd, A. M., 154, 169
Shepherd, J., 78, 95
Shih, C. Y., 272, 287
Shiraishi, Y., 229, 233, 266
Short, B. F., 385, 404
Short, R. B., 110, 143
Shutte, M. H., 114, 136
Silas, E. G., 248, 267
Silberberg, A., 60, 74
Silbert, J. E., 282, 287
Silk, M. H., 122, 143
Silvester, N. R., 155, 170
Silvers, W. K., 382, 400
Silverstein, R. M., 396, 400
Simon, C. R., 361, 371
Sims, R. T., 343, 351
Simkiss, K., 53, 57, 75
Singer, A. G., 396, 400
Singer, A. J., 361, 371
Singer, M., 272, 288
Siuda, S., 386, 404
Skaer, R. J., 2, 5, 134, 143
Skelding, J. M., 39, 74
Skelton, P. H., 226, 243, 267
Slais, J., 117, 143
Slater, T. F., 91, 95
Slayter, G., 336, 351
Sleigh, M. A., 65, 71, 206, 221
Sminia, T., 38, 75
Smith, C. L., 260, 267
Smith, D. F. G., 390, 402
Smith, J. H., 104, 106, 122, 125, 143
Smith, H. M., 147, 169, 245, 267
Smith, L., 157, 168
Smith, R. J. F., 229, 267
Smithers, S. R., 122, 141, 143
Smyth, J. D., 53, 75, 128, 131, 136, 138, 143, 349, 351
Snell, R. S., 91, 94
Snelson, F. F., Jr., 245, 267
Soderstrom, C. W., 361, 371
Sommerville, R. I., 165, 169
Southgate, V. R., 98, 99, 101, 109, 110, 114, 143
Southward, A. J., 195, 199, 201, 202, 204, 205, 208, 209, 210, 215, 218, 219, 221, 222
Southward, E. C., 195, 199, 200, 201, 202, 204, 205, 208, 209, 210, 211,

212, 214, 215, 216, 218, 220, 221, 222
Spannhof, L., 318, 333
Spearman, R. I. C., 228, 267, 269, 288, 297, 313, 318, 333, 336, 340, 341, 343, 344, 345, 346, 347, 348, 349, 350, 351, 352, 353, 354, 356, 357, 358, 359, 363, 365, 366, 367, 368, 370, 371, 372, 373, 404
Specian, R. D., 128, 144
Speed, J. G., 376, 382, 404
Speeg, K. V., 58, 72
Spence, I. M., 122, 143
Sprague, E. A., 360, 371
Steckoll, S. M., 78, 95
Stefano, F. J. E., 322, 324, 334
Stein, P. C., 113, 114, 122, 143
Steinman, R. M., 272, 288
Stenholt Clausen, H., 230, 250, 251, 253, 267
Stephens, G. C., 4, 5, 186, 191, 192
Stephenson, S. K., 336, 351
Stevens, C. E., 386, 404
Stevenson, J. M. J., 376, 404
Stewart, D. M., 39, 44, 74
Stockem, W., 293, 311
Stoktosowa, S., 231, 267
Storch, V., 104, 143, 190, 192, 216, 221, 222
Strauss, J. S., 397, 404
Strong, P. L., 114, 143
Sundara Rajulu, G., 173, 175, 192
Sunderman, F. W., 386, 404
Swain, T., 82, 95
Swan, G. A., 78, 95
Swanbeck, G., 358, 372
Sweeny, P. R., 272, 286, 298, 311
Swiderski, Z., 103, 104, 143, 335, 349, 352
Swift, R. W., 385, 401
Szabo, G., 92, 93, 319, 332, 332, 333
Szent-Györgyi, A., 88, 95

T

Takeda, T., 229, 233, 266
Talbot, N. B., 386, 403
Tao, Y., 243, 245, 264
Taylor, A. C., 272, 288
Taylor, A. G., 4, 5, 186, 191

SUBJECT INDEX

A

Abductin, 56, 406
Absorption through the skin
  absorbent surface in cestodes, 129
  calcium and other ions in molluscs,
    40–50
  glucose in flukes, 125
  ions in Amphibia, 297, 303
  organic solutes, 4, 43, 117, 205
  organic substances in pogonophores,
    205
  peptides and amino acids in cestodes,
    117, 132
  permeability in flukes, 113
  permeability in nematodes, 167
  permeability to water, 9, 33, 40, 79,
    167
  sodium pump in Anura, 309
Acid phosphatase, 113, 126, 278, 322
ACTH
  on hair growth, 387
  on moult in toads, 324–326, 331–332
Adrenal cortex, 386
Adrenocorticoids (*see also* Corticosteroids), 324, 326, 331
Alcohols (long chain), 9
Aldosterone (*see also* Mineralocorticoid
  hormones), 324
Alkaline phosphatase, 113, 126, 278
Amphibia, 269, 293–299
  adult skin, 275–285, 318–322
  changes in metamorphosis, 276–281
  larval skin, 272–275, 293, 299
Anagen, 382
Androgens (*see also* Testosterone), 399,
  407
Apocrine glands, 380, 390, 392
Arthropods
  characteristics of integument, 3, 7,
    336
  insects, 7, 33
  Merostomata, 14
Aspartyl residues, 17
ATPase, 60, 126

B

Basal lamina (basal membrane), 7, 36,
  99, 129, 198, 272, 281, 284
Breeding tubercles of fish, 225, 228,
  242, 243, 246
  control of development, 228
  functions of, 228
  value in systematics, 230

C

Calcification
  in keratinized structures, 349
  in molluscan shell, 57
Carbonic anhydrase, 59
Catagen, 382
Catechols, 26, 85, 87
Chitin, 3
  association with matrix proteins in
    arthropods, 12–19
  microfibrils in arthropods, 11–12
  in pogonophoran tube, 215, 336, 406
Cilia
  activity in relation to mucus, 61
  in amphibian tadpoles, 272
  in mollusca, 60–61
  in platyhelminth larvae, 99
  in pogonophores, 206
Collagen (cuticular)
  in annelids, 171
  in nematodes, 155, 336, 406
  in pogonophores, 201
Contact organs of fish, 239
  functions, 228
  relationship to ctenoid scales, 259
  value in systematics, 230
Cornification (*see* Keratinization)
Corticosteroids (*see also* Adrenocorticoids), 324, 325, 332, 357, 358
Covalent bonds, 26
Cuticle, 3
  amino acid composition in
    arthropods, 14
  Amphibia, 293, 295

423